BELIEF,
MAGIC, and
ANOMIE

BELIEF, MAGIC, and ANOMIE

Essays in Psychosocial Anthropology

by ANNE PARSONS

The Free Press, New York

COLLIER-MACMILLAN LIMITED, LONDON

Collier-Macmillan Canada, Ltd., Toronto, Ontario

Library of Congress Catalog Card Number: 69-11282

First Printing

For Anne's Friends and Colleagues

Contents

Preface   ix

Introduction   xi

part one:
FAMILY DYNAMICS   1
  1. Is the Oedipus Complex Universal? The
     Jones-Malinowski Debate Revisited   3
  2. Paternal and Maternal Authority in the
     Neapolitan Family   67
  3. Family Dynamics in South Italian
     Schizophrenics   98

part two:
SOCIAL ASPECTS OF
MENTAL ILLNESS   121
  4. Psychiatric Hospitalization, Social Class,
     and Immigrant Status   123
  5. Specific Patterns of Italian-American Life   135
  6. Some Comparative Observations on Ward
     Social Structure: Southern Italy, England,
     and the United States   151

part three:
CULTURAL THEMES IN EXPRESSIVE SYMBOLISM   175

7. Expressive Symbolism in Witchcraft
   and Delusion: A Comparative Study   177
8. Abstract and Concrete Images in
   Paranoid Delusions: A Comparison of
   American and South Italian Patients   204
9. A Schizophrenic Episode in a Neapolitan Slum   212

part four:
RELIGION AND SOCIAL CHANGE   237

10. The Pentecostal Immigrants, I: A Study
    of an Ethnic Central City Church   239
11. The Pentecostal Immigrants, II: Ritual and
    Culture Conflict   263
12. Dark Puritan   278

part five:
SOCIAL ASPECTS OF PSYCHOANALYSIS   283

13. Diffusion of Psychoanalytic Concepts   285
14. Cultural Barriers to Insight and the
    Structural Reality of Transference   295
15. On Psychoanalytic Training for
    Research Purposes   334

Index   359

Preface

Anne Parsons had much to say. But she was a craftsman with high standards of scholarship and therefore left behind several unpublished manuscripts when she died prematurely on June 9, 1964, at the age of 33.

We have assembled in this volume Anne Parsons' published papers, and those of her unpublished manuscripts that seemed to require only editorial revision. We have tried to make these revisions in a manner we judged, from our long associations with her in professional and personal friendship, would be her own. We hope that we have done justice to her fine mind.

The work of Anne Parsons that is reported in some of these papers was made possible through the cooperation of the staffs of McLean Hospital and Boston State Hospital, both in Massachusetts, and the Ospedale Psichiatrico in Naples, Italy. For the permission to reprint her published papers, acknowledgment is given to the American Medical Association, the International Universities Press, the *Journal for the Scientific Study of Religion,* L'Ospedale Psichiatrico, *Social and Economic Studies,* the Société Internationale d'Ethnopsychologie Normale et Pathologique, and the William Alanson White Psychiatric Foundation.

The teachers, friends, and colleagues here and abroad to whom Anne Parsons owed much in her work and thoughts were too many to be named. Among them were her French friends and colleagues, Serge Moscovici of the Ecole des Hautes Etudes and C. L. Pidoux of the Société Internationale d'Ethnopsychologie Normale et Pathologique; her Italian sponsors and friends, Piero Bontadini of the Institute of Social and Economic Research in Milan, Gustavo Iacone, Director of the Institute of Psychology at the University of Naples, and Manlio Rossi-Doria, Professor of Economics at that same University; and her American friends and mentors, the anthropologists Clifford and Hildred Geertz of the University of Chicago and Donald Pitkin of Amherst College, and the psychiatrist Alfred H. Stanton of McLean Hospital. To all of them goes our deeply felt gratitude in Anne's name. We also know that she would have wanted to express her warm thanks to Frances Merrill, her untiring research assistant for several years, whose devotion to her and her work deserves special mention.

We thank Grete Bibring, Talcott Parsons, and Harry Rand, who gave Anne Parsons professional and personal guidance, for having served as advisory editors for this volume. The responsibility for its shortcomings, however, is strictly our own.

THE EDITORS:
Rose Laub Coser
Renée C. Fox
Louisa P. Howe
Merton J. Kahne
Sidney Mintz
Jesse R. Pitts
David M. Schneider

Introduction

Anne Parsons was a map maker and interpreter whose meticulous attention to detail generates a clear appreciation of the continuities and relations among phenomena previously only dimly sensed as similar. She explored new frontiers; she created a conceptual base for the understanding of the uniformities of human psychology amid the cultural and social diversity which creates and is created by that psychology. A "clinical" anthropologist, she attempted to be for anthropology and psychiatry what the comparative anatomist is for biology and medicine.

Convinced of the relevance of psychoanalytic perspectives on the human condition and equally committed to the vital productivity of the classical anthropological tradition of field study, she freed herself very early in her professional career from the polemical concerns of partisan protagonists. The unique stance that she fashioned for herself made possible the conceptual syntheses that seemed to flow so easily and clearly from her pen. Her reluctance to depart from the truth as she found it took its inevitable toll in loneliness and estrangement from many of the very groups whose work she used as the foundation for building her own description of man. She was not unaware of the price she was forced to pay for maintaining, in the face of sophisticated argument, that Freud's anthropological hunches could not be simply written off because they might be found in particular instances to be substantively in error. Despite the formidable problems of documentation and construct formation, she vigorously insisted that both anthropological and psychoanalytic principles be given serious consideration in assessing any social event. Guided as she was by concern for empirical validity rather than for dogmatic opinion, it was a source of particular dismay to her when some psychoanalytic colleagues failed to grasp the constructive potentialities for their discipline of the anthropological point of view. It was Anne Parsons' personal triumph that she nevertheless persisted in her efforts to utilize, and to enrich, the teachings of psychoanalysis.

She had an exquisite understanding of the differences between a symbol and that to which it referred. Her dissection of the phenomena of delusions as they occurred in various social strata and cultural settings eventuated in the powerful, but as yet unexploited, concept of symbol equivalence, which makes systematic cross-cultural evaluation of the content of delusions feasible. Her painstaking elaboration of the social class and cultural determinants of the particular form of expressive symbolism imbedded in universal motivational structures provides the first usable system for analyzing delusional content that does justice to the hard-won insights provided by many disciplines.

To describe her as a participant observer is to caricature her actual enmeshment in the situations in which she found herself. Her involvement as a social scientist issued from the dual roles of social critic and political activist that her intellect and emotion demanded. Understanding was for something, and she had little patience with concepts that did not have some potentiality for social implementation. Her deliberate juxtaposition of Yankee and Neapolitan provided the sharp contrasts that revealed essential unities. These she intuitively recognized as the most relevant basis for man's urgent necessity to realize his kinship with all of his neighbors in a rapidly shrinking world. She herself talked with the studied sophistication of a Radcliffe graduate, but her hands spoke Italian.

Anne Parsons had a strong sense of man's need for an ethic which transcended his immediate biological and social imperatives. She also—for all her impatience with outmoded social forms—was a traditionalist at heart and understood the importance of ritual and formality in renewing one's sense of identity. And certainly she took uncomplicated pleasure in the sounds and sights of ceremony, be it in posing the South Italian slum dweller against the glittering pageantry of the celebration of a Catholic Mass or in the austere restraint of her New England Yankees.

Anne Parsons' research dealt with some of the most critical problems in the social sciences, problems of equal concern to anthropology, psychiatry, and sociology. Because she combined keen psychological insight with a firm grasp of the principles of the sister disciplines, she contributed significantly to our comprehension of the mutual influence of sociocultural and psychological processes. Though all of her research was ultimately concerned with questions of theory, she collected her own field data, concentrating upon subjects who were members of a clearly defined ethnic subculture.

Anne Parsons was particularly interested in the structural and psychodynamic characteristics of Neapolitan families of the working class, and she carried out fieldwork with informants of this background both within their original mileu and within an urban New World setting. The data with which she worked most tellingly were the thoughts, expressed feelings, verbal associations, and imagery of the South Italian men and women whom she studied, and she accumulated her field materials by observation, interviewing, and the use of projective techniques. Her unit of observation was the individual, but always in the full context of group patterns of interaction—at home, in church or, if very ill, in the setting of the hospital.

In her concern with the linkage of the psychic and the sociocultural, Anne Parsons dealt also with those persons who were psychologically disturbed. Thus, for instance, she studied in considerable depth a number of schizophrenic women of South Italian lower-class origin, demonstrating that "culture" and "personality," rather than referring to two disparate bodies of data, are really different ways of abstracting from the same concrete behavioral phenomena. She drew no sharp dividing lines between the normal and the abnormal, undertaking instead to reveal how behavior may be analyzed to expose a continuum of psychological variation within a small group. Here, as in much of her other work, she unified and refined the concepts of social science in new ways.

Anne Parsons' interpretations of certain "clusters" of attitude and belief typical of the South Italian subculture expose to our view a powerful, underlying psychocultural unity. In her phrasing, the bodies of belief and behavior centering upon courtship on the one hand and upon the Madonna on the other constitute "two contrasting sides of a global . . . South Italian cultural complex." She made clear in her work that these patterns operate importantly in the everyday social and familial interactions of the people she studied. But she also showed that they impart a particular psychological meaning to religious ritual (as in the ceremony of the First Communion for young girls); that they play a part in shaping unconscious conceptions of significant family figures; and that they noticeably influence the delusional materials generated by schizophrenic behavior among her South Italian subjects. Such interpretations are of considerable importance, tying together as they do the normal and the abnormal, the secular and the religious, and—perhaps most centrally—society, culture, and the individual.

In her work with "Pentecostal immigrants"—a group of South Italian men and women who had converted to Protestantism and founded their own church after their arrival in the

United States—Anne Parsons affords us additional illumination of the nexus of personality and culture. A whole generation after their migration, and in spite of their conscious assimilation of the beliefs, attitudes, and values of Protestantism, these converts continued to reveal the persistent power of their ancestral culture in the conduct of their church service, their pastors' sermons and oratorical style, and the nature of their collective prayer period. Once again, one is able to perceive that "culture," "society," and "psyche" stand for ways of viewing the same phenomenon.

Not content to suppose that culture and society are no more than the "conditions" under which psychological processes operate, nor to view personality as merely an epiphenomenon of society or culture, Anne Parsons progressed far beyond those who proclaim that one discipline is better equipped than others for the exploration of social reality. And she did not limit herself to affirming that culture, social structure, and personality are interdependent and to examining such interdependence in gross terms. By insisting always upon the need to weld together the insights of all of the social sciences in the analysis of human behavior, she was able to ask searching questions about some of the central concepts of these disciplines. Going beyond her fieldwork, she thought creatively about the Oedipus complex and the concept of *anomie,* stressed the need to reformulate these concepts into operational hypotheses, and sought to suggest workable research directions along these lines.

Her interest in psychoanalysis, tied as it was to her knowledge of the anthropological and sociological views of human behavior, led her to provocative interpretations of the premises of the psychoanalytic approach. Hence one comes most clearly upon the moral and existential concern that typifies Anne Parsons' view of the problems of social science. As an anthropologist and sociologist, she grasped the significance of cross-cultural variability and the relativistic implications of that variability for psychological theory. As a person in search of her own identity, she questioned the postulates of psychoanalysis and pondered upon the "new kind of religious role, based on empirical knowledge rather than dogma . . . that psycho-analysis is being asked to create."

Anne Parsons believed deeply in the social responsibility of the social scientist. She believed that it is the moral obligation of psychiatrists and psychologists, sociologists and anthropologists, to relate the ways of thought and the findings of their disciplines to contemporary problems. Her own research is marked by calm objectivity and careful insight, but at the same time she involved herself actively in such pressing current issues as disarmament and civil rights.

It was the special quality of Anne Parsons' intellect that, while she worked in great depth with individual informants, she was always able to address herself to important theoretical questions common to the social sciences: What factors account for uniformities in social, cultural, and personality systems and further their integration and stability? What factors contribute to their variability, disorganization, and change? How does the relative state of equilibrium of each of these three systems affect that of the others? The questions she asked of her materials, and the demands she placed upon her own comprehension, were never trivial or merely professional. The papers collected together in this volume exemplify both her approach to the materials, and her successes, both human and intellectual, in dealing with them.

BELIEF,
MAGIC, and
ANOMIE

part one

Family Dynamics

In writing on family structure, Anne Parsons refuses to limit herself to a one-sided analysis, whether of psychological, ethnological, or sociological factors. She shows the interplay of these variables and demonstrates, in the first paper reprinted here, that psychoanalytic concepts, far from contradicting social and anthropological explanations, become fruitful if integrated with them. Thus the Oedipus complex, initially seen as emanating from the triadic family relationship in the West, is seen as applying to other family structures as well, if it is redefined in its affective meaning within the family constellation.

It is again the total constellation of the family which preoccupies the author in the second paper. Authority relations in the Neapolitan family are depicted here from the vantage point both of social and psychological dynamics. The peculiar content of these relations is seen as dependent upon specific

1

economic conditions and in the context of the wider culture. From the analysis of typical family conflicts and relationships, Anne Parsons concludes that the type of family structure that is highly valued in Southern Italy is not viable under conditions of poverty. Paternal authority cannot be maintained without economic opportunities if this authority is based on the idea that the father be the family's provider. As a consequence, paternal authority loses its basis of legitimacy and hence its strength as a socializing force. Maternal authority, in contrast, though morally accepted, creates psychological conflicts of masculine identification and hence also fails to be socially effective.

In the third paper, Anne Parsons further explores problems of family dependence. She finds that South Italian schizophrenics tend toward a very close identity with family members rather than drifting away into isolation. She thus locates some sources of psychological pathology within the network of family relationships.

chapter 1

Is the Oedipus
Complex
Universal?*

The Jones-Malinowski
Debate Revisited

In the 1920's a famous debate took place
between Ernest Jones and Bronislaw Malinowski which set forth
some outlines of theoretical differences between psychoanalysis
and anthropology which are still unresolved today. On the
basis of field work in the matrilineal Trobriand Islands, Malinowski drew the conclusion that the Oedipus complex as formulated by Freud is only one among a series of possible "nuclear

* This paper is based on research carried out in Naples, Italy, in
1958–1960 on two grants from the National Institute of Mental Health,
Bethesda, Md. (M-2105 and M-4301) and was written during the term
of an interdisciplinary grant from the Foundations' Fund for Research in
Psychiatry. I am very much indebted to Merton J. Kahne, Donald S.
Pitkin, David M. Schneider, Alfred H. Stanton, and to my father, Talcott
Parsons, for many comments and discussions which have gone into the
formulation of the ideas in ways which would be difficult to acknowledge
specifically.

Reprinted by permission from *The Psychoanalytic Study of Society*,
III, eds. Warner Muensterberger and Sidney Axelrad (New York: International Universities Press, 1964), 278–328.

complexes," each of which patterns primary family affects in a way characteristic of the culture in which it occurs. In this perspective, Freud's formulation of the Oedipus complex as based on a triangular relationship between father, mother, and son appears as that particular nuclear complex which characterizes a patriarchal society in which the most significant family unit consists of mother, father, and child. The alternative nuclear complex which he postulated for the Trobriand Islands consisted of a triangular relationship between brother, sister, and sister's son, this in function of the nature of matrilineal social structure in which a boy becomes a member of his mother's kin group and is subject to the authority of his maternal uncle rather than the biological father. One of his most important observations was that in the Trobriand Islands ambivalent feelings very similar to those described by Freud with respect to father and son can be observed between mother's brother and sister's son. Relations between father and son, on the other hand, are much more close and affectionate; however, Malinowski felt that the father should not be considered as a figure in the kinship structure since the Trobrianders do not recognize the existence of biological paternity. The child is seen as conceived by a spirit which enters the mother's womb and later the father appears to him as the unrelated mother's husband.

In addition, Malinowski noted that the Trobrianders give a very special importance to the brother-sister relationship. While the brother has formal authority over the sister and is responsible for her support, their actual relationship is one of extreme avoidance, to the point that an object may be handed from one to the other by means of an intermediary. He characterized the brother-sister incest taboo as "the supreme taboo" from the Trobriand standpoint; while incest with other primary biological relatives and within the matrilineal kin group at greater biological distance is also forbidden, in no instance are the taboos as strict or surrounded by intense affects as in the brother-sister case. He also discerned, with his acute clinical eye, many evidences of the real temptations underlying the avoidance pattern, for example, in that while no Trobriander would admit to having such an incest dream, the questioning itself aroused a great deal of anxiety and often the assertion that "well, other people have such dreams, but certainly not me." He noted brother-sister incest to be a primary theme in Trobriand mythology, for example, in that love magic is seen as originating in a situation in which brother and sister actually committed incest and died as a result of it. He considered these variations from the European pattern of sufficient significance to uphold the view that the Oedipus complex is not universal.

Jones, in a 1924 paper,[1] upheld with considerable vehemence the classical psychoanalytic point of view that it is. Thus while he felt that Malinowski's field data were in themselves interesting, he came to the conclusion that they did not point to the need for any important theoretical revisions in the psychoanalytic framework. For the data on the Trobriand failure to recognize the biological relationship between father and son, he provided an alternative explanation, namely, that the nonrecognition was a form of denial covering affects originating in the Oedipus situation.[2] Much to Malinowski's dismay, this argument was carried to the point of the assertion that matrilineal social organization can itself be seen as a defense against the father-son ambivalence universally characteristic of the Oedipus situation. He also pointed out that Malinowski's observations of ambivalence between mother's brother and sister's son concerned adolescent and adult life, so that, theoretically, it is possible to see it as a secondary displacement in that there

1. Jones (1924) in a paper read before the British Psycho-Analytical Society first discussed three prior publications by Malinowski: "Baloma: The Spirits of the Dead in the Trobriand Islands" (1916) and two articles which were later published together as the first two sections of *Sex and Repression in Savage Society* (1927). The last two sections of this latter work were written in response to Jones's paper. For the most complete summary of the Trobriand field data, see Malinowski (1929).

2. Not all anthropologists have accepted Malinowski's observations on this at face value; however, the data he presents indicate that the Trobrianders had formulated a reasonably coherent and intelligent picture of the facts of biology for a people lacking in any scientific framework.

is an initial oedipal rivalry between father and son, but that in adult life the hostile feelings are displaced to the mother's brother. He also commented that similar patterns can be observed in Europe, for example, in that the hostile father figure may later be an occupational superior or rival, while the actual father remains a positive figure.

A re-examination of the debate in a contemporary perspective indicates that actually there are a number of intertwined issues. In the first place, it is characterized by a highly polemic character related to the newness and consequent defensiveness of both fields: for Jones "the" Oedipus complex appears as a kind of point of honor upon whose invariance psychoanalysis would stand or fall, and exactly the same is true of some elements of Malinowski's argument, in particular those which touch on the resemblance between Jones's views and those of the older evolutionary anthropology which he himself did so much to overthrow. Thus, concerning the question of whether matrilineal social organization can be seen as a defense against oedipal affects, it seems difficult now to see how a complex social pattern could be based on the "denial" of an affect which occurs in the individual. But on the other hand, one can regret that Malinowski, in his rebuttal, went into a tirade against the evolutionary implications of this view rather than attempting to answer Jones's much more cogent point, namely, that Freud's concepts concern infantile life, and in this perspective it is quite possible that the hostility toward the mother's brother observed in adolescent and adult Trobrianders might be displaced from hostility initially experienced toward the father. What is perhaps most regrettable of all, given his status with regard to the psychoanalytic theory of symbolism, is that Jones never discussed in detail Malinowski's observations concerning the special importance of the Trobriand brother-sister relationship and the integrally related material concerning dreams and mythology.

When we look at the present state of theoretical knowledge, we might come to the conclusion that the question of whether or not the Oedipus complex is universal is one which should not be asked in such a way as to create the impression that there is a yes or no answer. In the first place, the theoretical assumption that there are infantile sexual wishes is one which has proved so useful, and has brought together such a variety of clinical facts, that it seems simply foolish to abandon the general Freudian scheme until such a point when we have an alternative that appears scientifically more valuable. In retrospect, one might say that the major point that Jones wished to maintain was simply the idea that there is an infantile sexual life. Secondly, the main point which Malinowski was supporting is now also so well established that we need not any longer be defensive about it—that human societies do structure family patterns in different ways according to laws of kinship, or particular phrasings of the incest taboo, that by no means can be derived directly from the biological facts of mating and reproduction. These latter simply cannot explain facts such as the extreme significance given to the brother-sister incest taboo by the Trobrianders in comparison to ourselves.

Taking these two points for granted, we might then proceed to ask again the same questions which were asked by Jones and Malinowski and to re-evaluate some of the major points made by each in the light of contemporary psychoanalytic and anthropological knowledge. It is this task which we have set ourselves in this paper. After some general theoretical considerations, we will discuss a particular case with respect to the possibility of formulating a third distinctive "nuclear family complex" differing both from Freud's patriarchal one and from the Trobriand matrilineal case.

Theoretical Points

Much of the Jones-Malinowski argument centered on the evidence presented by Malinowski to the effect that Trobriand Islanders are unaware of the facts of physiological paternity. The main importance of this material to Malinowski lay in its value for demonstrating the independence of social from biological kinship; certainly one of the major points which troubled him and has troubled many other anthropologists since about psychoanalytic theory is the implication that these two must overlap. However, while Jones's formulation leaves itself open to just this objection, one might now wonder whether in fact psychoanalytic theory does presuppose such an equivalence. One of the fundamental tenets of instinct theory is that an instinct is displaceable according to source, aim, and object; but if we use the term "object" in a social sense, referring to either an external person who is the focus of a drive or to an internalized representation of a person, we might then say that the possibility of variant family structures is built into even Freud's earliest formulations. Moreover, Freud's theory, while it anchors affects and fantasies in biological concepts of instinct, might also better be seen as a psychological than a biological one; so that to the extent that it postulates universals, we should also see these psychologically rather than biologically.

Contemporary concepts of object relations and object representations[3] may make it possible to bring this point out more clearly than was done by Jones. Any clinician can cite from immediate experience a great many instances in which the object focus of oedipal affects has been a person other than the biological mother or father—an adopted parent, a more distant relative, or as in many cases today, a child therapist. Actually, Freud himself was very much concerned with the role played by domestics in the early sexual life of the Victorian upper-status child. We might then say that the question of the Oedipus complex has two sides to it, the first related to instinct and fantasy, and the second to identification and object choice. But it is hard to believe that the latter processes are not in some way directly dependent on social structure and social norms, or the available possibilities for object choice and object representation.

In this perspective, the idea of the distinctive nuclear complex for each society becomes much more compatible with the psychoanalytic idea that there is an invariant series of developmental phases which is rooted in instinct; the social factor need only influence the object side. Using this assumption, we might

3. See Jacobson (1954), T. Parsons (1958), and Stanton (1959).

interpret Jones's displacement hypothesis as saying that the passing of the Oedipus complex in the Trobriand Islands is equivalent to assimilating the polar distinction between two socially represented figures, the mother's brother and the mother's husband. Each of these then comes to have a differing or contrasting affective valence and one can even say that the boy identifies with both, but that each identification represents a different social function or aspect of personality. According to this view,[4] it is the social distinction which lies at the basis of the conscious representation, which could not even arise without the mediating effect of social exchange; if there were none, the biological drives would presumably arise nevertheless, but they would not give rise to a personality. Such a formulation seems much simpler and less awkward than to say that first the Trobriand child goes through an Oedipus phase centered on the father, somehow acquiring a knowledge of biological paternity which adults in his society do not possess, then represses this knowledge and displaces the affects to the mother's brother. What we are saying is rather that conscious representation of objects by definition depends on collective representation, though their affective charge or valence may be rooted in unconscious or instinct-based constellations which are prior to culture.

This formulation would permit us to say that it does not make much difference whether the relevant figure is father or mother's brother; psychoanalytic theory requires only that the small boy have some available figure for masculine identification. However, a second aspect of the Oedipus theory raises a more difficult problem. This is that, according to Freud, the boy's hostility to the father arises from the fact that the latter has sexual relations with his mother; in other words, the Oedipus complex is rooted in sexual jealousy. However, in the Trobriand Islands, it is the biological father and not the mother's brother who has sexual relations with the mother. In fact, though it is not impossible that the mother have other sexual involvements as well, the one person who could not be a sexual object for her

4. Which utilizes Durkheim's concept of collective representations (Durkheim, 1915).

is precisely the maternal uncle, since he is, of course, her brother.

Here it seems that we have reached an insoluble impasse; either we must abandon the Malinowskian attempt to isolate distinctive nuclear complexes, saying that the initial oedipal object must always be the father since he is the actual sexual rival, or we must take the more empiricist "culturalist" viewpoint which abandons the idea of infantile sexuality altogether and says simply that various role patterns are learned in direct relation to social interaction. But since neither solution seems satisfactory (the second because it does not utilize instinct theory), we might do better to look further. Perhaps in reconsidering some of the various possible phrasings of psychoanalytic theory, we may find that some are more compatible with Malinowski's attempt than others.

It is well known that Freud's thinking contains many, not always compatible, interwoven strands. One of his earliest conceptionalizations was the trauma theory; this is the one which most directly influenced Malinowski and, moreover, most of the early workers in the field of culture and personality. According to the trauma theory, specific sexual events or observations take place in childhood which then have crucial consequences for adult personality and attitudes. In much of Freud's writing about infantile sexuality (before he reached his more general structural and dynamic formulations), he acts as if he were taking the trauma theory for granted, for example, when he portrays the Oedipus crisis as the point when the child observes or becomes aware of the "primal scene," asks questions about sexuality and comes to some conclusion about this matter and his own future sex role. This formulation presupposes a highly rationalistic child and a very direct relationship between environmental factors and psychosexual development. However, over the course of psychoanalytic history, the trauma theory has gradually slipped into the background; much of it today might well be given the status of myth. The main reason for this may well be that it simply has not worked; we certainly cannot try to predict today, nor does anyone, complex adult personality patterns from specific and limited kinds of infantile events. Applied in the anthropological field, however, the trauma theory very readily lent itself to the view that almost any kind of cultural difference could give rise to variations in the nature of the oedipal situation, and many of Malinowski's own convictions, like those of the later culture and personality theorists, were certainly derived from this kind of rough empirical evidence.

However, here we are concerned with the question of global structures rather than with specific items of socialization or other kinds of cultural behavior. With respect to family structure, trauma theory would lead us to believe that if it is in fact the father who has sexual relationships with the mother, then he should be the object of oedipal jealousy. However, in a somewhat different framework we could also reach the conclusion that this need not be so. It is often said that psychoanalysis began precisely at the moment when Freud abandoned the trauma theory, i.e., when he began to consider the verbal productions of his hysterical patients as fantasies. At this critical point he became much less concerned with the environmental question of whether or not his patients actually had been seduced in childhood and much more concerned with the questions which were formulated and reformulated throughout his later life: what are the instinctual roots of fantasy, and what are the inhibiting factors which can prevent instinct discharge on the biological plane and how do they operate? The work on hysteria, of course, led Freud right into the problem of the incest taboo, since his explanation of the genital inhibition associated with it was precisely that later objects may represent tabooed incestuous ones; moreover, he, at this point, began to interpret the relevant genetic sequences and drive constellations retroactively from fantasy and symbolic productions, rather than to postulate environmental events *ad hoc*. This shift went along with very close attention paid to the actual mental content of patients in all its details. In this perspective, we might come to the conclusion that if the brother-sister-sister's son triangle is most emphasized by the Trobrianders themselves in mythology and dreams, that this one indeed has a primary unconscious significance in Trobriand culture. Jones's main methodological mistake would then be that he did not pay sufficient attention to Malinowski's clinical detail and rather postulated a paternal trauma on the basis of theory alone. On this level, his formulation is logical, but it is as if he had tried to apply the genetic theory of hysteria to a schizophrenic patient without having tried to modify it to fit what the patient actually had to say.

But if we abandon trauma theory, it might be possible to postulate a distinctive genetic sequence that does not depend on the actual sexual relationships of which the child may be aware. Lacking the necessary material, we can only make a hypothesis, but to do this we might begin by summing up the three major facets of the brother-sister-sister's son triangle as it operates in adult life. First, it is very evident from the dream and myth material that even though there is a strict taboo, or just because there is one, brother and sister are to each other very highly cathected libidinal objects. Second, not only is the expression of any wishes for sexuality or intimacy forbidden, but also the relationship is one of respect, so that the expression of aggression is inhibited as well; the sister must show deference to her brother as an authority figure, and he, in turn, owes certain responsibilities to her. Third, the sister's son comes into this relationship in that he also owes respect to the mother's brother, and for social continuity to be preserved, he must identify with him; for in time, of course, he will become a mother's brother with respect to his own sister's son.

Translating this into the genetic perspective, two difficulties arise. First, although this is not true in some other societies, the mother and father do share a habitation which is independent from that of the mother's brother. Second, as Jones points out, it may be difficult to conceive of the sister as a primary object (for example she may be younger and not present or an infant at the oedipal crisis), and later feelings about her may be displaced from the mother. In any event, one would expect the mother to form a part of the Oedipus triangle in almost any society since oedipal affects arise from the body closeness which is experienced in early infancy.

However, we can include the mother as a primary object

and also make the mother's brother into the primary focus of masculine identification if we presuppose that much of the boy's early feelings about him derive from the special place which the uncle, as her brother, occupies in his mother's eye. Presumably, at a very early age the small boy becomes aware of the special importance which he has to her, both as an authority figure and as a primary object in her fantasy life. In this perspective the idea of sexual jealousy can be built into the triangular situation involving mother, brother, and son in that we might say that, by some process which is not yet fully understood, the boy becomes aware of the strong affective importance which the brother has for his mother; and when his jealousy and anger are awakened, he deals with them by identification. The mother's brother then becomes the primary rival. Moreover, assuming that the passing of the Oedipus complex is equivalent to an assimilation of social representations of objects into the child's mind, we could also assume that much of his perception of his own mother is based on her role as sister, linked to the maternal uncle in the kin group to which he belongs. Having made this supposition, we could then suppose that the representations of the brother-sister relationship which are assimilated, in which the boy identifies with the brother role, then become transferred to the actual brother-sister relationship, within which the taboos are taught in the home very early in childhood. Such a formulation presupposes that identity and jealousy can both be transmitted through symbolic processes alone, without depending on particular observations or knowledge of parental sexual relations, but it would bring in the mother as a primary object, the distinctive aspect of the complex lying in the inclusion of her brother and the emphasis on her role as sister rather than father's wife.

Much of this is, of course, speculative since our knowledge of the possible range of perceptions of the oedipal child still has many gaps. However, such a formulation could reconcile the two assumptions with which we began, and moreover, could place the Oedipus complex in a more dynamic and wider social perspective, in that it would link up psychological knowledge with anthropological knowledge of kinship structure, given that we already know that this triangular relationship has a crucial status in the functioning of the matrilineal kinship system.

In a more general perspective, it should also be possible to say that each culture imposes restrictions on primary drives according to a particular pattern, and from the pattern of restrictions it should be possible to predict much of the cultural content from the assumption that symbols arise when a primary impulse is denied gratification. Such a possibility is found in the concept of repression, but perhaps comes out more clearly if we use the recent formulation of David Rapaport (1960), according to whom it is the fact of delay in drive expression which gives rise to the symbol, than in at least one facet of Jones's (1912) summary of the psychoanalytic theory of symbolism according to which there are biologically given types of primary symbolic content.

Returning to the Trobriand example, we could then say that the model for delay, or for the elaboration and maintenance of complex cultural productions, is provided by the brother-sister relationship. This latter would then be seen as the key relationship in a distinctive nuclear complex which can be used or interpreted on a number of levels: it is manifested directly in the myths of which brother-sister incest is the theme; it appears integral to matrilineal social structure; it presumably has genetic roots; and if we look to the actual experience of childhood and adolescence, we can see that quite concretely the brother-sister relationship is presented as the symbol of delay, for example, in that while infantile sexual games are generally rather freely permitted, this is not the case between brother and sister just as later in adolescence rather casual affairs are the rule, but between brother and sister the taboo is very strict. In other words, for the Trobriand Islands the brother-sister relationship has a special place on the borderline between instinct and culture; but it should also be possible to isolate such specially important relationships for other cultures as well.

Some South Italian Cultural Complexes

At this point, I should like to attempt the description of a third nuclear complex, resembling neither the matrilineal one of the Trobriand Islands nor the patriarchal one described by Freud. The material concerns Southern Italy, but descriptions by other researchers indicate the existence of similar patterns throughout the Latin world and possibly even in pre-Reformation Europe. My own concrete observations were made primarily in the city of Naples where I carried out a study of working-class families; however, the basic pattern does not seem fundamentally different in other areas of Southern Italy or in other social class groups, though, of course, there are many variations in details. What I shall try to do is to bring together a number of facts from quite diverse areas—general cultural patterns, intra-family behavior, and projective test material—in a way which depends on the framework sketched above.

The South Italian family system, similar in this respect not only to other Latin countries but also to much of the Mediterranean world, is in a certain sense intermediate between the kind of lineage system found in the Trobriand Islands and the discontinuous nuclear family characteristic of the industrial world. As we have seen in the Trobriand Islands, it is quite possible that units other than the biologically based mother-father-child one serve as the key axis of social structure; this is very often true of primitive societies where the latter unit usually is enclosed in some wider kinship unit which in turn defines patterns of social organization for the society as a whole. In industrial societies, on the other hand, it is often said that since there is such an elaboration of alternative nonkinship social structures (religious bodies, bureaucratic organizations, governments, etc.) the functions of the family have contracted to an irreducible minimum, i.e., the satisfaction of intimacy needs and the caring for small children. The family is discontinuous in the sense that it lasts only as long as particular individuals are alive; as children grow up they gradually move into a wider society and eventually form new families on their own rather than acquiring adult roles in a continuing social group. The world outside the family is seen in this perspective as a locus of positive achievement.

The South Italian family is an intermediate form in two senses. First, although there is no corporate lineage, since religious, economic, and political functions are handled by non-kinship organizations just as in any complex society, there is a rather loosely organized body of extended kin, the "parenti" which has some significance; one's "parenti," or relatives in a generic sense (usually meaning siblings of parents and their offspring), form the most immediate field of social relations and in theory at least are the persons on whom one can best count for aid in time of trouble. Second, while the family unit is the immediate biological one (with monogamous marriage, no legal divorce, and co-residence of husband, wife and minor children), this latter tends to be centripetal rather than centrifugal. In other words, parents, or in particular the mother, bring up children in such a way as to strengthen loyalties toward themselves rather than to move increasingly into a wider social context. This latter tendency is in turn associated with a definition of the world outside the family as hostile and threatening and very often as a source of temptations toward sexual or other forms of delinquency and dishonesty.

We can begin on the level of global culture patterns by examining a key complex of attitudes, namely, those surrounding the Madonna. The importance of the Madonna complex throughout the Latin world is evident to even the most casual observation; in the South Italian villages she stands in every church and along with the saints may be carried through the streets in procession, and in even the poorest quarters of the city of Naples she is likely to occupy some niche or other, decorated with the flowers or even gold chains brought by her children grateful for her favors. Moreover, every home has a private shrine, in which pictures or statues of the Madonna appear along with photographs of deceased relatives illuminated by a candle or lamp.

As a figure in Roman Catholic theology, the Madonna, of course, is only one element in a much wider religious complex.

However, popular religion in Southern Italy does not always conform to theological doctrine, for example, in that it has a considerable admixture of magical beliefs and in that the Madonna and the saints are conceived of more as persons of whom one can ask a favor (Italian *grazia,* or a grace) than as ideal figures in a moralistic sense. The Madonna may also be seen in characteristic folk manner as a quite familiar figure who is very much part of daily life. One older woman has said, "The Madonna must have had a hard time when she was carrying the Savior, because people couldn't have known about the Holy Ghost and they always gossip about such things." Religion in general is seen in this concrete and living way, and religious vocabulary as exclamations, for example, *Madonna mia* and *Santa Maria,* are very much part of daily conversation.

The most important characteristic of the Madonna is that her love and tenderness are always available; no matter how unhappy or sinful the supplicant, she will respond if she is addressed in time of need. Acts of penitence may be carried out for her, for example, pilgrimages or even licking the steps of the church one by one and proceeding to the altar (today only in the most traditional rural areas). Even such acts of penitence, however, are apt to be conceived of as means of showing one's devotion in order to secure a favor, such as the recovery of a sick child. In this sense, the Madonna complex is based on an ethic of suffering rather than sin; the devotee seeks comfort for the wrongs imposed by fate rather than a guide for changing it.

The Madonna is quite obviously the ideal mother figure, and the relationship of the supplicant to her is conceived of as that of a child. The other family figures in the Christian pantheon are, of course, not lacking, that is, the father and the son. However, God the Father is usually conceived of as being so distant that he is unapproachable except through the intermediary of the Madonna or a saint; in Naples, the first-cause theory of creation is very common, according to which God set the world in motion and then let it run according to its own devices. Christ, on the other hand, is perceived not as in many

Protestant denominations as a representative of moral individuality, or even as an alternative comforting figure, but rather
either as the good son who is truly and continually penitent or
else in the context of suffering; as dramatized in Lenten rituals,
the Madonna weeps when he dies martyrized by a hostile world.
Of the three figures, it is the Madonna who has by far the greatest concreteness in the popular eye. Moreover, of all her characteristics one of the clearest is her asexuality: she conceived without sin and so became mother without being a wife.

Not only is the most apparent deity a feminine one, but also
religion is defined as a primarily feminine sphere. Thus, while
small boys may attend mass regularly in the company of women,
as they approach puberty most of them are teased out of this
by their male peers or relatives. The level of participation in
religious functions (except for those touching on the secular
such as fiestas) is in general very low for adult males; but at
every Sunday mass one can observe crowds of young men
waiting outside the door. The reason they themselves give for
being there is that the girls are inside; thus, at the courtship
phase religious participation becomes an opportunity for escap-
ing surveillance, but with the difference that the girl's overt
devotion increases and the reverse is true for the boy. Moreover,
Southern Italy is noted for its anticlericalism, but, along with
some socioeconomic aspects, a major feature of this anticlericalism is a joking pattern whose main consequence is to raise
doubts concerning the ideals of purity which religion represents.
This joking pattern is an important part of interaction in the
male peer group which crystallizes around adolescence. It thus
seems as if religion and adult male sexuality are conceived of
as incompatible with each other.

The oppositional or skeptical trend which is represented
by anticlerical joking is seen in a number of other cultural
patterns as well; first, in swearing and obscenity which are
extremely widespread. The particular expressions used can be
divided into four groups: those wishing evil on someone else
(e.g., "may you spit up blood," from the extreme anxiety
evoked by the idea of tuberculosis); those reflecting on the

dead ("curse the dead in your family"); those reversing religious values (the most common oath being "curse the Madonna"); and those reversing the values of feminine purity. The latter group includes graphic expressions for a variety of possible incestuous relationships with mother or sister, anal as well as genital, and can also be linked with the horn gesture (index and little finger extended) implying infidelity of the wife. Cursing may be engaged in by women as well as men, but it is far more characteristic of the latter, particularly the last two types.[5]

The context and seriousness of insult and obscenity is extremely variable; one may curse the Madonna on the occasion of stubbing one's toe, but raising the possibility of the "horns" or using the incestuous expressions with enough seriousness may also lead to murder. It is this subtle distinction of style and context which differentiates Neapolitan patterns from those found in association with lineage systems where there are more formalized distinctions between those kin relationships which permit joking or obscenity, and those which do not because they are based on respect.[6] But the essential point is that the frequency of obscenity as used by men is such that one might talk of any positive value as reversible into a potential negative one; the reversibility relation is in turn confirmed by the particular content choices.

A second index of the same oppositional or skeptical trend is found in the style of masculine behavior and in social interaction within the male peer group. From adolescence on, an important segment of male life takes place on the street corner, at the bar, or in the club setting which at least psychologically

5. Women may in quarrelling with each other call each other prostitutes, but without reference to incest. They may also substitute euphemisms for actual curse words, such as *mannaggia alla marina,* literally "curse the seashore" for "curse the Madonna."

6. See Radcliffe-Brown (1952, pp. 90–116). For the Trobriand Islands, obscene jokes are freely exchanged with the father's sisters but not with the mother's brother, and there are obscene expressions referring to mother, sister, and wife. Of these the most serious insult refers to sexual relations with the wife, a fact which is not quite congruent with the emphasis we have placed on the brother-sister taboo (see Malinowski, 1927, pp. 104–108).

is quite separate from either the home or the church. But in this setting in contrast to the other two, it is masculine values which predominate over feminine ones. Not only are swearing and anticlerical joking characteristic, but most social interaction has a particular style which is partly humorous and partly cynical in quality; many features of both language and gesture point in the direction of skepticism. Moreover, attitudes toward all forms of higher authority, secular as well as religious, are far more negative than positive in emphasis. Much of this style has a ritualized quality to it, but again we have a further index of the reversibility in the masculine setting of values defined as positive in the feminine context. In addition, many male peer-group patterns, in particular the emphasis on gambling and risk, are such that they provide a kind of counterpoint to the extreme emphasis on protection and security found in the Madonna complex.[7]

The second cultural complex which we will describe centers on courtship. Courtship is highly dramatized, and in the very important tradition of Neapolitan drama one can find over and over again the same plot: girl meets boy, this is kept secret from the family, or in particular from the father, father finds out (by catching them or by gossip from others), there is a big fight in which the girl or the fiancé stands up for the couple's rights against the father, father gives in at last, and here the play ends. Sometimes there are attempts on the part of the parents to marry a daughter to an old and ugly man for reasons of *interesse* or financial gain, but they are apt to be frustrated and never go without protest from the daughter. Says Rita in the early nineteenth-century play *Anella* when her father tries to marry her off to a rich but effeminate rag dealer:[8]

You can cut me up piece by piece, but that Master Cianno, I'll never take him. Poor me! Even if I had found him while Vesuvius was erupting, I wouldn't have gone near him. If I weren't your daughter

7. See Vaillant (1958), Whyte (1943), and Zola (1963) for descriptions of relevant patterns.
8. Davino, Gennaro: *Anella: Tavernara A Portacapuana.* In: Trevisani (1957), p.125.

but your worst enemy, even then I wouldn't think of marrying that sort of man. What sort of life would it be?

The same play also serves to point up the very high degree with which courtship is romanticized and the particularly humble and supplicative position attributed to the young man. The following dialogue is addressed to Anella, standing in the balcony, by her suitor, Meniello:[9]

What sleep, what rest! What sleep, what rest can I have if I am in love, and the man in love is worse off than the man who is hanging on a rope and as soon as he gets a bit jealous, then the cord tightens. What sleep, the minute I close my eyes from exhaustion, jealousy makes me see my Anella up on her balcony surrounded by a crowd of lovers all looking up at her from below . . . what sort of sleep can you look for. And the worst of all is that I haven't even any hope of getting out of torment because I can't even ask her mother to give her to me as a wife because my dog's destiny made it happen that just to make a baker's dozen her mother is in love with me, too. You see what terrible things can happen in this world to torment a poor man in love!

(Anella appears) Oh, Menie, is that you?

(Meniello) Oh, beautiful one of my heart!

(Anella) What on earth is wrong? I haven't even dressed yet, and you are up already. Why on earth are you so early?

The dialogue continues between Meniello's supplications and Anella's much more self-assured and often more mundane reassurances against his jealousy.

Courtship is not only a theme of popular drama; it is also one of the major topics of conversation and joking in everyday life. In one sense, the social norms surrounding it are very strict, in that there are patterns of chaperonage, parents have many active rights of control, and the whole area is surrounded with an aura of taboo. Above all, it is considered highly important that the young girl keep her virginity until she is able to stand in

9. *Op. cit.,* Trevisani (1957, pp. 118–119).

church in the white veil which symbolizes it. Thus, there is a very sharp polar distinction between the good woman and the bad woman, the virgin and the prostitute. The assumptions underlying courtship are linked up in turn with a metaphorical image from which one can derive many specific customs and sayings: in a similar bipolar fashion, the home is defined as safe, feminine, and asexual, while the street is defined as inherently dangerous, tempting, and freely accessible only to men. Thus, a woman of the streets is one who has violated the taboos and in a sense has taken over masculine prerogatives. Coming into the girl's home is a very crucial step in legitimate courtship (popular terminology distinguishes between the often quite casual "so-so engaged" or "engaged in secret," and the more formalized "engaged in the house," i.e., with parental knowledge and approval), and the doorway occupies a particularly strategic intermediary position. Young girls usually become very excitable and giggly when they have the occasion for a promenade, and street phobias are a very common neurotic symptom in Italian women.

But a second aspect of the courtship complex is that in spite of the apparent strictness violations continually occur nevertheless, and the whole topic is treated with a particular kind of humorous ambiguity. Thus, while sexual matters are never referred to in serious or "objective" ways in everyday conversation, in a teasing or joking way they are an almost continuous focus of social exchange. The actual atmosphere or attitudes created by the strictness are far from puritan; it is rather as if the mothers and aunts and cousins who watch over the young girl with terrible threats about what will happen if she is "bad" are at the same time very much enjoying the possibility with her. One might by analogy to the many primitive societies in which there is a polar distinction between social relationships based on teasing or joking and those which are based on seriousness or formal respect, distinguish along the same lines between the Madonna complex and the courtship complex. For this reason, the distinction between the good woman and the bad woman is not as absolute as it might seem; often these may be alternative asexual and sexual images for the same woman, as when a father in anger calls his daughter a prostitute because she has come in late.

However, there is one point at which the sacred and the profane come together, and this is at the point of marriage, which almost without exception is symbolized by a church ceremony. Thus, while courtship is a secular process and while the idea of violation of chaperonage norms is often treated with humor, its more serious aim is nevertheless that it should end up in church with the young girl being able to stand "in front of the Madonna" in the white veil.[10] At the same time, marriage for the man symbolizes a kind of capitulation to the feminine religious complex, whose importance is denied in the male peer group setting by the pattern of sarcasm and secularization. In contrast to the girl, whatever prior sexual entanglements he has had lack significance. Thus, while at least in peasant areas even today the girl's "honor" may be verified by relatives after the wedding night, the whole question is seen as simply irrelevant on the sexual plane as far as men are concerned: said one informant, "How would anyone ever know if a man had it or not?"

There is, nevertheless, a sense in which the idea of honor is relevant to masculine identity as well as feminine. This is that the task of chaperonage is seen by the father (or brother) as a matter of maintaining his personal honor as well as the collective honor of the family. Thus, if a girl falls into disgrace, it will be said that the family honor has been lost, or that her father is also a *disgraziato* or lacking in grace. Moreover, whenever insults are cast at female kin, as in the oaths which reflect on the purity of mother, sister, daughter, or wife, the man is expected to consider this as a violation of his own personal integrity and to immediately come to their defense—in some instances with a knife. There are areas where the violation of the honor of a daughter or sister can lead to socially approved homicide, necessary to the defense of the family honor. This pattern is particularly characteristic of Sicily, where the brother's role is more

10. Voluntary abstention from public church ceremony sometimes occurs when wearing the veil would be a shame in front of the Madonna.

important than in Naples. In eighteenth- and nineteenth-century Naples the task of protecting the honor of slum women was taken over by the Camorra, the most highly organized form reached by the Neapolitan underworld, which was not averse to using knives in order to force a reluctant man who had violated virginity into marriage.

We can now try to sum up some of the respective implications of the courtship complex and the Madonna complex as two contrasting sides of a global cultural pattern. One of these we have seen as a joking pattern and the other as a pattern of serious respect and desexualization, although the two meet and cross each other both in the male peer-group rebellion against the Madonna and in the culmination of legitimate courtship in the church wedding. The symbol that unites them is that of virginity, or an initial asexual image of femininity that can only be violated in the appropriate social circumstances. These contrasting but interdependent patterns in themselves give us some of the elements of a distinctive nuclear complex; the two most important elements are that of the sublimated respect of children for the ideal mother and that of the game in which erotic temptations continually come into clash with this image of feminine purity. In the latter context, the most important actors, as Neapolitan drama would suggest, are the girl, her father, and the prospective son-in-law. The key value is that of virginity or honor, and the father seeks to preserve it against all comers; it is here that we can look for a distinctive triangular situation.

Family Structure

At this point, we can turn to the more direct consideration of the family. We noted earlier that the primary unit is the nuclear family but that it is embedded in a larger kin group, and there is a high degree of continuity to the mother-child tie. The family is close in a certain sense, at least in that family ties and obligations outweigh all others, but family life is also characterized by a great deal of aggression and conflict. One way in which conflict is handled is by various patterns for the separation of roles, a result of which is the extrafamilial male peer group. After marriage, as well as before, many of the man's needs for comradeship and mutuality continue to be filled by the male peer group and much of the time he is out of the home. The woman, on the other hand, continues in close daily exchange with her natal family (perhaps less in the city than in the villages, and neighbors may also be important) so that many needs for mutual sympathy are fulfilled by mother and sisters or by other women. The division of the sexes is such that the marriage relationship is not often a focus of continuous intimate or reciprocal affective exchange. After the courtship phase and the honeymoon, it more often than not becomes very conflictual, principally because of the emotional ties which both partners retain to the natal family.

In actual fact, of course, there are a great many varied families as well as the noted regional variations; however, many of the observable norms and patterns can be interpreted from the above structural givens. For example, there is a variety of possible balances to the husband-wife versus primary family conflict. For Naples, the most common type of residence is in the vicinity of the wife's family, but the husband as an individual is likely to maintain important contacts with his own. Sometimes the couple together becomes assimilated into one family or another; women, for example, who have had particularly unfavorable relations with their own families, or who have lost a mother by death, are more likely to accept the mother-in-law as a mother surrogate, thus achieving a better relationship with her than is generally expected. The same may happen in the case of the man who marries into a fatherless family or one consisting of girls alone who may take over male roles in that family with relative success. This is unlikely if there are competing figures. Quarrels concerning where the couple should reside are very common, and they are accompanied by a great deal of mutual projection; thus, a man may complain that his wife is much too dependent on her mother and pays little attention to him, and then suggest as a solution to the problem that

they move to the house next door to his mother. In extreme cases
the two families may end up with quite violent feelings about
each other; in studying schizophrenic patients, we found this to
be common, and many marriages, while maintained in form,
actually dissolved with each partner returning to his own home.
The uncertainties of the conflict are intensified by the fact that in
contrast to many simpler societies, there are no fixed rules of
choice or subordination. A result of this uncertainty is that in
situations of choice and conflict, it is more often the feminine
point of view than the masculine one which prevails, since it is
the woman who in daily life is most concerned with and most
emotionally involved in matters pertaining to the family.

It is also the mother who is the primary personage in maintaining family unity, and many results of this can be observed;
for example, ties with father or siblings are very likely to break
up or become more distant on the death of the mother. Another
consequence is seen in differential attitudes toward the remarriage
of widows and in differing consequences of the death of parents.
If a man is left without a wife, it is taken for granted that he will
need a woman, and whether or not he has children, he is likely
to find one, though often outside of legal sanction. Thus, many
persons who have widower fathers simply state that they have
drifted off somewhere, and the ties are no longer very real. On
the other hand, a widow or a woman deserted by her husband
may be condemned if she seeks alternative sexual attachments
before her children marry; it is assumed that her primary loyalty
is to them. Marriage, which in Naples is likely to take place
either in the late teens or not until the late twenties or thirties,
often in this latter instance follows very closely on the death
of the parents. Remarriages when both partners have children
are often conflictual on the grounds that each prefers his own
offspring, and the stepmother is seen as in the Cinderella legend.
She may do her best by the children, but even then the tie is
never the same; the best possible solution to the loss of a mother
is seen to be adoption by the mother's sister, who, because
related by blood, will come much closer to fulfilling the maternal
role. Marriage to the deceased wife's sister is not uncommon

in the case of widowers, though practiced more in rural than in urban areas.

The importance of the mother-child tie as the axis of family structure is seen in some additional patterns characteristic of lower-class Naples. Where illegitimacy occurs, the child is legally recognized and brought up by the mother in about 50 per cent of the cases; such status is not formally approved but it does occur.[11] Fathers very rarely recognize illegitimate children, but there are, on the other hand, certain forms of semi-institutionalized polygamy, according to which a father may have two distinctive families, one of which is legal while the other is not. In contrast to the pattern of the affair where it is assumed that if the relationship is not socially sanctioned, precautions will be taken to avoid reproduction, it seems that aside from prostitution it is usually assumed that children are the necessary and wanted consequence of any sexual relationship; thus, the rapid multiplication which often characterizes monogamous families also characterizes polygamous ones.

The major requirement for a husband is that he be able to feed and support his family. However, in the urban working class, it very often happens that he is not able to fulfill this task; thus, one common source of arguments is that the husband has not brought in any money. It is also the case in urban areas where the married woman often works in her own right; for example, women may be street vendors, artisans, domestics, etc. At the lower socioeconomic levels it is often the woman who has a better opportunity of earning money than the man. She is more motivated to work since she more willingly accepts a low-prestige or low-reward position because of concern for children, while for the man, peer-group relationships or a kind of pseudo identification with the higher status groups offers a more immediately rewarding proof of masculinity. One of the primary symbols of peer-group belongingness in Naples is the ability to

11. Of the illegitimate children born in Naples in 1956, 51 per cent were legally recognized by the mother alone, as compared with 9 per cent by the father alone, 10 per cent by both parents, and 29 per cent remaining unrecognized. See Office of Statistics of the Commune of Naples (1959, p. 22).

offer food or drink to others, so that the man is faced with an inherent conflict in that what he spends to gain status in relation to other men is bread lost out of his children's mouths. Thus, a vicious circle may be set in motion in which the wife accuses the husband of irresponsibility, and the husband in turn goes off in anger and tries to recapture his self-esteem by taking risks at cards or by treating his friends to coffee. It is, moreover, the way of dealing with this situation which differentiates male relationships with wives and mothers; the mother, if she has anything at all, will give it to her son, but the wife expects the husband to hand everything over to her in the interests of the children. Thus, financial conflicts are one factor which can push a married man back to ask for support at home.

A second factor is the degree to which intrafamily behavior is characterized by rivalry between husband and children for the attention of the mother in her food-giving role. One symbolization of the difference between South Italian society and the more truly patriarchal Victorian one can be found in the nature of eating patterns and their relation to family social structure; in contrast to the regular ritualized mealtimes of the Victorian epoch, with father taking a commanding position at the head of the table, there is a highly irregular eating pattern (space often makes a regular dinner table impossible) in which each member of the family may eat according to his own preference at his own time, but in which the mother is almost continually involved in the process of feeding. In this structure the superior position of the father, and of sons as they grow up, is symbolized by the right to demand what they want and the right to complain if not pleased. When a man complains, the woman will try to do what she can, and as long as she has anything at all, she will give it; but the pattern also puts the husband on an equal subordinate basis with his children.

Thus, the ties to the primary family, the high significance of the maternal role, and the very great difficulties in making a living which characterize most of the working-class groups are such that in spite of appearances the husband and father does not actually enjoy much prestige or authority in the home. From this standpoint the male peer group can be seen as an escape; the man who gets totally "fed up" always has the possibility of leaving. Likewise, many of the male rage reactions, which give the impression that the Italian family is patriarchal, though much more stylized, have the quality of the child who throws his plate on the floor when he has had enough. Moreover, many of the status-gaining activities of the peer group can be seen as identifications with the feminine feeding role, for example, the high importance attributed to offering food or coffee. However, a second aspect of the masculine role in the home and its relations to sex segregation should not be neglected. This is that male rage may be seen as truly terrifying to women, so that kicking men out becomes necessary, and this goes with an image of masculinity as a kind of threatening force which is a disruptive factor in the feminine circle; images used in daily conversation clearly suggest the idea of phallic intrusion.

A few details on socialization can serve to round out the picture of family life. Children become a center of attention as soon as they are born and receive a great deal of physical handling which does not undergo systematic interruption; moreover, as they are weaned, substitute gratifications are provided so there is no significant discontinuity ending the oral phase of development. However, it would be a mistake to conclude from this that they simply receive that much more of the "security" and maternal warmth which are currently so highly valued in the United States. In the first place, the mother may give little attention to any individual child, being busy and often having many; moreover, maternal behavior (in the sense of giving food and physical caresses) is so widespread that in actual social reality the maternal attachment is far from being exclusive. Rather, one might say that the circle of maternal objects progressively widens to include the family as a whole and in many respects strangers; along with this goes the learning of certain kinds of politeness and formality having to do with eating and giving.

In the second place, handling of children is often rough and unsubtle and includes a very high aggressive component.[12] As physical motility appears, it can be systematically frustrated by anxious adults who immediately bring back the wandering or assertive child to thrust a cookie into his mouth; one can see here the beginning of the forced feeding pattern which characterizes moments of tension in the family throughout life. An illustrative example concerns a three-year-old son of a gardener who picked up his father's tools and was immediately called back by mother with the tacit support of father. Children at this age may show considerable diffuse aggressivity and put on an unnatural amount of weight. Later, most of them learn to "talk back" with verbal rhetoric and gesture; these important components of South Italian culture might be seen as developed in counterreaction to muscular inhibition in that they become a major means for expressing individuality. A second relevant example concerns an eighteen-month-old girl who seemed hardly interested in learning to walk and was not yet able to talk; yet, held by her father she was able to perform fairly complex symbolic operations with her hands, such as snapping her fingers ten times when asked to count to ten.

For these early phases there seems to be little difference between the handling of the small girl and of the small boy, with the single exception that the small boy is more likely to go unclothed from the waist down and to have his penis singled out for teasing admiration.[13] This open phallic admiration is characteristic of the behavior of mothers to sons, and in teasing intrafamily behavior the genital organs may be poked or referred to with provocative gestural indications. Children may also share beds with their parents or with each other even at advanced

12. It is roughest among the poorest and here also may be quite erotically stimulating as well. I am indebted to Vincenzo Petrullo for the suggestion that this latter may be the case because when children have to go hungry, erotic stimulation may be a means of maintaining their interest in life.

13. This pattern is even more characteristic of Puerto Rico (see Wolf, 1952), where sex differences in modesty rules are also sharper.

ages (crowding often makes this necessary)[14] though precautions are taken to prevent their observing parental intercourse. One young man was asked what he would do if he saw this; the answer was "I would kill them." Except for small children, modesty taboos are very strict, and while physical proximity within the family is very close with respect to anything except genital activity, this latter is surrounded with some secrecy.

There are, however, two crucial points at which sex difference is more prominent. The first is in the ritual of First Communion which ideally takes place at the age of six or seven. Around this age the growing attractiveness of the little girl is the focus of considerable teasing admiration from father or older brothers, uncles, etc., though these have not taken much interest in the very small child. One Neapolitan informant, for example, told me how his seven-year-old daughter had taken to getting into bed with him in such a seductive way that he finally had to slap her and kick her out. It did not surprise him in the least when I said that a famous Viennese doctor had made quite a bit out of this sort of thing. However, once the small girl's oedipal affects have been excited to this degree, it is also necessary that the culture find a resolution for them which it does in the ritual of First Communion; the small girl is dressed as a miniature bride, and at this point it must be impressed on her fantasy that she must delay fulfillment of her wishes until such a time as she can again appear in church in a white veil. Thus, a particularly elaborate cultural symbolization is provided for feminine oedipal wishes.

For the boy, on the other hand, there is much less in the way of such cultural elaboration of the Oedipus crisis, nor for that matter is there any ritual symbolization of masculine status at adolescence, as there is in many other cultures where socialization at earlier stages is so exclusively in the hands of women. First Communion does take place, but masculine emphasis and

14. I know of examples of mothers sharing beds with adult sons, and also of a case of a mother who lost a child in infancy whereupon she asked a thirteen-year-old son to take the milk from her breast; he, however, refused on the grounds that "she was my mother and I was ashamed."

degree of symbolization is simply less. Moreover, in many ways the boy's position at home is much more passive than that of the girl; the beautiful warm-eyed docility which one can observe in many boys in the Neapolitan slums might make for the envy of the American mother in the Hopalong Cassidy phase. The same degree of aggressive tension does not appear to be present, nor for that matter is there as much elaboration of the phallic "I want to be when I grow up" type of fantasy. What does differentiate the small boy from the girl is, first, the open admiration which may be shown for his purely sexual masculine attributes, and second, the fact that he has much less in the way of home responsibility and is in many ways favored by the mother; but since the father is so often out of the home, his socialization is placed in feminine hands almost as much as that of the girl.

In other words, while cultural ritual can be seen as providing a complex symbolic framework for feminine oedipal wishes, this is not true in the case of the boy, who may receive special privileges and an open acknowledgment of his physical masculinity, but no such elaborate social symbolization of it. Presumably, this should result in much stronger motivation for the delay of sexual wishes in girls than in boys. This kind of differential in turn becomes extremely important in adolescence, at which point the pattern of sex differentiation becomes a much sharper one, for it is then that chaperonage rules begin to apply to the girl, and the boy in turn acquires a special freedom to move out into the inherently dangerous and sexualized world of the street.[15] It is at this latter point that the prerogative of adult masculinity crystallizes, especially with respect to the quasi taboo on feminine inquisitions concerning masculine activities which take place outside the home.

15. Boys are of course outside earlier too, the actual age and amount of time depending on the specific social milieu. The street gang in the slums may include girls and in some groups much of the family income may come from small boys. The important fact is the lack of any very formalized masculine authority over the boy.

Projective Test Material

One of our initial assumptions was that culture appears in the individual in the form of object representations which crystallize in the conscious mind at the time of the passing of the Oedipus complex. In this perspective, the norms of intra-family behavior should be reflected on the psychological plane in the form of more or less uniform representations of the significant family figures in relation to the self. This dimension is one which can be measured through the use of projective tests. Such material will be presented as a supplement to the cultural and social observations which we have already made.

In two separate studies, a number of cards from the Murray TAT were presented to working-class informants in Naples. Four cards (6GF, 6BM, 7BM, 7GF) will be discussed here. They were presented to the informants with the specific directive that they represent family scenes (mother-daughter, father-son, father-daughter, and mother-son), and they were to describe the scene as it appeared to them. Though few very elaborate stories were given, the subjects saw the cards in an amazingly vivid way with a high degree of sensitivity to the immediate perceptual and gestural details of the figures.[16] The high degree of uniformity of response is in itself a proof of the psychological reality of culture. This uniformity was greatest for the mother-son and father-daughter scenes.

MOTHER-DAUGHTER CARD

The mother-daughter card was presented to twenty-six female informants with a specific directive: "The mother is advising the daughter, what do you think she is telling her?" Additional questions such as "How does the daughter feel about it?" were also asked. Thus, we purposely biased the situation in the direction of emphasis on maternal authority. However, only to a certain extent was this the major theme; rather, the

16. "Stories" more often took the form of "well, from the way his eyes are you can tell that , , , ," followed by a conclusion about motivation or feeling.

responses fell into three distinct groups, of which the first is most directly relevant to the question of authority as such.

For eleven subjects, the mother appeared as giving some very definite form of censure or advice. In only one such instance is the reaction of the daughter to this seen as wholly positive; in one other instance the reaction of the daughter is openly rebellious, and in the remaining nine, the daughter accepts the advice as "for her own good" but with expressed resentment; however, the mother is finally vindicated since "things don't turn out well in the long run":

The mother is giving good advice to the daughter; the mother tells the daughter to behave well, not to go out much, to pay more attention to things at home. She has to help her mother to do the housework. The picture is beautiful because there is nothing bad in it.

The mother is yelling at the daughter because with the excuse of the child who is her little brother she goes out walking and comes in late. The daughter talks back to her mother saying "What do you want with me? You made this baby and now you go around finding out bad things about me."

The mother is moralizing. The daughter is a bit fed up with the mother's words. . . .

The mother tells the little girl that she has to do housework and the daughter is not looking at the mother as if she had not heard and did not want to do this work. . . . Things won't go very well because the daughter won't listen to the mother.

The first reaction is particularly interesting in that by implication it so clearly brings out the asexual nature of the home in contrast to the outside world where there may always be "something bad." The second is equally interesting in that where there is open rebellion on the part of the daughter, the mother is also portrayed as a sexual being. The remaining responses show a very classic pattern of internalized but ambivalently accepted authority; the mother is clearly a superego figure, but considerable rebellion and resentment are experienced toward her.

For the next group of subjects, the card itself provided a particular difficulty. The Murray card shows a girl in the latency period being read to by her mother and holding what could be either a doll or a live baby. The situation of a mother reading to the daughter is, of course, somewhat out of the ordinary in this group, but in addition a number of informants were led to comment from the girl's age that this could not actually be an authority situation since "the girl is too young to be given the most important advice."

Thus, these responses were limited to fairly factual and emotionally neutral kinds of advice ("the mother is telling the daughter how to bring up her little brother"), and more crucial attitudes of mother and daughter were not made clear. The responses are important principally for their value in pointing up just how crucial the courtship situation is as compared to any other area of performance with respect to the question of authority in general.

For the third group of three respondents this was true as well, but they simply ignored the age of the girl on the card and perceived the situation as involving a mother, her daughter, and the latter's illegitimate child :

The mother talks with the daughter that is married and has a child, no, I mean the daughter is not married. The mother tries to help her and get her married, the mother is good and does not throw her out of the house.

The girl is not married and it seems to me that her mother gives her advice on how to bring up the child. It seems that the mother has forgiven her and tells her to treat the child well. The mother gives advice to the daughter about how to behave and how not to fall a second time. Because the mother is understanding she says to the daughter to be careful because the mother should try not to say to the daughter that she is guilty because the girl could do something to hurt herself, she could commit suicide or fall into the same error again thinking that she doesn't have anyone who cares.

This is, of course, a crucial and dramatic situation where norms have actually been violated. The responses make clear that fear of loss of maternal love is a major threat preventing more frequent violations; but also in the actual crisis situation the mother may not really kick the girl out of the house. Another evidence of the internalized nature of maternal authority is seen in the respondent who conceived of suicide as a possibility in the event that such forgiveness did not take place.[17]

FATHER-SON CARD

The father-son card was presented to ten men and ten women in a second study. No specific directives were given beyond the statement that the scene involved a father and a son. Authority, however, turned out to be the most important theme, found in the responses of seven men and three women, but in contrast to the mother-daughter responses the specific content of the advice or censure given by the father to the son was left indeterminate. However, there is no doubt but that fathers were seen by the majority of men as censuring figures :

. . . the father reproaches the son . . . the son is a delinquent, you can see from his face that he is not a nice person and I think he will not listen to the father's advice. . . .

The son is bitter and the father displeased because the son would like to talk about something and doesn't. During the family life, the father asks the son what trade he would like to have while the son takes the matter unhappily. He would like to be a chauffeur and the father makes him learn carpentry and the result is that he practices his trade against his own will and cannot succeed in it. After a few years he begins to hate the father and so he remains without any trade at all. The son on his side would like to be a chauffeur. As a result father and son fight, the son curses the father, the father says "you ought to listen to me."

17. Low suicide rates are often taken as evidence of the lack of internalized superegos. However, material from Southern Italy, including the fact that depressive symptoms are not at all rare, might suggest that instead there are secondary social mechanisms (i.e., the possibility of forgiveness) which alleviate guilt whose subjective intensity may nevertheless be very great. The high suicide rates found in modern industrial countries may result then from the lack of these, or what Durkheim (1897) calls anomie.

The second response was stated to be an autobiographical one; the respondent was the son of an artisan and, as the result of having gambled away his youth and refusing to learn a trade, was at the time I saw him a very despondent man, father of eight children whom he tried to support as a street vendor. Moreover, while all the male respondents were themselves fathers with children, they seemed not to take the perspective of the father. The exceptions to the rule that both were seen negatively were only partial ones; one respondent did unconvincingly portray the father as affable while another (particularly intelligent and outward seeking) was the only respondent to think of the possibility of positive rather than negative assertion against the father :

The son is affable and absolutely convinced of the father's counsels.

The father is decided and authoritarian, ugly. The son *might* be bad, he has an independent spirit and does not want to listen to the father. The son follows something else, as if the father's wisdom were something annoying, not very important for him.

Two of the remaining three men saw the situation as one of shared sorrow for the death of a woman and the third presented an alternative comradely view of their relationship :

There is a close friendship between the father and son, they confide in each other.

But for women it was themes of common sorrow and depression which took precedence over those concerning authority. Thus, three saw authority themes and three a common sorrow over death; but the remaining four show the two as sharing a common sense of helplessness with respect to the (primarily economic) external reality :

They are desperate (for money)—they worry. Nothing more.

They are worrying about something, the office, work, because they are melancholy.

What a shame, the father is completely blind! Don't you see he has his eyes completely closed and an absent expression? The son is as if he were listening to something, it must be a radio, but the father has the look really of a blind man. (Don't they say anything to each other?) No, the father minds his own business, really with the look of a blind man, and the son on the other hand is listening, he must be listening to the radio.

In this the women seem to be able to portray a socially very real aspect of their relationship, that it is hard for a man to be an effective authority when he cannot provide anything for his son, which the men themselves have to deny.

The most striking features of the responses to the father-son card are, thus, the lack of a clear social agreement concerning the nature of this relationship, and for the men the lack of effective internalization of paternal authority. By the latter, we mean that sons are simply seen as "bad" or "delinquent" in relation to the father, without, as was the case in the mother-daughter situation, there being a view of how the son ought to accept the authority for his own good. One might say that this provides further evidence that the society is not patriarchal, and masculinity is defined more in terms of rebellion than positive identification. In simplest terms, the conflict is that portrayed by one informant who says, "They seem against each other."

FATHER-DAUGHTER CARD

For a contrast with responses to the father-son scene, we might again quote the street vendor, who turned to this card with considerable relief and pleasure :

This case here defines a father, he is sociable. Here it is no longer a job problem, the girl must know a man and he knew from the information that he has been a delinquent. He says "look for another path, there are millions of men." The father wants happiness for his daughter, he wants her to marry someone who will give her something to eat. (Q) The daughter answers "it's my business," no daughter ever listens to her father. (Q) They get bitter but then they make peace after a child is born.

Unfortunately, we do not have enough male answers to this card to analyze quantitatively; however, this one indicates that while the father does have authority over the daughter, its overthrow is to be expected even by the father himself and while they may "get bitter," the bitterness is nothing like the real hostility of the father-son antagonism. The same card was administered to thirty-two female respondents, and it was among these that the highest degree of uniformity was found. Twenty saw the situation as conflict between father and daughter related to courtship :

The father does not want the daughter to get engaged to a man he knows and does not want this man to marry his daughter. The father is making her ashamed. The father seems bad to me. He is jealous of the daughter and does not want her to get engaged. The daughter is a beautiful girl. She cares a lot about this man that her father doesn't want to give her to and she wants to get married at any price.

The father is mortifying the daughter. The father is having it out with the daughter because other people have told him something. He makes her ashamed and she remains surprised and amazed. The father wants to know the story of his daughter's engagement. She does not want to tell about her affairs and probably the father heard about this engagement from other people. The father wants to know if it is a good marriage for his daughter.

The daughter seems like an actress. The father is reasoning with the daughter. They are probably talking about the daughter's fiancé ; the father wants to know how things are going in her engagement. The father is happy and the daughter is a bit fed up because her father wants to know many facts about her relationship with the fiancé. For this reason she is not answering spontaneously.

Nine of the remaining twelve respondents gave generally very inhibited answers or denied that the scene could actually be father and daughter in such a way as to suggest some neurotic inhibition.

I don't know how to say anything about this picture. The father is mad and the daughter is calm. They are talking about not very important problems that have to do with family life.

(Informant says that the test seems a bit complicated here.) The father is upset because the daughter didn't do something in the house; she should have done some errand and didn't do it. The father says to the girl, "You got dressed up to go out and didn't do the errands." The father doesn't let her go out but the relations between father and daughter aren't bad.

And finally three informants saw the scene as one in which the father was making seductive advances toward the daughter.

The father is looking at the daughter in a strange way, that is more like a man than like a father. She looks at him perplexed and almost struck dumb. The father will not succeed because the daughter has understood his intentions, she will control herself unless he attacks her. The father is not behaving very well; he has gone astray . . . maybe because the girl is attractive.

All three saw the girl as able to control the situation. An additional two among the above nine, while denying that the scene could be father and daughter, saw, respectively, a husband and wife, and an older Don Juan boss seducing a secretary.

As far as we know the incest responses were not given by seriously disturbed women and they show fewer signs of inhibition than the respondents who did not perceive any shame or conflict between father and daughter at all.

For the first group there was not a single informant who failed to perceive the situation as a conflictual one in which the conflict lay between the father's censure or possessiveness and the daughter's wish to have a boyfriend. Moreover, the card typically evoked a complex of affects which included pleasure (blushing and giggling), shame, and embarrassment. When we look for the outcome of the conflict, we find one element in common with the father-son card, namely, the tendency is in the direction of expected rebellion rather than internalized acceptance of paternal authority. In ten out of twenty instances the daughter is specifically stated to win the battle with father, while in only three does she concede; in the remaining cases the fact of conflict is simply stated. In other words, the TAT responses repeat the same dramatic pattern which we have already seen in the play *Anella* in which the courtship situation is a triangular relation between father, daughter, and prospective son-in-law, and the expected outcome is the ritual termination of the father's possessive relation to the daughter.

MOTHER-SON CARD

The most important characteristic of these responses is the extent to which they show a close correspondence to the Madonna complex, just as the father-daughter card corresponds to the courtship one. One theme occurs over and over again, more frequent among male than female respondents, namely, that of the penitent son who is returning to the mother:

. . . the son is asking forgiveness of the mother, repenting of the evil he has done. . . .

The mother pushes the young man away and he asks for something insistently. Or maybe he did something very serious, probably he went away, and so now he has come back to ask her forgiveness and the mother no longer wants to receive him.

The mother has a son she has not seen for many years . . . he returns after having done many bad things, stealing and other things. He returns to the family to ask forgiveness. Who knows whether or not the mother will give it to him but I think she will.
The son is asking forgiveness for something . . . a mother would always forgive her son, even if he were an assassin, even if he were Chessman.

The penitent son who returns to the mother and the mother cannot or does not know how to forgive him.

In comparison to the responses concerning the father, what is most striking is the extent to which the son places the burden of guilt upon himself, in that asking for forgiveness implies an internalized sense of wrongdoing.

There was some variation among the respondents as to whether the mother was seen as certain to provide forgiveness or not; the fact that some expressed doubt or uncertainty is evidence that maternal love is not conceived of as wholly unconditional. In two instances informants were known to have marked difficulties in their actual relationships with the mother. One of these is the informant who states that "the mother cannot or does not know how to forgive"—but he portrays the son as the saint who forgives the mother unable to forgive. The second, recently kicked out of home, is the only one who saw the mother as acting aggressively ("The mother pushes the young man away," etc.), but after in a sense blaming the mother, he changes pattern and like the others puts the burden of guilt on the son.

For ten male and ten female respondents, what we call the penitence response was given by seven men and four women. Among the other responses, three portrayed simple sadness ("The mother is sad because the son will leave"), and three anger. All of the anger responses were given by women, who, on the whole, presented a less romanticized view of the relationship. One response given by a beggar is particularly interesting in that it shows a relation between psychic abnormality and open anger and sexual deviance on the part of the mother:

As if he (she?) were all upset. You can see the son is arguing with the mother, he has turned his back, maybe they had a family fight. (About what?) Mama and son because the mama you can see made a lot of scandals and the son wants to find out something, who knows what, and so mama and son are arguing . . . because you can see that the mother is a bit off in the head because she turns her back on the son. (Yes, you can see that she is a bit angry. But how does the son feel about it?) The son has an enraged face, he has his nerves out of place too. (In response to further questions, she shifts subject.)

In many instances the fact that the American card portrays a mother looking away from her son was sensed as disturbing but that it could imply psychic distance was denied. Thus, while it may be perceived by women, there seems to be a taboo on perceiving anger in the mother-son relationship by men. In this respect there is a very clear contrast with respect to the father-son relationship.

Conclusions

We began, with reference to the Jones-Malinowski debate, by considering the possibility that each culture is characterized by a distinctive nuclear complex whose roots lie in its family structure. Our subsequent task has been to pull together various orders of data concerning Southern Italy in such a way as to portray such a nuclear complex which differs both from the brother-sister-sister's son triangle characteristic of the Trobriand Island and from the patriarchal complex isolated by Freud. In the South Italian data we have found that two cultural complexes, the sacred one centered on respect for the feminine Madonna figure and the secular joking pattern surrounding courtship and embodied in popular drama, also have their reflections in the actual patterning of family life and childhood experience and in the intrapsychic life of the individual as seen in projective tests. It is this continuity which has led us to the conclusion that it is possible to define a single global complex which can be perceived simultaneously either as intrapsychic or as collective, the representations which are passed on from generation to generation on the social level coming to be internalized in the individual in the form of representations of the self in relation to objects. The task which remains is the more precise summary of the outlines of the South Italian nuclear complex, comparing it with Freud's patriarchal one, and the drawing out of some more general implications with respect to research methodology and application.

Our principal supposition is that the two most significant among the biologically given family relationships are those between mother and son and between father and daughter. In the former instance the son occupies a subordinate position in the sense that authority stemming from the mother is fully internalized, and violations of it are subjectively sensed as inducing guilt, in comparison to the father-son relation where the son may openly express hostility or rebellion in such a way as to put the father in a negative light. In other words, respect for the mother is much stronger than respect for the father. We do not mean by this to say that women dominate in any simple sense, since it is evident that many other taboos, such as the barring of feminine interference in areas of activity defined as masculine ones, act against this result, not to mention the open admiration and permissiveness which women usually show toward the masculinity of their sons. However, in many ways the mother-son relationship is qualitatively different from that of our own society or that of Freud, most notably in the continuation throughout life of what might be referred to as an oral dependent tie, i.e., a continual expectation of maternal solace and giving rather than a gradual or sudden emancipation from it.

It is this fact that might lead an American observer to speak of an "oral" culture, or one based on feeding as the dominant mode of libidinal interaction, in contrast to a hypothetical "anal" or "phallic" based one. However, this type of formulation we would consider quite inadequate both with respect to theory and the empirical facts. It is evident that types of interaction based on the exchange of gifts and food do have an extremely important role, though these result in very complex types of adult interaction which can by no means be derived directly from infantile roots. More important, however, is the theoretical postulate which would lead us to believe that the phallic phase of development nevertheless occurs. In other words, although he may not give up oral types of gratification, the boy nevertheless passes through a phase at which the wishes he experiences toward the mother are sexual and masculine in nature, and that, moreover, this phase will be associated with aggressive reactions against the subordinate feeding position. We can then trace some of the implications of these postulates rather than simply stopping with the "oral culture" formulation.

In this perspective we can better see some of the more general consequences of the fact that the masculine role is so little emphasized within the home and that cultural values center on the feminine image. From the genetic standpoint, we might say that while oral gratifications do not have to be renounced (although they do come to take more complex social forms), this is not true with respect to phallic and aggressive wishes toward the mother; these in fact must systematically undergo repression as they arise. In fact, to characterize the relation to the mother as one based on respect, in social language, is exactly the same thing as to say in psychodynamic language that sexual and aggressive wishes cannot be expressed directly. We then can ask what happens to these wishes, assuming that in some form they persist, and arrive at three kinds of formulation, each of which is relevant to the understanding of culture patterns. Through all of them the important contrast with Freud's formulation lies in the greater continuity of the relationship with the mother and the lesser continuity of that with the father.

First, referring back to the concept of the symbol as arising in precisely those areas where a culture both exploits (by actual affective closeness) and inhibits (by imposing of taboos) primary drives, we can say that the erotic wishes of the son toward the mother come to be sublimated, and it is precisely this fact which gives rise to the representation of the Madonna figure. Moreover, in her characteristics we can see both derivatives of the actual cultural reality, e.g., in that the dependent relationship of the penitent to the maternal figure is preserved, and some unrealizable aspects of fantasy, e.g., in that the Madonna became a mother without being a wife. This latter is, moreover, the characteristic which in itself represents oedipal repression, in that the Madonna is perceived as an asexual maternal figure. But in addition, and in contrast to the "oral culture" view which might say simply that mothers are more permissive, the Madonna is a "superego" figure; she could not be forgiving if she did not have a concept of sins which have to be forgiven. In this perspective we can say that oedipal wishes are repressed in such a way as to give rise to an internalized representation of the tabooed object, who then comes to play the role of conscience. However, the complication in this case is that the internalized object is in the case of men a feminine one; it is this which we mean by speaking of a matriarchal rather than a patriarchal "superego." What it leads to then is a masculine identification with a set of cultural values identifiable as feminine, or even as very concretely perceived according to a feminine body image. The most important of these is the respect for virginity, shared by men and women alike and manifested in the courtship taboos on entering the home of the girl who is sought before the relation is formalized. The identification of the girl who is legitimately courted with the idealized mother is seen in the similar submissive relation adopted by the male; the infantile wishes underlying the image of the pure woman are also seen in a sometimes extreme degree of defensiveness concerning the issue of whether or not the purity is real and to be believed.

Second, however, impulses which are repressed can also be dealt with by displacement. It is in this respect that the significance of the masculine peer group and the definition of the sphere of life outside of the home, i.e., the sum total of masculinity as defined by the rebellion pattern which we have discussed, become apparent. Many of the patterns of the outside peer group are distinctively phallic in nature. Moreover, in many more concrete senses one can conceive of the outside world as the focus for aggressive and phallic wishes which must be displaced outside the home, e.g., the common situation of the male in anger who simply picks up and leaves, or the great importance of cursing. Thus, aggression which arises within the home may be dealt with by displacement outside it. One characteristic of the Madonna is that she is an ideal figure; ordinary mothers of course rarely approach her, in that they may not forgive, they may very often get angry or impatient, or they may in fact dominate in a very aggressively matriarchal way and in this event the recourse of the male is the privilege of exit. Women in turn support this form of expression of masculinity by respecting the taboo on interference and often by direct admiration and encouragement of even delinquent extrafamilial activities. In addition, anger which arises in a mother-son relationship conceived of as exclusive in fantasy may also be dealt with in a complex series of intrafamilial rivalries and jealousies within which the affective consequence of reality frustration vis-à-vis the mother may be expressed with respect to other family objects. Thus, displacement both within and outside the family is used to deal with aggressive impulses whose direct expression toward the mother is tabooed.

Third, erotic wishes may be displaced as well as aggressive ones, and it is here that we can find the source of the bipolar distinction between the good woman and the bad woman. The contrary image to the Madonna is, of course, that of the prostitute, and the close intertwining of the two images is seen at a great many points, e.g., in the obscenity patterns that reverse the values of feminine purity and in the family quarrels where even closely associated women may be accused of promiscuous impulses. The persistence of the early sublimations in later life is manifested in two crucial assumptions: first, that the sexualized woman may be appreciated in a naturalistic way but she is always perceived as on a lower spiritual plane than the pure one; and second, the idea of sexuality is almost inevitably associated with the possibility of betrayal and pluralization of the relationship, i.e., in that wives, sweethearts, and mistresses are continually suspected by men of wanting other partners than themselves as soon as the idea of sexuality comes into play.

It is facts such as these which lead us to postulate an underlying and persistent fantasy of an exclusive maternal object as a theoretical assumption. Because of repression, we cannot, of course, acquire direct information concerning the sexual aspect in most cases. One particularly important area of research, however, is found in schizophrenic cases where one may see gross breakdowns of cultural sublimations. One of two South Italian schizophrenic men whom I have seen intensively showed the sexual aspect of the mother-son relationship and the associated Madonna complex in a very transparent form. He had many religious delusions; while praying to the Madonna he had open and bizarre erotic experiences and he was unable to distinguish consistently between maternal and erotic objects. The early history was probably one in which prolonged nursing merged into the awakening of genital feelings. However, the second case points up the need for care in separating local and individual variations from global patterns. Coming from a mountainous area where patriarchal patterns and a lack of sentimentality are more typical, the patient showed a much more autistic form of pathology of which the most conspicuous elements were warded-off homosexuality and an extremely submissive identification with the father. He rejected the breast of a wet nurse at an early age, and a crucial traumatic experience was a childhood seduction by an older brother.

One consequence of such a relationship, which fits many of the data we have concerning the South Italian family, is that it acts against social mobility in the broadest sense of the term by making for a very strong centripetal tendency. In other words, if a key axis of family structure is the relationship between mother and son, and if this relationship tends to maintain itself by the preservation of an infantile fantasy which is then dealt with by a complex series of social sublimations and displacements, rather than by attenuating its significance by dispersal or replacement by other objects, then we should have no theoretical basis for explaining the formation of new families. Rather we should expect each mother-son combination to simply continue until the death of the mother; the incest taboo alone does not seem sufficient for explaining the process of change, since nothing in South Italian norms prevents the adult son from obtaining immediate sexual gratification outside while continuing to occupy the emotionally more important position of son. It is at this point that we might turn to the examination of the father-daughter relationship, which can be seen as complementary to the mother-son one in defining a total structure.

The most important difference between these two lies in the dimension of continuity. The father is not continually and lovingly interested in his daughter as the mother is in her son, but rather his interest becomes particularly important at two points in the daughter's life history: the oedipal phase and the courtship phase. At both of these points the father is highly sensitive to the daughter's femininity, and the daughter is given considerable scope for exploiting this sensitivity in what is often a very active way. Moreover, while the taboo on incest between mother and son is as in all societies a very deep-lying one, it is very easy to come to the conclusion that the desexualization of the father-daughter relationship is not nearly as complete. Thus, in particular in instances where the mother has died, father-daughter incest is not an unheard of phenomenon and the possibility may be referred to even rather casually, as in the many stories about "that case in our village" that go around. We noted this on the TAT responses. In an American setting an openly incestuous perception might be taken as an indication of serious pathology, but we have no reason to believe this was the case for our informants. Their counterpart in the normal case where the taboo is preserved is found in the teasing behavior or embarrassed avoidance which characterizes the relation between the father and the sexually mature daughter or in the giggling embarrassment which women associate with the idea of being found out in their love relationships.

In other words, the incestuous impulses in the father-daughter relationship are quite close to the surface, in such a way that we might speak of a lesser degree of repression than is implied in Freud's concept of the Oedipus complex. There is of course a taboo but one might well speak of a persistence of the incestuous impulses on a preconscious level in such a way that they are openly expressed in cultural idiom, as in the frequent use of the word jealousy to describe the father's feelings about the daughter's suitors, and transformed into the joking pattern which is characteristic of the courtship complex.

The major significance of the triangle involving father, daughter, and prospective son-in-law, moreover, lies in the fact that it is to a much greater extent with respect to the daughter than to the wife or mother that the man plays an active role. When he himself is courting, he has to beg at the balcony for a well-protected woman whose virginity he has to respect, but in the case of his own daughter it is he who does the protecting and whose consent has to be sought by the prospective suitor. Thus, the most fully institutionalized masculine role in Southern

Italy, one which is defined positively and not by rebellion, is that of the protection of the honor of the women who are tabooed. In turn, if the sexual affects felt toward these are quite close to the surface, considerable fantasy satisfaction must take place in a way which is active and masculine in contrast to the mother-son relationship, which in so many ways spreads into the marital one, where the male role is passive.

But in addition it is in the father-daughter relationship that we can find a mechanism of change which acts against the centri-petal family tendency. The courtship situation not only gives the father an active role but also has a particular affective style, namely, that of a sudden explosion in which erotic impulses break out with a dramatic intensity which suggests some under-lying dynamic force. Moreover, in spite of the chaperonage norms, the behavior of young women at this point is not such as to suggest much innocence or ignorance of sexuality; they just as well as the young men seem propelled to rebel against the taboos, and they are very often teasers. We have also commented at length on the ambivalent nature of the taboos themselves, in that while violations may be severely condemned explicitly, it often seems as if they were just as much encouraged. It almost seems as if the entire pattern of restriction and parental control were a kind of cultural fiction whose actual purpose is to cover something else; this is what we mean in characterizing it as a joking pattern.

In this perspective it is not at all difficult to postulate that much of the actual source of tension lies in the socially exploited incestuous tie between father and daughter. Thus, the South Italian girl does not appear as inhibited or naïve for precisely the reason that even though carefully kept away from outside men, she has in a great many indirect ways been treated as a sexual object by father (and brothers or other male relatives) both at puberty and during the oedipal crisis. Within the family the incestuous tension may be handled by joking (or avoid-ance[18]), but to the extent that the wishes generated seek a

18. Casual joking and teasing between men and women within the family is characteristic of urban areas; in some country ones (where

biological outlet, the daughter has to seek an object outside of the family—and the father has to rid himself of a woman whom he perceives as very desirable but cannot possess. We would then say that it is the strength of the incestuous wishes which accounts for the dramatic and explosive quality of the courtship situation; and the father-daughter relation, by accentuating incestuous tension and at the same time by imposing a taboo, acts as a kind of spring mechanism which running counter to the strong centripetal forces inherent in the mother-son tie has sufficient force as to cause the family unit to fly apart, resulting in the creation of a new one. In this context the insufficiency of the oral culture view again becomes apparent.

One can then see the father's role in defending the honor of the daughter as the masculine counterpart of the Madonna identification; the father's incestuous impulses are sublimated in the active role which he plays toward the daughter in competition with her suitor. Since the sexual wishes cannot be fulfilled, the symbolic assertion of authority is much more important than the actual outcome, a consideration which can explain the ritualized nature of the father's control over courtship and the gracefulness with which he eventually backs down. As the street vendor stated, his real wish is for his daughter's happiness, but in order to show that he is a man he has to be able to demonstrate the power he has over her, and over the still subordinate prospective son-in-law. The principal means he has at his disposal for doing this is by being obstinate in such a way as to increase the excitement of the drama—of which one could say the most important member of the audience for him is the daughter. Likewise, the complementary wishes of the daughter are sublimated in the pleasure which she experiences over the fact of being controlled, a pleasure which is evident in the courtship descriptions of women, however much they may verbally express resentment or rebellion. Moreover, just as the Madonna fantasy provides a feminine identity for men, so the

courtship taboos may be taken more seriously), there is more likely to be embarrassed avoidance, or *vergogna* (shame), between father and daughter.

courtship complex provides masculine modes of expression for women, in that in participating in an active teasing pattern the daughter may also identify with the father, as seen in the great importance which women attribute to their own capacity to make a stand in front of him which demonstrates that they really want a suitor.

In other words, while the mother-son tie acts primarily as a centripetal one, in that it maintains itself in such a way as to make for an unbroken continuity of the primary family, the father-daughter tie acts in the inverse sense in that the incestuous tension, being much closer to the surface, has to seek an external outlet so that a kind of spring mechanism is generated. The two together make up a viable structure which can be differentiated from our own on two counts: first, it emphasizes the romantic cross-sex ties within the family far more than same-sex identifications, and second, it preserves incestuous fantasies in such a way that they may never be fully replaced by the actually sexual husband-wife relationship. Thus, though courtship is based on the idea of individual romantic love, this latter does not appear as a prelude to an intimate emotional interdependence between husband and wife, but rather as a temporary suspension of an equilibrium in which intergenerational ties are in the long run more significant. One might say that after the wedding the supplicant suitor returns in fantasy to his own mother, and at the same time comes increasingly to resent the maternal aspects of his wife in such a way that he is again driven outside, much as in adolescence. The wife on the other hand may experience a parallel disillusion when she discovers that the husband is not the father of fantasy, and she comes increasingly to transfer her own affective needs to her son, and so the pattern repeats itself. The husband will of course have a reawakened interest in the family later, namely, when he has a daughter.[19] Thus, on both

19. The importance of the father-daughter relationship becomes particularly apparent when we contrast South Italian patterns with those seen in other cultural groups where the rule is the matrifocal family, in which there is no stable husband-wife attachment and the only constant relation is between mother and child. The matrifocal family (found throughout the Caribbean and among working-class American Negroes)

sides, it is having children, and in particular children of the opposite sex, which provides the principal affective source of commitment to the family.

We have up to this point given little systematic attention to the mother-daughter and father-son relationships, which we have conceived of as having a lesser cultural significance than the cross-sex pairs. This is, of course, not to say that they are inexistent or unimportant; but what we mean by a lesser cultural significance might come out more clearly if we draw a few brief contrasts with our own society and with the Oedipus complex as formulated by Freud.

The TAT responses for the mother-daughter card indicate a pattern that is quite classic in that the daughter appears to internalize maternal authority but she does so in an ambivalent way—contrasting with the romantic internalization found in the case of the son. Moreover, the actual mother-daughter relationship corresponds to that found in most societies; it is the mother who teaches the daughter the routine techniques of daily life. However, an additional feature of the TAT responses was that the informants themselves often stated that "these counsels are not very important," implicitly by comparison with those given during the courtship phase. But this comment gives us the possibility of tying together one global feature of South Italian values with the family nuclear complex: utilitarian accomplishments, notably in contrast to Protestant value systems, simply do not receive much emphasis. As our society sees the Oedipus complex, its outcome is that the child gives up the sexual fantasies centered on the parent of the opposite sex and then identifies with the parent of the same sex, whom he or she takes over as an ego ideal. Thus, the small girl wants to grow up to be a

---

seems regularly to appear where masculine identity cannot be easily maintained on the basis of some real occupational achievement. The same conditions hold in Southern Italy and should be seen as underlying the matriarchal trends which we have described; however, with a few exceptions the monogamous family is nevertheless maintained. But the active role which the father has vis-à-vis the daughter must be one of the primary reasons for this, a view which should be considered by social agencies that often too readily seek to save daughters from fathers whom they see as acting solely from cruelty.

woman like her mother, and fantasies that when she is, then she too will have a husband, this depending on how well she learns to carry out womanly tasks. But in small girls or young women in Southern Italy there is remarkably little in the way of the ego ideal, or the superior person one hopes to emulate. The necessary tasks are taken for granted, but the affectively more important matter is not becoming something one is not yet but rather guarding something one has already, namely, virginity. This in turn can be related back to the fact that the infantile wish is dealt with to a greater extent by symbolic replacement (the First Communion enactment of the role of the bride) of the cross-sex fantasy than by identification with the same-sex parent. In other ways the mother-daughter relationship acts as a centripetal force in much the same way as that between mother and son, and the two go together in defining a somewhat static social tendency rather than an active accomplishing one.

The father-son relationship on the other hand seems to constitute an unresolved cultural problem, a fact which may have roots in economic conditions which make continuity of identity from father to son through occupational or social achievement very difficult to attain, though the nature of the family may in turn help to create such conditions. It is in examining the father-son relationship that the contrast between South Italian patterns and those described by Freud becomes clearest. The TAT responses do indicate that the father may be perceived by the son as a judging or condemning figure. However, when we have said that this does not give rise to an internalized paternal superego figure, what we meant was that on the whole our male informants did not present any social values going beyond their immediate relationship which the father represents, e.g., according to a pattern of "well he was tough but he did it to teach me to act like a man." Moreover, although they were adult men, they identified with the son figure far more than the father, and they saw the outcome as a simple mutual antagonism in which the father accuses the son of delinquency but the son justifies himself and his own rebellion, rather than channeling the rebellious forces into any kind of sublimated form.

In other words, father-son hostility simply leads to fights and antagonism rather than being restrained in the interest of higher social goals or symbols. The clearest case in this respect was that of the street vendor, who very explicitly relates the kind of decreasing social energy with respect to occupation—for which he is one of a great many representatives—to a failure to solve the problem of antagonism with the father in any creative way. But for Freud, of course, the exact opposite is true : in perceiving the great importance which hostile wishes against the father on the part of sons may have in psycho-dynamics, he also provides a cultural resolution in his view of repressed father-son rivalry, and its many derivatives in adult life, as a dynamic which can underlie superior creative achieve-ments—including his own creation of psychoanalysis which resulted from his reactions to the death of his father and the contemporaneous intellectual competition with Wilhelm Fliess.

In this perspective it is possible to look at Freud's formula-tion of the Oedipus complex in its wider cultural context in such a way as to bring out some of the contrasts with the South Italian complex. First we might sum up some of the essential characteristics of the latter in such a way as to make a compari-son possible. We have seen the mother-son relationship as the primary axis of family continuity and emphasized the degree to which the son maintains a dependent position vis-à-vis the mother, dealing with sexual and aggressive feelings in a variety of ways among the most important of which is an identification with the feminine values of purity; we have also brought out the extent to which the father-daughter relationship provides a counterpoint pattern by a failure to repress deeply the incestu-ous element. We have also noted that cross-sex relationships are emphasized more than same-sex ones and have suggested that this may build both romantic and conservative elements into the social structure, in that the strength of intergenerational ties wins out over individually formed ones and in that the cross-sex emphasis acts against the creation of ego ideals which the individual seeks to achieve. Both the conservative and feminine emphasis are summed up in the importance given to virginity as a social symbol : virginity is something which is given and not acquired and it is given to women and not to men.[20]

But in discussing the Oedipus complex Freud is quite explicit about the fact that oedipal wishes are given up in such a way as to be replaced by identifications with the same-sex parent; where this does not take place the resulting phenomena are seen as pathological. Moreover, his formulations start from the assumption that the primary factor is rivalry between father and son; these two struggle with each other for the possession of a woman whose background position is taken for granted, just as is that of Sarah who waited until the age of ninety-nine for a son with only one outbreak of skeptical laughter and then did not complain when Abraham took Isaac off as a sacrifice to a patriarchal God. And finally he assumes a very high degree of capacity for delay or sublimation which takes the form of an ability, based on identifications, to turn instinctual impulses into future-oriented creative achievement. This in turn in his own thinking primarily takes the form of masculine imagery, e.g., penetrating reality in the interests of scientific conquest and overcoming resistance, whether in patients or in any other facet of reality.

What differentiates his view of the father-son relationship is then the very high degree of sublimation which he assumes to characterize the conflict : identification with the father, in his view and in his own life, even if ambivalent, does not result in the kind of open hostility and decreasing social energy which we saw in the case of the street vendor, but rather in a complex identification with a continuing tradition. As opposed to the South Italian view, it is the feminine sphere which is the lower and more naturalistic one, while father-son conflict gives rise

20. At least from the South Italian perspective, where the body referent is very clear: as a humorous response to the assertion that Freud defines femininity in terms of a lack of masculinity, we could again refer to the Neapolitan informant who, when questioned about the double standard, replied, "But how could you ever tell if a man had lost it or not?"

to the most complex social sublimations, e.g., the many intellectual ties based on a patriarchal model which characterize Freud's life. This is not to say that he was insensitive to other human possibilities—the work on hysteria, and in particular the paper on transference-love, bear witness to a kind of paternalistic but subtly seductive appreciation of women, in many ways a more sophisticated variant of the South Italian father-daughter pattern; and of course his fantasy view of Rome as a romantic opposite to the active competition of his Viennese life is well known. But it is hard to doubt that Freud was a patriarch with a patriarchal view of man.

The sources of his patriarchal bias can be seen as twofold : the first in the Hebraic tradition which, as discussed in *Moses and Monotheism* (Freud, 1939), was of considerable symbolic importance to him, and the second in elements common to Western society since the Reformation. From both perspectives one can see ways in which the Oedipus complex formulation ties in with broader cultural features. The historical importance of Moses lies in his having organized what was initially a series of patrilineal kin groups into a larger collectivity. The Old Testament makes many of the specific taboos and perceptions of the patrilineal kin group very clear : in the image of the thundering patriarchal God (which we can think of as arising when demands for respect taboo the expression of aggression against the father), in the emphasis on rivalry between brothers, in the tracing of lines of descent solely through men, and in the strong taboo against homosexuality (as seen in the story of Ham who was cursed for looking on his father's nakedness, and perhaps in the extreme anxiety which surrounds the idea of seeing God). From the second point of view, Freud does nothing more than reinforce and deepen our genetic understanding of values of active accomplishment and mastery of external reality, which in the degree of emphasis contrast post-Reformation Western society with many others and which can be thought of as masculine in style. In this perspective, moreover, the continuity between Freud's society and that of the contemporary United States becomes apparent—the common elements being the emphasis on active mastery, the delay of gratification for future rewards by means of identification and ego ideals, and the emphasis on separation from early feminine attachments.

However, questioning of some of Freud's more narrowly patriarchal bias has been characteristic in this country and has had many reflections in psychoanalytic thinking, for example, in the much greater emphasis given to the mother-child relationship. This must certainly be related to the more egalitarian concept of the family, and one might say that psychoanalysis itself has been crucially involved in the elaboration of some new cultural values and images which are feminine in quality: the terms "warmth," "security," and "support," with all of their psychological and social ramifications, are evidence of this, and they in turn serve in the definition of norms for intimate relationships, for example, that the mother should send the child into the outside world, but not in such a sudden or traumatic way that he loses the sense of support of security.[21] In the same way, the ideal wife furthers her husband's extrafamilial activities by giving her support, in a way which may imply far more submissiveness than the Italian image of an intruding male presence which may on occasion be kicked out, and this goes with the positive rather than negative definition of the extrafamilial world. In addition, family patterns may in many ways make for a lack of differentiation between maternal and erotic aspects of love, in that the latter are not defined as "bad" or forbidden in themselves, but rather, in current American morality, tend to be legitimized precisely to the extent that they are assimilated to qualities such as "warmth" or "security." Thus, in contrast to many societies, we perceive no inherent conflict between family continuity and the sexual instinct. The details of this pattern and its cultural ramifications have yet to be described, but while it certainly involves major changes from nineteenth-century ideals of discipline and control or emphasis on masculine authority in the direction of a higher cultural valuation of the feminine role, it also seems likely that values such as warmth

21. Cf. the harsh separation characterizing early school life both in the Puritan and Orthodox Jewish traditions.

and security will nevertheless remain subordinate to the primary social goal of mastery; we would not see these changes as working in the long run in the direction of matriarchy.[22]

In conclusion, we should like to say a few words on the subject of research methodology. Psychoanalysts who have continued to base their work on Freud's theory of instinct have often commented that work based on the concept of culture is likely to deal with motivation in a way which is behavioristic or even superficial. That many of the potentialities of Freud's theory were overlooked in much of the early work on culture and personality is, we believe, quite true. Among the reasons for this is a too hasty attempt to take over the trauma theory in such a way as to postulate uncertain and often mechanical relationships between specific features of child training and adult personality or culture patterns, e.g., culture X is oral because it has a long nursing period, and culture Y is anal because toilet training is surrounded with anxiety. At the same time, in particular where it has not hesitated to deal with cultural patterns of meaning as expressed in symbolic form—for example, Mead and Bateson's (1942) attempt in *Balinese Character* to relate an entire ritual sequence to infantile experience—the field of culture and personality has also produced some quite new modes of thought. Similarly, beginning with Malinowski's work, the use of the psychoanalytic concept of affect and the emphasis on the more intimate dynamics of the family have added an entirely new dimension to the comparative study of kinship, the field which makes up the most solidly founded and scientifically based area of social anthropology. In contrast to the field of culture and personality, this latter is almost completely unknown in psychoanalytic circles, a fact which can lead one to believe

22. Grete Bibring (1953) has commented on some differences between European and American family patterns as reflected in comparative analytic case material. While noting important matriarchal trends in the latter setting, she comments that these are nevertheless not congruent with the total social context and may become pathogenic for this reason. One could add that matriarchalism in the sense of uncompensated female dominance in the family may be quite common as the result of various processes of social change, but that in the long run compensating social mechanisms should appear.

that the assertion that the "culturalist" approach is a superficial one is as much based on attitudes concerning differences on theory and technique which have arisen within the psychoanalytic movement as it is on serious study of the actual work of anthropology.

Moreover, at the present time psychoanalysis is facing a crisis as the result of increasing pressures both from without and from within for more careful scientific demonstration and elaboration of its conceptual apparatus. One of the potential dangers of this situation is that psychoanalytic research will itself take an increasingly behavioristic direction, i.e., attempt to reduce concepts whose initial orginality derived from their immediate perception of meaningful or symbolic phenomena to a form which is quantifiable or experimentally testable in a way which is independent of the interpretive sensitivity of the observer. But this latter, for the anthropologist just as much as for the clinically oriented psychoanalyst, is a factor which cannot or should not be left out of any attempt to create a truly human science of human behavior, however sophisticated we may become concerning the inevitable emotional or normative bias of individual observations. In this perspective the moment when Malinowski, alone in the Trobriand Islands, had to turn to the Trobrianders themselves for companionship—because in his isolation he had lost interest in the questions concerning evolution and the nature of primitive man which he had so heatedly debated with his colleagues in London—is to modern anthropology what Freud's discovery of transference is to psychoanalysis: both make the observer's sensitivity to what is happening around him a primary instrument of research, and both focus research on living human situations rather than artificially created ones.

But today one might say that the initial supposition of Malinowski and numerous other anthropologists that comparative work provides a particularly important means of testing and elaborating psychoanalytic concepts is no less relevant than it was a generation ago, both in that the variety of living cultures provides a natural laboratory setting and in that participant observation, or the attempt to at least hypothetically adapt the framework of a culture different from one's own, may provide an antidote for that part of observer bias that stems from the taking for granted of particular cultural suppositions, i.e., normative bias. In the latter respect, in fact, one might say that comparative work is perhaps all the more necessary now that psychoanalysis, rather than being an isolated and badly misunderstood field of endeavor, has in itself become a source of social norms. One of the dangers of the latter situation is that personality attributes favoring psychoanalytic investigation may be postulated as components of an ideal "human nature" and in turn may be built into a theoretical apparatus. Many qualities common in Southern Italy, for example, may well appear as "ego weakness" from the standpoint of a therapist, but if we look at them in their own setting we may find ways in which they are adaptive and in turn use such observations to enlarge our concepts of the ego and adaptation.[23] A great variety of concepts and postulates also takes on new meaning or leads to new questions if they are applied in the comparative framework.

This paper in itself, moreover, raises many theoretical questions which we have not even tried to answer; for example, can one really say that some kinds of incest wishes are closer to consciousness in one society than in another, and if so, what does this imply for the concept of repression? Or, what are the theoretical consequences for concepts concerning psychopathology and delinquency of what we have called the lesser internalization of paternal authority in Southern Italy and its related social consequences such as the importance of negativism in the peer-group setting? It is clear that failure to show a positive masculine identification in the occupational sphere cannot in itself be taken as an indication of psychopathic personality, if by the latter we mean the lack of any superego restraint, because it is by no means incompatible with a fully internalized respect for women and family norms: witness the affirmative role played by the Neapolitan underworld in the protection of virgins. But such facts should in turn lead us to seek a more careful

23. See A. Parsons (1961).

definition of the superego, which, if it is indeed a universally found psychic apparatus laid down in early infancy, should be definable independently of variations in norms relevant to adults.

In other words, in a great many areas more careful and self-conscious comparative thinking might help us to tighten up some of our theoretical concepts and in particular to separate that which refers to early infantile life from that which defines normative expectations for the adult. Such attempts can in turn have immediate clinical implications for matters such as diagnosis and prognosis. Many social scientists have pointed out the ways in which normative bias may appear in diagnostic judgment when there are social differences between psychiatrist and patient; moreover, such biases follow some fairly consistent and predictable patterns. Thus, diagnoses such as "character disorder" and "psychopathic personality" are certainly overused for Italian male patients; when the neurotic acts out his difficulties outside the family, or even within it (as in the common example of the depressed and dependent man who beats his wife), he quite often gets into trouble with the law. Similarly for women, "oral" elements are commonly overemphasized (in the sense that significant areas of competence or of genital focus in intrapsychic conflict are overlooked) in the light of the greater restriction of life to the family setting. It would be our view that in this group one can individualize the major genetically rooted personality structures predictable from psychoanalytic theory (schizoid, depressive or cyclic, obsessional, and hysteric), but that the overt differences in phenomenology can be such that even the experienced diagnostician may have difficulty if he does not know the cultural expectations. Such difficulties in turn may have important implications for the evaluation of the depth of pathology or for treatment decisions.

In summary, we believe that comparative research has a potentially very important contribution to make in the light of the current need for further testing and elaboration of psychoanalytic concepts with respect to a variety of materials. Moreover, this is the case both for general social or cultural formulations and for more specific studies of psychopathology in ways which are relevant to the understanding of personality dynamics and which can have immediate applications for diagnosis and treatment. For the original question of whether the Oedipus complex is universal or not, we would sum up by saying that it is no longer very meaningful in that particular form. The more important contemporary questions would rather be: what is the possible range within which culture can utilize and elaborate the instinctually given human potentialities, and what are the psychologically given limits of this range? Or in slightly different terms: what more can we learn about what Claude Lévi-Strauss (1949) has characterized as the "transition from nature to culture"? To answer fully questions such as these will require the equal and collaborative efforts of psychoanalysis and anthropology.

BIBLIOGRAPHY

BIBRING, G. L. (1953), "On the 'Passing of the Oedipus Complex' in a Matriarchal Family Setting," in *Drives, Affects, Behavior,* ed. R. M. Loewenstein. New York: International Universities Press, pp. 278-284.

BUSHNELL, J. (1958), "The Virgin of Guadalupe as Surrogate Mother in San Juan Atzingo," *Amer. Anthropol., 60*: 261-265.

CANCIAN, F. (1961). "The Southern Italian Peasant: World View and Political Behavior," *Anthropolog. Quart., 34,* 1: 1-17.

DE JORIO, A. (1832), *La Mimica degli Antichi investigata nel Gestire Napolitana.* Naples: dalla stamperia e carteria del fibreno.

DURKHEIM, E. (1897), *Suicide.* New York: The Free Press, 1951.

——(1915), *The Elementary Forms of the Religious Life.* New York: The Free Press, 1958.

FREUD, S. (1900), *The Interpretation of Dreams.* New York: Basic Books Inc., 1955.

——(1939), *Moses and Monotheism.* New York: Vintage Books, 1958.

HARTMANN, H., KRIS, E., & LOEWENSTEIN, R. M. (1951), "Some Psychoanalytic Comments on 'Culture and Personality' in *Psychoanalysis and Culture,"* eds. G. B. Wilbur & W. Muensterberger. New York: International Universities Press, pp. 3-31.

JACOBSON, E. (1954), "The Self and the Object World: Vicissitudes of Their Infantile Cathexes and Their Influence on Ideational and Affective Development," in *The Psychoanalytic Study of the Child, 9*: 75-127, eds. R. S. Eissler *et al.* New York: International Universities Press.

JONES, E. (1912), The Theory of Symbolism. *Papers on Psychoanalysis.* Boston: Beacon Press, 1961, pp. 87-145.

——(1924), "Mother-Right and Sexual Ignorance of Savages," in *Essays in Applied Psychoanalysis, 2*: 145-173. New York: International Universities Press, 1964.

LEVI-STRAUSS, C. (1949), "L'Analyse structurale en linguistique et en anthropologie," *Word, 1*: 35-53.

——(1949), *Les Structures Elémentaires de la Parenté.* Paris: Presses Universitaires de France.

MALINOWSKI, B. (1916), Baloma: "The Spirits of the Dead in the Trobriand Islands," *J. Royal Anthropolog. Inst., 46*: 353-430.
——(1927), *Sex and Repression in Savage Society.* London: Routledge & Kegan Paul, 1953.
——(1929), *The Sexual Life of Savages.* London: Routledge & Kegan Paul, 1953.
MASTRIANI, F. (1871), *I Vermi: Studi Storici Sulle Classe pericolose in Napoli,* 4 Vols. Naples.
MEAD, M. & BATESON, G. (1942), *Balinese Character: A Photographic Analysis.* New York: Special Publication of the New York Academy of Sciences.
MOLLER, H. (1951), "The Meaning of Courtly Love," *J. Amer. Folklore, 73,* 287: 39-52.
——(1959), "The Social Causation of the Courtly Love Complex," *Compar. Stud. Soc. & Hist., 1,* 2: 137-163.
MOSS, L. W. & Thomson, W. H. (1958), "The South Italian Family: Literature and Observation," *Human Organiz., 18,* 1: 35-41.
OFFICE OF STATISTICS OF THE COMMUNE OF NAPLES (1959), *Annuario Statistico del Commune di Napoli: Anno 1956, 21.* Naples: Stabilimento Tipografico Francesco Giannini & Figli.
PARSONS, A. (1960), "Family Dynamics in South Italian Schizophrenics" [this book, Chapter 3].
——(1961), "A Schizophrenic Episode in a Neapolitan Slum" [this book, Chapter 9].
PARSONS, T. (1958), "Social Structure and the Development of Personality: Freud's Contribution to the Integration of Psychology and Sociology," *Psychiatry, 21,* 4: 321-340.
PETRULLO, V. (1937), "A Note on Sicilian Cross-Cousin Marriage," *Primitive Man, 10,* 2: 8-9.
PITKIN, D. (1959), "Land Tenure and Family Organization in an Italian Village," *Human Organiz., 18,* 4: 169-173.
PRATT, D. (1960), "The Don Juan Myth," *Amer. Imago, 17*: 321-335.
RADCLIFFE-BROWN, A. R. (1952), *Structure and Function in Primitive Society.* New York: The Free Press.
RAMIREZ, S. & PARRES, R. (1957), "Some Dynamic Patterns in the Organization of the Mexican Family," *Int. J. Soc. Psychiat., 3*: 18-21.
RAPAPORT, D. (1960). "The Structure of Psychoanalytic Theory," *Psychological Issues,* Monogr. 6. New York: International Universities Press.

SCHNEIDER, D. & GOUGH, K., eds. (1961), *Matrilineal Kinship*. Berkeley & Los Angeles: Univ. of California Press.

STANTON, A. H. (1959), "Propositions Concerning Object Choices," in *Conceptual and Methodological Problems in Psychoanalysis*, 76:1010-1037, ed. L. Bellak. New York: Annals of the New York Academy of Sciences.

TREVISANI, G., ed. (1957), *Teatro Napoletano dalle origini*, 2 Vols. Bologna: Tip. Mareggiani.

VAILLANT, R. (1958), *The Law*. New York: Knopf.

VERGA, G. (1953), *Little Novels of Sicily*. New York: Grove Press.

WHYTE, W. F. (1943), *Street Corner Society: Social Structure of an Italian Slum*. Chicago: Univ. of Chicago Press.

WOLF, K. R. (1952), "Growing Up and Its Price in Three Puerto Rican Sub-Cultures," *Psychiatry, 15,* 4:401-433.

ZOLA, I. K. (1963), "Observations of Gambling in a Lower Class Setting," *Soc. Prob., 10,* 4:353-361.

chapter 2

Paternal and Maternal Authority in the Neapolitan Family*

This paper examines the authority structure of the Neapolitan family. Although it is generally accepted that authority in the traditional Italian family is invested in the head of the household, it seems fruitful to examine the conflicts his authority generates and the economic conditions under which it is exercised, as well as its effects on the personality of son and daughter. This is an attempt, therefore, to examine the social

* The research on which this paper is based was carried out under a research grant from the National Institute of Mental Health, Bethesda, Maryland, M-2105. Many of the ideas were derived from seminars on the problem of authority in the peasant community held in Rome and Naples in 1959–1960, and I should particularly like to acknowledge the contributions of Francesco Campagna, Donald Pitkin, and Manlio Rossi-Doria.

Published in Italian, "Autorità Patriarchale e Autorità Matriarchale Nella Famiglia Napoletana," in *Estratto dai Quaderni di Sociologia,* XI (#4), 1962.

structure of the Neapolitan family and to relate it to economic conditions as well as to some psychological processes at work.

The traditional family in Southern Italy generally has been considered to be patriarchal, in the sense that there is a hierarchy based on age and sex and with the father having formal authority over wife and children. On a psychological level, a patriarchal family system should produce perceptions of the father as a severe and somewhat distant figure, to be treated with respect rather than intimacy and affection. These latter needs are more likely to be fulfilled by the mother, who is seen as giving and as softening the father's authority, as the Madonna in the Catholic religion is gentle and forgiving and intercedes before God the Father for the penitent sinner.

Most empirical studies of the Southern Italian family have been carried out among peasants. They have shown that in peasant families male superiority and paternal domination are indeed normative. However, they have also pointed out some problem areas or ways in which the image of Southern Italy as a patriarchal society needs qualification. Pitkin, for example, has noted that in contrast to many other peasant societies, the continuity of the father's authority over the son may be somewhat tenuous, because so many peasants work as day laborers; thus at work both father and son are subject to the authority of an unrelated third person, just as is an industrial laborer.[1] Likewise, Moss and Thompson attribute an important role as power-holders to peasant women, as a result of their frequent control and apportionment of a pieced-together income.[2] And Tentori has observed that in any case traditional models may be inadequate to fit the changed situation of peasants in the modern world.[3]

Moreover, these authors have raised important questions

1. Donald Pitkin, "Land Tenure and Family Organization in an Italian Village," *Human Organiz.*, 18, 1959.
2. Leonard W. Moss & Walter H. Thompson, "The South Italian Family: Literature and Observations," *Human Organiz.*, 18, 1959.
3. Tullio Tentori, *Il Sistema di Vita della Communita Materana*, Rome, 1956.

concerning the congruence of the patriarchal family system with the economic and historical conditions of Southern Italy. They suggest both that the traditional family may already contain many elements of built-in conflict, in that subordination of son to father at work may be economically difficult or impossible, and that social change is producing additional modifications. Thus the concept of patriarchality needs to be reinvestigated with some of these questions in mind.

There are many grounds for maintaining that the rural-urban contrast is far less sharp in Southern Italy than in many other areas. This blurring of the lines can be accounted for in two ways. The economic status of the peasantry corresponds in many respects to that of an urban proletariat because of the lack of individual property holdings. Conversely, the economic status of the Neapolitan proletariat resembles that of an agrarian population in that Naples has never succeeded in becoming an effectively operating city with a specialized occupational structure independent of family enterprise. Rather, the external social structure is highly unstable and the family preserves a compensating degree of importance. This makes its structure more similar to that of an agrarian than to that of the typical industrial urban family. One consequence of the lack of occupational differentiation appears to be that in Naples there is a high degree of continuity in family ties, so that questions concerning both subjection to parental control and dependency on parents for economic or psychological support are far more real in the lives of adolescents or young and even married adults than in the cities of Northern Europe and the United States. In these highly industrialized countries the family tends toward a discontinuous nuclear type in which both support and authority between parents and offspring rapidly become less relevant as the latter come increasingly to participate in extrafamilial groupings. The Neapolitan family, however, is not fundamentally different in its patterning from the surrounding peasant family, and does not resemble the "democratic" or "egalitarian" family which tends to accompany urbanization in advanced industrial areas.

The second way in which the Neapolitan material may be useful for an understanding of the peasant world concerns questions of social change. It is well known that urban patterns have great prestige throughout rural Italy at present and that rural areas are increasingly being drawn into the national orbit through the penetration of bureaucratic agencies, extensive migration, the spread of mass communication, and so on. Thus even to the extent that there are now significant differences between rural and urban family structure, one can expect the rural patterns progressively to approximate urban ones. Such a process already becomes apparent with respect to courtship norms; although chaperonage is now much more strictly enforced in villages than in Naples or Palermo, a gradual loosening is underway and in a few years' time one may expect the difference to be sensibly diminished. From this standpoint, data concerning the present-day Neapolitan family, which has already experienced the impact of certain pressures toward change, may have value in defining the direction which the changing rural family is likely to take. Moreover, since the economic marginality common to peasant and Neapolitan is unlikely to disappear in the near future, such material might provide a more accurate predictive index than the too hasty extrapolation of patterns found in New York or Milan.

Empirical Investigation

Two studies, one in 1959 and the other in 1960, were aimed at uncovering the social dynamics of the Neapolitan family among the proletariat and sub-proletariat—so designated because it is difficult to characterize this population as working-class because of their failure, for the most part, to hold stable occupations. Each study entailed the interviewing of approximately twenty-five informants, all of whom were between eighteen and forty-five years of age and married.[4] Most had not

4. The interviewing for the first study was done by Miss Autora Benvignati and for the second by myself.

studied beyond elementary school and a few were illiterate; none had completed the *scoula media* (middle school) or held a white-collar position. The occupations ranged from a beggar, on the lowest economic level, to a skilled workman, on the highest.

The focus of the first study, in which all of the informants were women (interviewed on a maternity ward), was on court-ship and marriage; informants were asked to tell the story of their own courtship in relation to the overall family setting. In the second study a roughly equal number of informants of both sexes were interviewed under a variety of circumstances: office, hospital, slum residences, and so forth. The goal of this study was the very broad one of obtaining an idea of the meaning that the concept of family had for the informants.

In neither study was I primarily concerned with official norms concerning authority, but rather with gaining an overall view of family structure and process. In both studies a projective test was used (the Murray Thematic Apperception Test (TAT) in which the subject is asked to relate stories about a series of interpersonal scenes).[5]

The results of the projective test provide data concerning attitudes which it would be difficult to secure by direct question-ing. Those cards from the TAT which are most relevant and

5. In addition, in the second study, uniform questions were asked concerning the respective uses of *tu* (familiar *you*) and *voi* (formal *you*, indicating respect or social distance) within the family. Patterns found in family dialogue in Neapolitan drama indicate that the *voi* pattern became established about the eighteenth century, with the reciprocal *tu* being used in the sixteenth and seventeenth. The results of this latter survey will not be presented in detail, but briefly they indicate that the reciprocal use of *tu* between parents and children is becoming more common. Informants who addressed their own parents with *tu* rather than *voi* were a minority, while those who are addressed with *tu* by their children have become the majority. This would suggest a current change in the concept of the family according to which an emphasis on hierarchy, or the formal submission of children, is giving way to an emphasis on intimacy or intrafamilial solidarity. This was indicated by the informants' justifications for their own usage according to which those who used *voi* saw it as indicating respect or "education," while the reciprocal use of *tu* was valued for its implication of greater intimacy or trust. The latter usage, of course, is more congruent with patterns found in the modernized segments of Italy or Northern Europe.

which were presented to most subjects in the second study portray the four dyadic relationships into which the nuclear family can be divided: father-son, father-daughter, mother-son, mother-daughter. The first section of this chapter will be devoted to the responses to the TAT, specifically, to the perceptions that various family members have of authority within the family. The second will deal with the interpretation of these findings with the help of case reports, specifically in relation to socioeconomic factors..

The Murray Thematic Apperception Test consists of a series of cards portraying a variety of scenes, and which are given to the subject with the simple request that he tell a story about them. However, since my goal was the securing of social perceptions of specific family relationships, I gave more specific directives, presenting the relevant scenes with comments such as, "This is a father and son, how do they seem to you?" At certain points, after the subject himself had provided the theme, stimulating questions were asked, such as, "How does the situation end up?" or, "How does the son react [to whatever the father is saying]?" For three of the four cards to be discussed here—father-son, mother-son, father-daughter—the choice of theme was left entirely to the subject. However, the theme of authority was directly suggested for the mother-daughter scene, which was described as "a mother advising her daughter."[6]

6. A few complicating factors did arise in administering the test. First, many subjects feared that they were incapable of producing interesting responses because of a lack of schooling, although all possible attempts were made to reassure them on this point. Their timidity seemed to restrict the elaboratedness of their responses. However, it is precisely because of the lack of formal education that many of the stories are direct expressions of the subjects' own experience, and thus a better index to family structure than if the informants had wider knowledge to call on. The majority of the stories are very simple ones; the subjects revealed an ability to seize on direct perceptual clues—eye focus, body position, gesture, and the like—to a degree I doubt one would find in the more educated population, where the test has been used most frequently. In the second place, since the test was designed for American rather than Neapolitan use, some features of the cards have cultural

FATHER-SON CARD

The father-son card was presented to ten male and ten female informants in the second study. Since the directives stated only that the scene portrayed a father and son who are standing together, the frequency with which authority situations are evoked can be used as an index of the importance of this theme.[7] Authority themes were in fact the most common among male but not among female respondents.

Male responses were more likely to show a hierarchical relationship, and the son was never portrayed as attempting to control the father's behavior (Table 1).

Table 1—Reference to Hierarchical Authority in Father-Son Relationship by Sex

	Male	Female
Mention of Authority Relation	7	3
No Mention of Authority Relation	3	7

The specific content of censure or advice was in most instances left indeterminate and the majority attributed a negative or rebellious reaction to the son:

. . . The father reproaches the son . . . the son is a delinquent, you can see from his face that he is not a nice person and I think he will not listen to the father's advice . . .

. . . A scene from La Traviata of the father who reproaches the son. The son is bad . . . the father has the eyes of a judge, of one who has much wisdom . . .

. . . The son must have had a reproach from the father. You can tell from his face that he [the son] is a bit angry . . .

---

meanings which are not initially intended. Where these are relevant, they will be discussed with respect to the specific card.

7. Any response in which the father was seen as attempting to direct the son's behavior, whether by giving counsel or judging character or past actions, was classified as referring to authority.

Among the nonauthority responses the most common ones concern a shared situation of sorrow, e.g., the father and son are both sad for the death of the mother.[8] In only one instance are father and son simply shown as comrades for whom the question of authority does not enter:

There is a close friendship between the father and son, they confide in each other.

Although the father-son situation is perceived as involving a hierarchically defined authority for the majority of male respondents, this is not true for the majority of women. One seemingly obvious response by four women did not come from a single man, namely, that father and son are comrades in distress because of shared economic problems.

They are desperate—they worry, nothing more.

They are worrying about something, the office, work, because they are melancholy.

Another woman pointed to a lack of communication between father and son, which was hinted at also by others.

What a shame, the father is completely blind. Don't you see he has his eyes completely closed and an absent expression? The son is as if he were listening to something, it must be a radio but the father really has the look of a blind man. [Don't they say anything to each other?] No, the father minds his own business, really with the look of a blind man, and the son on the other hand is listening, he must be listening to the radio.

For the men, at least, it seems clear that an authority hierarchy usually is perceived as essential to the father-son relationship. However, the nature of the paternal authority needs further exploration. If one takes a hierarchically defined relationship as

8. Both men on the card wear black ties and one informant interpreted this explicitly as a sign of mourning. [It is clear that some ambivalence of feeling toward the mother is also being expressed in this response. — *Ed.*]

a point of departure, one can arrive at two hypothetical outcomes for conflict between father and son (and all the informants in the authority category perceived the situation as conflictual!): either the son will successfully rebel against paternal authority and create an independent identity or he will submit to it, identifying with the father in such a way that his dictates become part of the son's personal self-image. In the latter instance guilt should be experienced for rebellious impulses. One of the responses goes far in the first direction:

The father is decided and authoritarian, ugly. The son *might* be bad, he has an independent spirit and does not want to listen to the father. The son follows something else, as if the father's wisdom were something annoying, not very important for him.

Two respondents, in contrast, show at least partial acceptance:

. . . I think he will not listen to the father's counsels, or he will listen to the father's advice and put himself on the good path.

In the remaining four authority responses given by men, this uncertainty is much more vividly portrayed, so that actually the most common tendency is for a portrayal of the father-son situation as one of unresolved ambivalence; the two simply remain in a state of conflict, with neither of the above two possible resolutions being attained:

They seem against each other [no further elaboration can be elicited].

The son is bad . . . the father has the eyes of a judge. [But the son neither finds "something else to follow" nor accepts the father's judgment as legitimate.]

One subject elaborated the theme at considerable length in direct relation to his own life,[9] but he nevertheless concluded nothing beyond the existence of conflict:

9. This subject was the forty-year-old son of a transportation worker whose self-confessed ambition was to become a chauffeur. He

The son . . . would like to be a chauffeur and the father makes him learn carpentry and the result is that he practices his trade against his own will and cannot succeed in it. After a few years he begins to hate the father and so he remains without any trade at all . . . As a result father and son fight, the son curses the father, the father says "you ought to listen to me."

In sum, the responses indeed indicate that the father is perceived by men as a real source of social control. However, some characteristics also point to a need for a further elaboration of the concept of patriarchal authority. Considering the two possible solutions to the hierarchically perceived authority situation, one might distinguish between an external and an internal acceptance of the commands of the father. If paternal authority becomes internalized so that it is an essential component of the son's self-image, it can then be effective as a mechanism that ensures social continuity, for the son will himself try to realize the values represented by the father.[10] An alternative, of course, is that the son will attempt to differentiate himself from the father, seeking an independent identity from other sources, and although the first solution may be sufficient for social continuity in a traditional setting, the second is increasingly required in a more dynamic society or in any situation of social change.

However, the data indicate that neither of these two mechanisms works effectively. The respondents show neither a "traditional" acceptance of paternal dominance nor, except for the one who "follows something else,"[11] an individualism predisposed to change. Rather, father and son seem to remain in an unstable compromise with each other so that the father retains

attributes his actual position of *venditore ambulante* (person who sells goods in the street), which is highly depreciated in his own eyes, to having failed to take the problem of the "trade" seriously in his younger days.

10. Rebellion might nevertheless be characteristic of certain phases in the life cycle, e.g., adolescence or early manhood. However, I doubt that the age of the informants here can explain away the failure of the cards to reveal positive identification with the father. All were fathers and the age range is well past adolescence (twenty-eight to forty).

11. This man showed much hostility against his real father, but also an unusual capacity for self-discipline and self-education.

his right to control the son and the son his right to rebel against the father. Moreover, the fact that authority was not the predominant father-son theme in the eyes of the women might make one wonder whether paternal authority is actually the mainspring of the maintenance of family integrity.

MOTHER-SON CARD

If the mother is perceived as complementing the father's authority by means of pacification and softness, we should expect themes concerning understanding, feeding, comfort, and the like to appear in response to the mother-son card. That this aspect of the maternal role is clearly defined is shown by one informant who made explicit comparisons between the two cards:

The difference is here [son with mother] the son is good and there [with father] he is bad . . . The father says less, as long as his son keeps going he doesn't say anything, then he reproaches, while a mamma understands more, she cries, she wants her son to be like other people . . . The father gets fed up if one makes a mistake, the mamma is different, she says "can my son really do that?"

The theme of the mother as a person who is less demanding than the father, more likely to love the son regardless of what he does, is conspicuous throughout the responses to the mother-son card. However, the most surprising finding is that the mother nevertheless has a very real place in the son's self-judgment. Thus when authority is taken in the wider sense of social control through moral judgment of action, the theme of authority appears in response to the mother-son card just as frequently as it does in response to the father-son card (see Table 2).

Table 2—Reference to Moral Authority in Mother-Son Relationship, by Sex

	Male	Female
Mention of Authority Relation	7	4
No Mention of Authority Relation	3	6

It would be gravely misleading to understand these results as implying that the role of the mother is regarded as similar to that of the father. The mother-son relationship is not hierarchically defined. It is not the mother's principal task to impose her judgment upon the son. Rather, the most frequent theme is that of penitence: the son voluntarily humbles himself to ask his mother's forgiveness. This theme does not differ substantially according to whether the informant is male or female, although it appears somewhat less frequently in women's responses.

. . . The son is asking forgiveness of the mother, repenting of the evil he has done. . . .

. . . Maybe he did something very serious, probably he went away and so now he has come back to ask her forgiveness and the mother no longer wants to receive him.

The mother has a son she has not seen for many years. . . . He returns after having done many bad things, stealing and other things. He returns to the family to ask forgiveness. Who knows whether or not the mother will give it to him but I think she will.

The son is asking forgiveness for something. . . . A mother would always forgive her son, even if he were an assassin, even if he were Chessman.

The penitent son who returns to the mother and the mother cannot or does not know how to forgive him.

In most cases it was assumed that the mother would forgive her son but there were two exceptions, both from respondents who were estranged from their own mothers. One referred at first to a cruel mother who pushed her son away, but the respondent was unsatisfied with this story and produced another in which the burden of responsibility was placed upon the son, who left. The other respondent was estranged from both parents, but although in interviews he expressed hostility against his father with little reticence, he simply failed to discuss his mother, and on the test showed the son as trying to take over a saintly role himself by forgiving the mother who "cannot or does not know how to forgive." Thus even in situations of overt antagonism the son is not shown as having aggressive impulses against the mother; in this respect there is a very clear contrast to perceptions of conflict with the father.

The fact that the card portrays an elderly mother whose back is turned to her son was explicitly mentioned by many subjects as if it were disturbing; a mother is expected to turn toward rather than away from her son. Male respondents handled this in some fashion. They might deny the implication of her turning away, as in the following:

The mother has her back turned. What does that mean? It means she loves him.

Another male respondent ingeniously rationalized the mother's turning away by portraying her as calling on a saint:

The young man is bitter, you can see that he must have lost some money gambling . . . The son has his eyes to the ground and an abandoned-looking face, and the mother looks into the distance as if she did not know what saint to turn to in order to convince him.

Among the themes other than that of penitence, three referred to simple sadness and three to anger:

The mother is sad because the son will leave . . . [male respondent].

As if he were all upset. You can see that the son is arguing with the mother, he has turned his back, maybe they had a family fight. . . . Mama you can see made a lot of scandals. . . . The son has an enraged face, he has his nerves out of place too . . . [female respondent].

(Puzzled, hesitant) The mother is turning her back. Why? They are fighting, the mother and son [female respondent].

All three responses concerning quarrels were given by women. The fact that no male respondent drew the conclusion from the picture, in which the mother was shown as turning away, that the relationship was an openly angry or disturbed one (in spite of the fact that anger or disrespect is the conventional meaning of turning one's back in Naples) goes to confirm the existence of an implicit taboo: the father may be perceived by the son as unfair or unjust but the mother may not.

In other words, it appears that the mother is indeed perceived by the son without the harshness of the father but that, contrary to initial expectations, this by no means results in a removal of the mother-son relationship from the sphere of social control. Rather, the structure of the commonly evoked penitence myth—according to which the son returns to the mother to ask forgiveness for actions which he himself considers wrong—implies that maternal authority is accepted as a legitimate source of control.

MOTHER-DAUGHTER CARD

A mother-daughter scene was presented only to female subjects in the first study. Since the scene was presented as "a mother advising her daughter," the question of authority was suggested and the percentage of responses in this category cannot be taken as a valid index of the significance of this theme. Moreover, difficulties were again encountered with respect to the objective stimulus situation. The Murray card portrays a girl of ten or twelve holding a doll or baby while the mother is reading to her from a book. The women were often bothered by the unaccustomed situation of reading and in addition many stated that "the daughter is too young to be given the most important advice." However, this latter is in itself illustrative with regard to the social definition of a mother's authority over her daughter: the most crucial area is that of courtship and marriage, which is not relevant before adolescence. Many subjects simply ignored the card and treated the situation as if the girl were older, invoking sexual themes. Otherwise the majority of responses concerned routine household matters of child care, e.g., "the mother is telling the daughter how to take care of her little brother."

With respect to the nature of authority, the mother-daughter responses show a pattern which resembles both that of the father-son and that of the mother-son relationship. First, the women show a much greater willingness to express reactions of hostility or annoyance toward the mother than the men:

The mother is moralizing. The daughter is a bit fed up with the mother's words . . .

The mother is yelling at the daughter because with the excuse of the child who is her little brother she goes out walking and comes in late. The daughter talks back to her mother saying, "What do you want with me? You made this baby and now you go around finding out bad things about me."

There is also a more beneficent conception of the mother, paralleling the male's attitude, but it is rarer and less romanticized:

The mother is giving good advice to the daughter ; the mother tells the daughter to behave well, not to go out much, to pay more attention to things at home. She has to help her mother to do the housework. The picture is beautiful because there is nothing bad in it.

In one particular context the theme of forgiveness also appears, namely for three women respondents who saw the scene as a young woman with her mother and illegitimate child:

. . . The daughter is not married. The mother tries to help her and get her married, the mother is good and does not throw her out of the house.

The girl is not married and it seems to me that her mother gives her advice on how to bring up the child. It seems that the mother has forgiven her and tells her to treat the child well. . . . The mother should try not to say to the daughter that she is guilty because the girl could do something to hurt herself, she could commit suicide or fall into the same error again thinking that she doesn't have anyone who cares.

The internalized nature of authority in this context is made very clear in the last story in which the respondent conceives of suicide as a possibility for the girl who loses her mother's esteem.

The mother-daughter responses differ from the father-son responses in that even when hostility or resentment is expressed, most of them nevertheless come to a definite moral conclusion favoring the mother's point of view.

The mother tells the little girl that she has to do housework and the daughter is looking as if she had not heard and did not want to do this work. Things won't go very well in the end because the daughter won't listen to the mother.

The little girl will not follow the mother's advice but it would be better if she did because she is too small to decide for herself.

Moreover, there is an emphasis on the necessity for serious planning for the future, which implicitly is a justification for the mother's advice. This theme was not present in responses to any of the preceding cards.

The daughter has a doll in her arms, the mother says she should think about other things [work] and not about dolls. . . .

The mother says to the daughter: it's better that you think about your future, if I tell you this it is for your own good. . . .

Acceptance of maternal authority as distinguished from paternal authority becomes clear in a comparison between stories in which parental advice is portrayed as good or justified and those indicating either a situation of unresolved conflict or a rejection of parental advice because it is seen as bad or irrelevant. More often than not, paternal authority is rejected or produces conflict (Table 3).

Table 3—Acceptance of Parental Authority for Father-Son and Mother-Daughter Stories

	F-S	M-D
Authority Accepted	2	9
Authority Not Accepted	5	1

In other words, it is the mother-daughter relationship that seems to provide the most effective mechanism of social control, since it is almost always conceived of as being legitimate. Though they did not significantly differ from the male respondents in age, the women showed a far greater capacity to identify with the maternal perspective.

FATHER-DAUGHTER CARD

The father-daughter card was administered to twenty-six women in the first study and to an additional six women and four men in the second.[12] Taking all of the subjects together, by far the most common theme is that of courtship behavior or marriage: it accounts for all four male responses and for twenty of the thirty-two responses given by women. Of the remaining twelve, three perceived the situation as one in which the father was making incestuous overtures toward the daughter. The other nine gave diversified but generally rather inhibited or fragmentary responses. Since the question of authority is not relevant to most of these,[13] they will not be considered in the thematic analysis that follows.

For the twenty-four responses concerning courtship or sexual behavior, authority is the central issue; none of them failed to perceive the situation as a conflictual one in which the father is either censuring or attempting to control the daughter. Three standard stories appear: the father has discovered something about the daughter's romantic life, the daughter wishes to go out and the father opposes her, or the father disapproves of the daughter's marital choice:

. . . The daughter does not want to tell about her private business and probably the father learned about this engagement from other people. The father wants to know if it is a good marriage for his daughter.

12. More male subjects would have been desirable but the card was unavailable at the beginning of the second study. The number of male responses is so small that I have not tried to analyze them.
13. Except for the incest responses, where all three (women) saw the daughter as imposing control over the father.

The father calls the daughter to ask what she is doing. The daughter answers that she is going out for a walk. . . . The daughter is waiting for the father to go away to continue to walk with a girlfriend.

The girl is engaged to someone the father doesn't like. The father is saying that he is not the right man for her because he isn't a serious person. He might be a thief or a playboy.

The tests point up the crucial part which the control of sexual behavior plays in the father-daughter relationship.

In this respect the father-daughter results differ from those concerning the father-son relationship: in regard to the latter, the specific area in which authority is applicable is not well defined. However, the two are similar as to the very high frequency of conflict situations described. I have classified those concerning courtship into three categories. There are those in which paternal authority is accepted, as in the following:

. . . The father wants to make her leave her fiancé because according to the father he isn't the right man; he's a delinquent. The daughter is very unhappy; however, she will leave the fiancé because her father insists on it every day to make her leave him and the father is right.

In other responses, the existence of conflict is stated without taking sides:

. . . She cares a lot about this man that her father doesn't want to give to her and she wants to get married at any price.

In a third type of story, the outcome is the successful overthrow of the father's objections by the daughter:

. . . the girl is hurt by the father's reproaches and does not want him to reason this way because she is very much in love with her fiancé. However, she will get married anyway and act in such a way as to convince the father.

Rebellious responses are by far more frequent than accepting ones:

Acceptance	Unresolved Conflict	Overthrow
3	11	10

In other words, it appears that the father's use of authority over the daughter rarely evokes outright acceptance. The conflict either remains unresolved or the father tends to be won over to the daughter's wishes.

The conflict with the father as well as its lack of resolution would seem to have its source not in the dynamics of the family situation but in the cultural norms prescribing courtship, which are ambiguous if not actually outright contradictory.

The father formally has authority in regard to both the daughter's sexual behavior and her marriage choice, over which he has the right of veto. This authority is, of course, an integral part of a courtship pattern in which few social contacts between unmarried men and women are officially permitted. Yet, marriage is not based on formal arrangement by the parents; individual choice and the romantic element are positively emphasized. Thus the courtship system involves a built-in contradiction: the girl is not supposed to have any contacts with prospective suitors before the formal engagement—but at the same time she *must* have such contacts if she is to make an individual choice.

The result is that the supposedly very strict norms for the closeting of young girls are widely violated. The frequency of violations and the ease with which these can be admitted jokingly make it appear as if these norms are not held with the degree of seriousness one might expect from the overt content.[14] Among the twenty-six Neapolitan informants seen in relatively casual interviews, eight stated they had been "engaged in secret," six that they had been out unchaperoned after formal engagement, and six confessed or implied they had been married without the traditional white veil. The largest number, ten, first met their husbands by being followed in the street, an area symbolically taboo for the "good" woman. Actually, the more significant

14. There may be a gradually diminishing degree of seriousness of adherence to norms as one moves north from Sicily or in from the more isolated villages.

taboo seemed to apply to *interesse,* rather than romance, determining the marriage choice.

In sum, conflict and a general tendency for the daughter to resist paternal authority or to succeed in overthrowing it characterize the courtship responses. However, these responses differ from the father-son responses. The father-son situation is depicted as truly difficult and conflictual, while the father-daughter card provoked much blushing and laughter among the women, almost as if the conflict were only apparent, or more a game than a reality. There is an implication that father and daughter understand each other rather well, because both know he will eventually give in and allow her to marry the man of her choice. The difference is illustrated in the response of the *venditore ambulante* who turns to the father-daughter card saying: "Here it is no longer a job problem."

This case here defines a father, he is sociable. Here it is no longer a job problem, the girl must know a man and he knew from the information that he has been a delinquent. He says, "Look for another path, there are millions of men." The father wants happiness for his daughter, he wants her to marry someone who will give her something to eat. [Q.] The daughter answers "it's my business"; no daughter ever listens to her father. [Q.] They get bitter but then they make peace after a child is born.

Thus the father is seen as having legitimate authority over the daughter, even though he lacks the power to do much to improve his daughter's life chances. The daughter's rebellion seems to be seen as much less serious a threat to male self-esteem than that of the son.

Discussion

Up to this point I have been principally concerned with psychological variables, with only token acknowledgment of their socioeconomic context. However, the initial questions concern the viability of the patriarchal family system in an urban environment and the effects of social change on family structure.

In spite of the many very evident tensions and fractionating tendencies in the Neapolitan family, there is far less gross disorganization of the family as a social unit in Naples than has often occurred in lower-class urban groups in other areas, at least if such disorganization is interpreted to mean isolation of individuals from any effective family ties. Moreover, what instability there is appears principally in the marriage relationship, while the ties between parent and child, and in particular between mother and child, have much more resilience and durability.

Actually, the concept of family disorganization is one which should be used with caution. Although some aspects of a family may be seen as disorganized, for example when norms concerning monogamous marriage or the continuous residence of the father in the home are violated, other features of the structure may be effective in fulfilling the essential functions of the family, namely ensuring that young children are fed and socialized. One deviant pattern is for a man to form one family, having a number of children by a legal wife, then desert it and form a second and even a third equally large family. However, this pattern is quite different from random promiscuity in that it does presuppose the creation of a family unit based on monogamy even if it is not permanent. In such cases the ties of the children with the father may be somewhat tenuous[15] but those with the mother much stronger and effective. Such a pattern has been found to occur in other economically underprivileged groups on the margins of modern society, where children are brought up in a primarily feminine unit, e.g., by the mother in cooperation with the maternal grandmother or maternal aunts. Among low-status American Negroes such a family form has been found to be

15. Two of the thirteen men interviewed (but no women) said they were illegitimate, in both cases the offspring of such arrangements. Both had negative relationships with the fathers, who, however, were real social figures; in both cases there was a very intense attachment to the mother, although in one the mother eventually expelled the son as well as the father from the home.

widespread and to receive little or no social condemnation, so that many children are illegitimate and may not even know their father's name.[16] This is probably a consequence of the low economic rewards and instability of male occupations in this social stratum, which leaves the man with little incentive for staying in one place and raising a family. Hence, the principal burden of responsibility remains with the woman who, as in Naples, may often more easily find a job, e.g., in domestic service.

Thus one might easily expect to find in the Neapolitan subproletariat a family where authority resides with the maternal figure. Not only does the economically independent woman acquire power, but also the mother's mother-mother-daughter unit may function more effectively from an economic and from a social standpoint than the husband-wife unit. In such families there is not simply a disappearance of social order, for definite social rules govern family relationships. For example, one of the rules is that one does not strike one's own mother. M. C., a professional beggar and mother of eleven children, reported quarrels with the mother-in-law as follows:

We fought, and then my husband said to his mother, "One of these

16. Munro S. Edmunson & John H. Roher, *The Eighth Generation: Culture and Personalities of New Orleans Negroes* (New York, 1960), pp. 126–185.

The illegitimacy rate is 218 per 1,000 for nonwhites in the United States in 1957 as compared with 50 per 1,000 for the Commune of Naples in 1956. The illegitimacy rate for Naples probably is somewhat higher than surrounding rural ones, but not enough to contradict the assumption that gross disorganization of the nuclear family does not take place. That illegitimacy is indeed associated with a matriarchal family system is indicated by the fact that 51 per cent of the illegitimate children born in 1956 were recognized by the mother alone, as compared with 9 per cent by the father alone, 10 per cent by both parents, and 29 per cent remaining unrecognized. See *Vital Statistics of the United States, Dept. of Health, Education, and Welfare* (Washington, D.C., 1959) I Table BO, LXXXIV; *Annuario Statistico del Comune di Napoli*, Anno 1956 (Naples, 1959), XXI, 23; and *Annuario Statistico Italiano*, Istituto Centrale di Statistica (Rome, 1957), p. 47. The latter gives 31 per 1,000 as the illegitimacy rate for the Campania and 40 for primarily rural Calabria in 1955.

days you are going to make me go through some real trouble and I will blame it on my wife, and you'll see, my youth will be spoiled because I will have to spend ten years in jail. . . ." He wanted me to listen to what his mother said and I didn't give a damn and talked back . . . so he took it out on me and hit me . . . he said to his mother: "At least the two of you could do me the favor of not letting me know about your quarrels because I, in sum, I love you and I love my wife and when the two of you fight, who should I beat, you or my wife?" [Husband answers himself] "I always have to beat my wife because you are my mother."

The ideal of respect for the mother that prevails in such families entails two complementary norms: in return for the respect she receives, the mother will always defend her children against outsiders; she will accept the obligation not only to feed them as children, but to give them whatever they ask for throughout life if this is at all possible. The first principle appears in descriptions of street fights, which usually begin between children, with the respective mothers subsequently intervening and fighting with each other, each automatically taking the side of her own child. When a Neapolitan drawing entitled "Rissa di Donne," portraying a street fight, was administered to a number of subjects as a projective card, the majority of respondents characterized it as a fight over children, with a number of mothers each protecting or being protected by their own children. Male interpreters considered the scene as irrelevant to themselves; several pointed to the one man in the drawing as an amused observer.

The second, namely the obligation to feed and to give, again is well illustrated by M. C. Lest it be objected that the predominant preoccupation with "giving" is associated with her "occupational self-image" as a beggar, it must be stressed that this role attribute determines a series of relationships within the wider family unit. She does perceive herself in a rather optimistic way as a constant receiver of gifts from others and as deserving them not only for herself but for her children. Although there are other potential sources for receiving gifts—sisters, brothers, sons-in-law, and indirectly mother's brothers—the usual channel for giving runs between mother and daughter. Even though contacts with M. C.'s own—now bedridden—mother are infrequent and casual, they appear to be fruitful:

My mother had five brothers and now out of five she has two . . . Every once in a while they bring something to Mama, they don't give anything to me but they do to Mama . . . Mama, you know what she does? . . . when she has something she gives it for my children . . . the brothers give it to Mama and she puts it into my hands for the children. I have my brother who has a job and he drinks wine, he has four or five children, what can he give me? Not even a lira comes out, Miss.

The interviews indicate that the mother's obligation to feed her children gives rise to a series of cooperative relationships of which the dominant axis is the matrilineal line—mother to daughter to daughter's daughter—and that these relationships are of key importance for family structure in the Neapolitan setting.

The next question is that of the role of the husband-father in the home. Although M. C. verbally accepts the view that the father should be the dominant figure, a number of conflicts are apparent, as in her account of her husband's failure to provide at least some of the food:

This morning he saw that the weather was good and he said to me, "Now this morning I am going to get a couple of clams at the beach." . . . Then this morning it rained, it's my misfortune that he couldn't get the clams at the beach, I had thought about them, I had already said to myself: tonight when I get home I will get a couple of clams to eat . . . but this morning it rained so he couldn't even go to dig clams.

The husband's inability to provide was also mentioned in response to the TAT card representing the father-son situation: "The son asks the father for money and the father is embarrassed at not being able to give it."

The father's failure to achieve strong authority also appears related to the importance of outside agencies of social control. M. C. describes an occasion on which her husband did severely punish one child for withholding money to buy herself candy; but another child was so troubled that she called the police, and the husband had to stay in jail until forgiven by the punished child.

The picture of family life is far from that of the traditional patriarchal family; and the relevant modifications would seem to follow from the dual problems of economic insecurity and the involvement of other agencies in family life. First, family structure is modified by the simple failure to live up to traditional customs: neither the informant nor her daughter had dowries or celebrated their weddings with festivities. With respect to the problem of authority, the economic factor acted so as to augment the authority and power of the mother. Under conditions of scarcity, the food-giving maternal role gains overwhelming importance.

The family picture presented by M. C. stands in sharp contrast to that presented by G. R., the thirty-four-year-old stevedore in a stable job, who came from a family in which the father had wielded considerable authority, and whom the sons continued to visit. Until G. R.'s marriage, the relationship with his father was one of formal subordination. During his adolescence the father set definite curfew hours, and would beat his son or lock him outside the home for failure to meet them. Marriage symbolized independence and gaining of an adult male status; for G. R. it followed six years of formal engagement during which chaperonage rules were enforced, and it was celebrated with important festivities—200 friends, relatives, and *compari* were invited. G. R. stated that when he was younger his father's severity provoked many rebellious reactions. However, being a father himself now, he understood that severity is necessary with children and planned to use similar discipline with his own son. He explained:

I've seen the American sailors at port. They have no discipline at all and one day one of them is going to light a cigarette at the wrong moment and blow up an oil tanker.

The mother, and his wife and sisters, appear in the role of

protectors. He remembers his mother having let him in when he was locked out of the house by the father. In the hospital where he was interviewed, his wife and a sister came regularly to bring him special food. G. R. also stated that he would not let his wife out without his permission. On Sundays he either went out alone or took his wife, depending on his own pleasure. The penitence theme did not appear on his TAT; the mother was simply perceived as sad because her son was departing, and the father was perceived as joining his son in mourning.

It must be stressed that the strong patriarchal ideal presented here is associated with a rather secure occupational status; the stevedores in Naples are organized, and there is a high degree of job stability, with a scalar system for advancement by seniority. In no other case was the father's authority presented so clearly. Of the twelve men interviewed, the father was a strong figure and object of positive identity only for three. Six showed the father as a vague figure, and the parental home was seen as "the house of my mother," even though the father was present and living; three showed the father as a strong figure, but he stood out as an object of negative identity.

Even though a pattern of clear-cut maternal authority is not widespread, there are strong tendencies in that direction within the Neapolitan family. These in turn can be related to a number of social phenomena such as the tendency of men to become unsatisfied with one family and to found a second. There is also a continuous fearful preoccupation with marital infidelity, and frequent temporary wanderings on the part of married men. Almost without exception, the informants of both sexes perceived the husband-wife TAT situation as one which the husband was attempting to leave, either for another woman or to fight with another man, while the wife was trying to restrain him. Of particular importance was a tendency noted with respect to residence choices and marital quarrels: the marriage unit appears unstable partly because both husband and wife are likely to retain strong ties to their mothers, so that when the two loyalties come into conflict, it is often loyalty to the mother which prevails. In this sense, the family structure tends toward matrilinearity in that the strongest social tie is likely to be that between mother and child rather than between father and child or husband and wife. Actually, the mother does not have formal authority over the grown child; marriage gives individuals official status as independent agents. However, the strength and continuity of the mother-child tie are such that the mother actually retains a great deal of power—partly because of her self-defined role as someone who cannot refuse requests for help from her children. Since such help is so often necessary under adverse economic conditions, the strong link already established with her tends to retain its strength.

On a psychological level, such a system can be seen as favoring an identification with the mother, since she appears as the stronger and more important figure. As noted, for nearly half the men interviewed, it was the mother who stood out as by far the more prominent of the two parents, in three instances because the father was not a permanent resident in the home. Although the data are incomplete on this point, they also point to a clear relation between this phenomenon and the occupational instability of both father and son, together with a greater prevalence of both working mothers and working wives. Where the father's occupation is more steady (e.g., where there is an artisan family tradition), paternal authority seems to be more effective in producing an impression for the son that father is the stronger figure. In other words, the matrilineal tendency seems most closely associated with the sub-proletariat.

That such a strong matrilineal family system should create personality problems for men is not surprising. While a girl can easily learn to take over a maternal role with which she has ample opportunity to become acquainted, for a boy after early childhood the family system poses a problem in masculine identification.[17] That such a problem actually exists is indicated by the TAT results, from which the mother's authority appears to be much more comprehensible to the daughter than that of the

17. Roger V. Burton & John W. M. Whiting, "The Absent Father: Effects on the Developing Child," Laboratory of Human Development, Harvard Univ. Unpublished Ms.

father to the son. There are social mechanisms available for dealing with such problems, as when the "gang" offers boys an opportunity for masculine learning. Studies in the United States have indicated that belonging to an extrafamilial all-male gang in adolescence or early adulthood is very commonly associated with having been brought up in a matrifocal household.[18] The gang can be seen as a social compensating device in that it accentuates masculinity for the boy, often by defining it as participation in group-encouraged delinquency or otherwise physically aggressive action.

Such a self-reinforcing masculine society exists in Naples at present and used to exist in the now extinct Camorra. The Camorra provides a classical example of the organized delinquent group that emphasized aggressive masculinity. This was symbolized by the requirement that a member be willing to defend his honor with a knife, and by an initiation rite in which he was presented with a dagger and welcomed into the society only after giving his own blood and ritually refusing a glass of wine presumed to be poisoned.[19] At present physical violence is less characteristic of Naples than in the past and there is no such formally organized masculine society. However, the fact remains that masculine power and prestige are based to a far greater extent on activities in a male extrafamilial world than on an authority role within the family.

In place of the Camorra, one now finds a rather loosely organized network of masculine friendships in which persons at the lowest social level seek connections with those above who hold out potential economic benefits. This network cannot be seen simply as a consequence of the matrifocal family; in a much

18. Edmunson & Rohrer, *op. cit.*; Walter Miller, "Lower Class Culture as a Generating Milieu of Gang Delinquency," *J. Soc. Issues, 14* (1958).

19. Although not only deception and stealing but also murder could be justified for the ends of power and prestige, the Camorra exerted social control with respect to the maintenance of the family system and the protection of women by providing pensions for the widows and children of those jailed or killed in action, and by exerting pressure on seducers of virgins to marry. See Francesco Mastriani, *I Vermi: Studi Storici sulle Classe pericolose in Napoli* (Naples, 1877), IV, pp. 172–76.

broader sense it defines the power structure of the city.[20] However, it does have a particular circular relation to the family in that the father who lacks power in the home is able to find male companionship outside it. His absence from home in turn increases the power of women and perpetuates the matrifocal system. The son, lacking a father figure in the home, in turn is attracted by outside groups in his search for a masculine identification. Thus a series of vicious circles are set up. When a wife criticizes her husband for not bringing home enough money, he will find opportunity to revive his self-esteem by treating his male friends to wine or coffee; as a consequence he must again be reproached by his wife for having forgotten the problem of bread. Although the masculine friendship network may have political and economic functions, at times these are not clearly evident. Rather it often seems that the goals of the male peer group—to acquire friends and wealth, to seek amusements, to make oneself respected as an important figure—have taken on important significance in their own right.[21]

My hypothesis is that one significant source of anxiety in the matrifocal family has to do with masculine identification. The importance attributed to virginity, the cult of the Madonna, and the penitence myth as presented in the subjects' TAT responses all point to the key importance of women in the maintenance of moral standards. The male friendship network by contrast often tends toward delinquency; it does not sharply condemn violations of norms when these are a means of attaining power, or prestige, or personal pleasure.[22] Latent hostility toward the mother, revealed, it will be remembered, in male subjects' denial that the mother had "turned away" in one of the TAT pictures and also in the perception of father and son as

20. Gaetano Salvemini, "Lo stato italiano e la vita politica meridionale; Un episodio: le lotte amministrative a Napoli nel biennio 1878–80," in Bruno Caizzi, *Antologia della Questione Meridionale* (Milan, 1955). The politicoeconomic aspects of the Camorra and its present-day equivalent have also been emphasized by Francesco Campagna.

21. Herbert J. Gans, *The Urban Villagers* (New York: The Free Press, 1962).

22. Edward C. Banfield, *The Moral Basis of a Backward Society* (New York: The Free Press, 1958).

mourning the mother's death, points to a source of ambivalence with regard to these same moral standards.

One is in fact led to wonder whether delinquency may not be a psychological necessity for a boy if he is to avoid thinking of himself as a saintly and self-sacrificing woman in a culture that emphasizes the Madonna and the penitence myth. When the son is with the mother, as on the TAT card, he is seen as "good"—like the mother or the Madonna, but his "goodness" is tinged with ambivalence, and carries with it the threat of failure to be fully masculine. The father-son relationship, which the son tends to perceive as more external and as of secondary importance, does not seem to offer the socially more constructive possibility of being "good" like the father and being nevertheless a man.*

Conclusion

Although Neapolitan family structure shows many of the individualizing effects of urbanization and considerable democratization of relations between the sexes and between generations, I doubt that it could be considered as very close to the discontinuous nuclear family characteristic of the advanced industrial countries, in which the lack of emphasis on hierarchy within the family is closely related to the presence of more stable authorities outside it.[23] Rather, the sometimes extreme individualism of the Neapolitan family might better be seen as a negative consequence of certain incongruent aspects of a hierarchized patriarchal structure which is still strongly sanctioned as legitimate.

Thus with some allowance for status variations or changes in time, I would conclude that the basic family form for the Neapolitan sub-proletariat is strongly matrifocal, sometimes be-

23. Talcott Parsons, "The Kinship System of the Contemporary United States," in *Essays in Sociological Theory, rev. ed.* (New York: The Free Press, 1954).

* *Editor's note*: Certain further implications for the male of being "good" (*buono*) are made clear in the case of Mr. Calabrese, presented in Chapter 14.

coming the pure matriarchal family in which paternity is only a biological and not a social fact, but more often remaining in an intermediate position in which, within the family, the father's role is minimized. At the upper reaches of the proletariat, where occupations are more stable or the family has roots in the artisanate, the patriarchal tradition is evidently less subject to strain.

Put more concretely, one hypothesis is that male occupational instability gives rise to a matrifocal family structure in Naples. Growing up in such a family creates problems in masculine identification for the boy which can be relieved in part through his participation in the male peer group. At the same time, the various forms of delinquency and self-indulgence which the peer group encourages further tend to weaken motivation for gainful economic activities on the part of the man.

Considerations such as these would be of direct use to the social planner who is interested in the "human factor" in that they should lead him to include a new range of variables in his plans. Family structure is not necessarily unmodifiable, and the cost of serious incongruence within this structure is high. This cost is clearly evident when a husband must wait for his wife in the evening in order to buy cigarettes. "Like a soul in Purgatory, he waits for me with his mouth open just like the children when they cry for bread." It is evident as well to the woman herself, who is not sure that her family's only problem is hunger: "It's total insanity because there are so many of us. One yells, another screams, it's a problem, Miss, we are always blind, what should I tell you, we are always stuffing ourselves in our house and we are always full of troubles."

chapter 3

Family Dynamics
in South Italian
Schizophrenics*

Recently a number of studies have indicated
that a closer analysis of the associated family dynamics may
make an important contribution to the understanding of schizophrenia [Refs. 2, 4, 5, 7, 8]. This viewpoint has for the most
part been an outgrowth of the increasing use of psychotherapy
in hospitals: as attempts have been made to coordinate treat-

* The research for this chapter was supported by a grant from the
National Institute of Mental Health (M-2105). I should like to acknowledge the help of Miss Aurora Benvignati in the family interviewing and
Drs. Theodore Lidz, Domenico Ruosi, and Alfred Stanton for their
numerous contributions to the formulation of the material. A briefer
version of this paper was presented at the meetings of the Eastern
Sociological Society, April, 1960.

ment programs on a psychosocial level, the observations of personnel concerning the patient's intimates have been given increasing weight and in some instances treatment has been modified so as to focus on the family as a unit rather than on the individual patient. The material gathered has in turn come to serve as a focus of research, so that at present the search for generalizations concerning the mode of pathology characteristic of families of schizophrenics is now well underway. With a few exceptions, such studies have been carried out by psychiatrists or other therapeutic personnel.

In another perspective, sociologists and anthropologists have long been concerned with the family as a particular microscopic social structure. In this respect, the major contribution of social anthropology has been that of the comparative method. As a wide range of societies has been observed, it has become apparent that although all societies have some moderately consistent social arrangement for the regulation of sexual desires and the raising of children, the particular way in which these problems are handled is subject to considerable variation. Even among the minority of family systems in which monogamous marriage and the independent coresidence of husband, wife, and minor children is taken for granted, there is considerable variation in mate choice patterns, extent of contact between family members, parental control over children, etc. Thus, the anthropologist is inclined to think that no knowledge concerning the family is complete unless it is comparative.

With respect to studies of the families of schizophrenics, the comparative approach raises a new set of problems. Because they are so closely associated with psychotherapy as practiced in the present-day United States, these studies have generally taken for granted the norms of family behavior as relevant to American middle-class society. However, we know at the same time that schizophrenia is not limited in its occurrence to the middle-class United States; although there are still many uncertainties as to sociocultural variations in incidence, it is at least established that schizophrenia does occur under a wide variety of social conditions [Refs. 1, 6, 17]. Thus, if family factors do play an etiological role, it is necessary to study them comparatively before general formulations can be worked out. Moreover, such studies may help to eliminate biases according to which the observer may see intra-familial behavior as pathological simply because not congruent with his own norms.

In this paper, some data concerning schizophrenic women studied in Southern Italy will be presented. Studies carried out in the United States have already indicated that there may be variations between patients coming from different class levels or ethnic groups both in the symptons and personality of the patient and in the associated family patterns.[5, 15, 16]. In comparing Italo-American and Irish-American male schizophrenics, Opler and Singer [Ref. 16] discovered that the Italians were less prone to elaborate fantasy or delusional development, more likely to act aggressively on the ward, and more likely to have had histories of overt homosexuality; the latter is related to freer attitudes concerning sexuality and to an acute conflict with a powerful father figure. The writer's observations of Italian-born schizophrenic women in the United States indicated parallel cultural particularities. Perhaps the most significant of these is that to the contrary of the widespread image of the schizophrenic as a lonely and isolated person lacking in any real identity, Italian female patients often appear to have a very deep subjective involvement in the ongoing process of family life. Two cases encountered in the United States can be presented as examples.

A. C. was the youngest daughter of a lower-middle class Sicilian family, inhabiting a Boston slum at the time of hospitalization. The psychotic break took place on the occasion of her older daughter's marriage and first pregnancy after she had successfully survived long separations from her husband, emigration, and widowhood. The principal symptom was a delusional fear that some harm would come to the daughter and hospitalization was provoked by the family's inability to keep her from troubling the latter with her intense anxieties. This problem was never resolved, but over 10 years in the hospital the patient's social facility in other areas was maintained. Family visits were regular and a sister or the less involved younger daughter took her home as a matter of course for all important festivities in which she participated fully. She was noted to have been very much spoiled in her natal family as the youngest child and in marriage received the same devoted attention from her lower-status husband. When seen after many years' residence on the "back wards," she appeared neither inhibited in her demands for attention nor unable to reciprocate by constant gift-giving to both relatives and strangers.

C. P. was a middle daughter in a large peasant family, considered to have been a very shy and dutiful person. She emigrated as a young adult after marriage had been arranged with the father's sister's son who with her brother was already established in the United States. The psychosis began after the brother's marriage and involved intense quarreling with the sister-in-law; after her brother actually wrote a letter threatening to send the Mafia if the two women could not come to terms, she became confused and openly paranoid with the fear that the Mafia was coming to kill her and her brother would poison her. During the first 9 years of a recurring psychosis, she retained her home role and continued to bear children during the intervals between hospitalizations, but after this point social agencies intervened, the family was broken up, and she became a chronic patient. Strong guilt and anxiety on the part of the brother undoubtedly played a role in the breakup and the husband was later hospitalized with paranoid delusions centered on his cousin-brother-in-law. As a result she has never been visited in 25 years of hospitalization. But the significance of family belongingness for her identity is seen in the fact that she has remained continuously on the disturbed ward because she believes she hears her children outside and wishes to escape to them, and in her introduction of herself as a member of the P. family she stated, "*We* are seven sisters, two are dead and Carmella is in the insane asylum."

In both these cases, respectively, 12 and 34 years after the events, it was possible to recapture a vivid image of the relevant family tangles and the patient's position in them. This is so because in neither case did psychosis involve detachment from an immediate social context. In one case the family functioned in such a way as to permit the patient's retaining considerable ego integrity while residing in a hospital where the language barrier alone prevented any very effective social participation. In the second case the family as a whole broke down, one cannot say whether primarily from internal pressures or because of the intervention of social agencies with differing value orientations. However, even in this family the psychosis can be better related to a kind of "folding in" of the family structure as a consequence of the cousin marriage than to forces isolating individuals from social participation.

In the light of the South Italian family structure, none of these features is particularly surprising. The South Italian family appears as a highly centripetal system when it is compared with the American middle-class one: The major social expectations center on loyalty to persons related by birth rather than on independent initiative and achievement. This is particularly true for the young woman who, in contrast to her American counterpart, is expected to wait at home until she is seen standing in the doorway (the demands for control of sexual impulses are much stricter for women than for men) and asked for in marriage rather than making a diffuse range of social contacts with males. Marriage, of course, involves a realignment of family relationships but does not usually sharply interrupt the close tie to the natal family and, as seen in the case of A.C., a mother may expect close involvement with a daughter even after the latter marries. Cousin marriage is disapproved by the Catholic Church, but in some areas it is not popularly condemned and occurs frequently enough so that it could be attributed the status of preferential marriage.

From this standpoint, it is not surprising that intense dependency should be such a prominent feature of the schizophrenic cases and this, as well as extreme isolation, has at times been given a pathogenic significance [Refs. 10, 11]. With respect to childhood schizophrenia, Margaret Mahler [Ref. 12] has distinguished between 2 polar patterns, the autistic type seen in the child who treats people as if they were things and the symbiotic type in which the child is unable to differentiate himself from his intimates. For adult schizophrenia, the polar distinction may be more difficult to make since a higher level of ego development makes possible a greater internal complexity. However, it nevertheless seems worth considering the hypothesis that of these 2 patterns, it is the symbiotic one which should most often occur among South Italian patients. This appears to emerge clearly in the case of A.C.; her apparent stability was dependent on her very close involvement with the daughter and when the latter became more distant upon marriage, she was unable to maintain it.[1]

Thus, the cases investigated in Italy were studied with this hypothesis in mind. In particular, it was predicted that we would find very close reciprocated relationships of dependency between patients and their mothers and that psychotic episodes would often occur on the occasion of the latter's death or some other physical separation. However, in one respect it is necessary to qualify this hypothesis. It was constructed in an attempt to bring together psychodynamic and social variables, i.e., it assumes that one type of family structure favors a particular psychodynamic pattern over another possible one. However, one is not justified in consequence in attributing a general causal significance to the family structure. In other words, we do not wish to say that South Italian family structure per se favors "dependency" and therefore pathology, because for one thing there is no conclusive evidence to the effect that there are more schizophrenics or potential schizophrenics in Southern Italy than in other quite different societies. Rather it seems important to make a precise attempt to differentiate normal from pathological patterns taking specific social variables into account; one would suppose that the Sicilian girl who settles happily into matrilocal residence has more areas of freedom than A.C.'s very rebellious and disturbed daughter.

1. Most of her delusions seemed to be based on an identity with the daughter; when she felt anxious and hostile she believed her daughter was in great danger and needed special protection.

Italian Data

In order to obtain a better view of family patterns which occur among South Italian schizophrenic women, a sample of 25 patients hospitalized in public hospitals in Naples and vicinity was investigated. Each patient was observed on the ward over a period of at least 3 weeks and interviewed at least 4 times by the writer while from 3 to 10 interviews with close relatives were held by an Italian-trained social worker. The majority of the patients came from economically marginal groups and had little education; about half were acute first admissions and none had over 4 years total hospitalization at the time of study. Cases were carefully selected for diagnosis, and agreement between 2 senior consulting psychiatrists was required for inclusion of doubtful cases. In some instances, contact with the patient continued intermittently over periods up to 18 months, and in some, family visits to the hospital were observed or the writer or social worker played the role of intermediary between patient and family or between family and hospital.

The observations relevant here concern principally those relatively stable patterns in the family which had crystallized by the patient's adolescence or young adulthood; in some instances earlier patterns may have been different and in many the patient's acute psychotic behavior was out of character relative to the more stable patterns. Fifteen patients had married, but in most instances the marital pattern which crystallized appeared closely related to the initial family situation and in many cases marriage had little effect on the continuity of natal family ties. It would have been impossible to consider marital relationships alone without reference to the latter.

The relevant patterns fall into 4 more or less distinct subgroupings, as follows:

EXCLUSIVE DYADS

Four patients had extremely close ties to one parent at radical cost to all other family relationships—in 2 cases with the mother and in 2 with the father. One case in the latter group is that of G. S. who also married her father's sister's son and was so closely involved with her father as to separate from her husband and return to live with him in what may have been an actually incestuous relationship. The single brother appeared as totally excluded although present as a shadowy figure.[2] The situation was such that the patient might be seen as having taken over the mother's role in the home and it followed the latter's death in the psychiatric hospital; her complaint on admission was that her husband and daughter were in league to get rid of her. The marriage was probably directly engineered by the father over strong opposition from the mother and the patient's first psychotic break took place soon after it. The second case was very similar and may also have involved overt incest. Both patients were considered extremely jealous and capricious personalities before psychosis.

The two patients closely involved with the mother presented quite different personality types in that both were very quiet and dutiful, like C. P. mentioned previously. In both cases, rather than a progressive disintegration of other families ties, the patient's intense involvement with the mother was favored by the lack of any effective father figure in the home from the beginning: One was an illegitimate child brought up by her mother alone[3] and the second an only child as a result of the father's death during the mother's only pregnancy. Both married, but both marriages suffered from interference on the part of the mother and seemed to be disintegrating at the time of study; one husband justified the large family he had no means to support by saying that every time he made a child, his mother-in-law took it away.

Two other features are shared by these 4 patients. First, in all 4 instances not only were other ties within the nuclear family nonexistent or tending toward disintegration, but also significant disruptions or attenuations of the wider range of family

2. Maternal relatives reported him as having suffered from severe psychic inhibition from the death of the mother.

3. With two full siblings, but both had migrated out of the area by the patient's adolescence.

ties were discovered where they were initially present. Thus, G.
S.'s maternal relatives, who had cared for her extensively in
childhood, stated at the time of study that they no longer
wished to retain contact with her because she was so closely
attached to the father for whom they blamed the mother's
psychosis. Likewise on the paternal side kin ties were disrupted
by the failing cousin marriage, since the father's sister supported
her own son just as the father supported the patient. Second,
the psychoses were of longer duration and greater severity than
was generally true in the Italian group: Two had spent 3 years
in the hospital without discharge; discharge seemed unlikely for
one at the time of study, and the fourth (G. S.) usually recovered
quickly from acute episodes but repeatedly returned to the hospital.

IMBEDDED DYADS

The exclusively dyadic cases on the whole are those for
which family breakdown is most severe. For the next 5 cases
exclusivity did not reach the same proportions and on the
surface families appeared to function as normal units. However,
on closer examination it appeared that the patient had a special
attachment to or received special favors from one parent at
some cost to other relationships even though the dyads remained
embedded in the larger collectivity. In 3 cases the patient very
noticeably idealized the mother or a mother-figure; 2 were
effectively only daughters in rural families in which sex role
divisions were very sharp ones. Two others, both urban, were
very close to the father and both identified with him to the
extent of working outside the home in an occupation closely
related to his.

In the first group, the case of O. L. is typical. As a child
and adolescent in a small village she was noted to have been
very good and somewhat tied to her mother's apron strings.
After her mother's death, she compensated a routine existence
in a convent with a highly idealized memory of her, so that
when she arrived at the hospital she spent much of the time
anticipating the imminent moment when mother would arrive in

an airplane "to take me up there." When asked about her father, she expressed conventional attitudes of respect and affection, but her face never lit up as it did everytime her mother was mentioned. In the second group is the case of D. F., who was from a somewhat more prosperous Neapolitan family. The businessman father appeared to be a chronic schizophrenic and it was the patient who was most closely involved with him while considerable balance was maintained in the rest of the family (several sisters) by a much more stable mother. D. F. was given a small store as a dowry and began to develop a delusional system when this store failed and father and husband came into conflict as a result. Although the conventions of the mother-daughter relationship were maintained, there appeared to be very little intimacy.

All of these patients were noted to have been quiet and good before psychosis. No disruptions were noted in the wider range of kin ties where they had significance. Only one patient was hospitalized for more than 6 months; this was not associated with seriously disturbed behavior but could probably be explained as a result of the extreme poverty of the family.

COMPETITIVE AND UNSTABLE SITUATIONS

An additional 4 patients show seemingly more complex patterns in which it is very difficult to judge one intimate as of more significance than others. Rather the patients had a much wider range of affective ties and showed pronounced and chronic instability within this range. Three showed a common pattern: All had relationships with the mother which at times were openly conflictual; also all had close relationships with maternal relatives who were higher in social status than the immediate family, and all were upwardly mobile by marriage. The fourth showed conflicting but equal identification with both parents.[4] Three had sisters who were more closely identified with the mother than they.

All 4 patients were characterized as jealous and capricious

4. This case has been described at greater length elsewhere [Ref. 17].

and all had the capacity for taking considerable social initiative. None remained over 6 months in the hospital although one was repeatedly readmitted for failure to come to some equilibrium outside; none succeeded in ordering natal and marital family ties after marriage, so that collective warfare between the families was part of the hospitalization situation for all of them.

A variant on this pattern is furnished by 3 much more restrained patients all of whom had stuck quite closely to the natal family home. All in certain respects were treated as special favorites, but by the family as a whole or by both parents rather than by one parent alone. In 2 instances the patients were only girls and appeared to be the focus of parental competition for their affection, and in one case the patient was the baby of a large family. However, although all 3 showed jealous and capricious traits at times, none developed the conspicuously jealous and capricious personality. Only one of these patients married and she did so in a situation in which both families approved the marriage and the couple continued to live close to her parents.

ISOLATES

The final group consists of 7 patients who all showed the quiet and good personality type and in certain respects fit the view of the schizophrenic as an isolated and inhibited person much better than the others. Three at the time of study were unmarried and still living in the natal family; all 3 stood out in the home as those who were most willing to assume responsibilities and to accept controls. However, although past patterns might have been different, at the time of study all seemed to lack any intense reciprocated closeness even in the family. Four others had moved outwards appearing to seek major satisfactions elsewhere. Three had worked as living-in-maids beginning in adolescence and 3 had married (2 after working for many years), but in contrast to the openly conflictual or natal-family-centered marriages of the other groups, all seemed to increase the distance from the natal family by utilizing the husband's relatives as a social center of gravity. All 7 patients came from large families.

Typical of the first group is the case of A. A., the second of 8 siblings. In the interim periods between several brief hospitalizations she remained home and kept the family dirt-floored one-room habitation impeccably neat while her widowed mother and sister worked outside. Her attempts to find a boyfriend were hesitant ones and far more subject to inhibition in the face of censure than those of the other adult unmarried sister. Typical of the second group is the case of T. F., the first of 5 siblings, who left the rural family home at 15 to work as a maid in town while her sister and brothers remained. The psychosis began after 10 years of satisfactory work and several more of a marriage in which she accepted domination from her mother-in-law without overt protest, at the point when the parents and siblings also moved to the provincial capital. Both patients could be easily contacted and had appealing girlish qualities, but neither took the initiative in social relationships.

Five of these patients were discharged within 6 months with considerable improvement, but two had had earlier brief hospitalizations. No significant disruptions of extended kin ties were noted although in the majority of cases they were never known to have been particularly crucial in the family picture. In at least 4 cases, siblings are known to have been better considered or have had more intense involvement with parents.

The 2 final cases could not fit easily into any of these groups because of lack of information or special complicating factors.

Comment on the Symbiotic Hypothesis

When considered in the light of these data, it is evident that the symbiotic dependency hypothesis needs a number of qualifications. First, with the exception of the group of patients who went out to work at an early age, it does seem that their lives were principally bounded by the home role and that this role provided considerable meaning and in many cases intense attachments to others. However, at the same time the range and depth of intimate family relationships is subject to considerable variation (and moreover, this brief study undoubtedly left many aspects unexplored), and an examination at closer range leads one to think that South Italian schizophrenics are no exception to the rule that such patients do show profound disturbances with respect to the most crucial of intimate ties. In 9 cases, this disturbance appears in the form of an inability to extend or maintain intimacy to persons beyond the single significant parent. In 4 it consists of an inability to maintain any stability or hierarchization of object relations and in 7 of an inability to form relationships on any but a docilely submissive, although affectionate, basis.

It is the first 2 groups for which the symbiotic hypothesis seems most appropriate in that the patients quite clearly move toward people rather than away from them. However, in its most rigorous form, not even these cases clearly confirm the initial hypothesis, for we expected to find a number of patients whose prepsychotic adaptation was relatively untroubled and who became psychotic only because of the death of the relevant parent. But, in fact no patient first became psychotic after the death of the mother and only one, probably in the isolate group, after the death of the father. Moreover, we did not as we expected find the majority of patients showing very close dependency on the mother as opposed to other intimates and in a number of instances, even where the conventional expectations for the relationship were maintained, there was considerable psychological distance between mother and daughter. And, finally, even in the group of patients where exclusive dyadic relationships crystallized, life history material and psychotic material indicate that the patients had very strong ambivalencies about their situations and that all made real attempts to escape, even if direct parental pressures or unconscious needs prevented their realization.[5]

5. For example, the husband of R.M., the illegitimate child closely bound to her mother, was quite amazed that she began to speak pure Italian during her psychotic episode since only Calabrian dialect was spoken in their town. It turned out that she did so in order to express a highly romantic individual view of their courtship which she had derived from pulp novels, i.e., "that charming maiden who passed by you one day in April."

Several reasons for the inadequacy of the initial hypothesis come to mind. First, it neglected the intense ambivalence which is probably better conceived of as an inherent characteristic of the schizoid personality than as the consequence of any specific family constellation. Both in the exclusive dyadic cases and more conspicuously in the unstable and competitive situations, aggression acts as a force pulling the patient away from the exclusive relationship even if the symbiotic need acts in the opposite direction. Second, it did not to a sufficient extent consider the family as a whole. If a patient's symbiotic needs are to be reciprocated, another person must be available and willing to play the complementary role. But this availability depends on the total balance of intrafamilial relationships and (although this aspect could not be dealt with within the limits of this study) on the internal needs of the partner.

However, we do think that a modified version of the initial hypothesis can be retained, namely, that all other things being equal, South Italian schizophrenics tend towards a very close identity with family members rather than a drifting away into isolation. There does appear to be a greater variety and complexity of forms this identity may take than was initially predicted, but the hypothesis can nevertheless account for many particularities of psychotic behavior in this social setting.[6] Phrased in this way, the hypothesis raises a new question, namely, what features of the family as a whole might account for the variations in form. This question is a particularly important one because as appears in the above material the subpatterns appear to be related to other factors, i.e., personality type and severity of illness.

As has been noted, the patients tend to fall into 2 quite distinct groups with respect to prepsychotic personality pattern:

6. Including many not discussed here, for example, that even when thinking is grossly disorganized, South Italian patients usually appear to be concerned with concrete persons and events rather than the impersonal abstractions so often found among psychotics in other countries. Moreover, even those patients whose life histories revealed some distance from the natal family tended to return toward it in thought or reality during the psychosis.

those characterized as "jealous and capricious" and those characterized as "quiet and good." Actually there was a surprising amount of agreement concerning these characterizations; over and over again we got the same terms from relatives without trying to elicit them. When one looks at the patterns of socialization and family life in Southern Italy, in one sense it is the jealous and capricious pattern which appears as the most expectable one. Although discipline may be firmly imposed in certain specific areas, systematic discipline and control are not typical. Rather considerable emotional instability is tolerated within the family (and outside it) and socialization tends to take an alternating course, i.e., at one moment children may be scolded because parents feel aggressive impulses and at another given concrete tokens of affection. Many social relationships take the form of competitive attempts to gain special attention, and jealousy, both in sibling and heterosexual relationships, is a constant preoccupation for adults as well as children. Thus, although they may show extremes which are not typical, the traits of jealousy and capriciousness are so much taken for granted that short of gross delusions or seriously threatening aggressive behavior, the patients in this group were not seen by intimates as inherently disturbed.

However, it is necessary to explain the "quiet and good" pattern as well since it is the quantitatively most frequent one and bears the closest resemblance to schizoid personality patterns as described elsewhere. In order to do this, it is necessary to call on factors other than the amount of permitted emotionality or the gratification given to children. Actually, when one considers the family as a social whole, it becomes doubtful whether it could persist in this or any society if norms and socialization practices were such as to make constant capriciousness possible for everyone, for the result would be chaos. Rather there must be some other limiting factors which impose some kind of order or hierarchy. One such factor which comes to mind is that of family size. Although competition for parental attention may not be systematically limited, when there are 8 children numbers alone (as well as poverty) must limit the amount of gratification any one child may receive. But, if in fact it is the pressure of competing siblings which puts limits on the patients' searches for exclusive attention, there should be a relationship between family size and the prominence of jealous and capricious traits.

When the data were examined with this hypothesis in mind, the results[7] were as follows:

Table 1—Character Traits Among Patients, by Number of Siblings

	Number of Siblings	
Character Traits	Less than 4	4 or More
"Jealous and Capricious"	7	0
"Quiet and Good"	5	10

In other words, it appears that when the family is large, the patient tends to fall to the bottom of the totem pole and when it is small to rise to the top. This appears in a very sharp difference between the nature of family identity between the 2 groups. For the jealous and capricious patients, identity is conspicuously not with the family as a whole (much of their behavior was very destructive to family unity) but rather with particular persons from whom many satisfactions were secured (or nearly secured). For the quiet and good patients on the other hand, it is precisely family unity which has the greatest importance, i.e., they act according to the official norms and tend to sacrifice their own interests in favor of the interest of the collectivity.[8] But the extreme pattern, i.e., a wholly exclusive relation to one parent, seems to result in more severe and prolonged illness than any other possibility.

The only group of patients which provides an exception is

7. Including only full siblings living past 6 years. Three patients could not be classified for lack of information or because both elements were prominent.

8. E.g., A. A. who kept the family home neat and accepted censure of her attempts to find a boyfriend, as compared to her sister who was more rebellious and discovering an interesting world outside.

that of the 5 quiet and good patients in small families. Two factors seem to be involved here. First, all 3 patients who were only children (one adopted) were of the quiet and good type. One of these grew up in an extended family situation which was actually a large one because cousins took the place of siblings and another and 2 additional patients had very close dyadic relationships with the mother. Close involvement with the mother would thus seem to constitute an additional variable which regardless of family size works in the direction of restraint. One particulary interesting case in this respect was that of the youngest child in a large family with a very mothering mother. In consequence she was breast-fed until age 4, at which point, as the mother remembers it, she weaned herself; already quite verbally fluent, she announced "just one more sip and then I will give it up," whereupon she did although she continued to caress her mother's breasts occasionally until age 10. In spite of this unusual (even by South Italian standards) amount of oral gratification, guilt was a more prominent aspect of her personality than for most patients in the sample. Guilt feelings about taking things which come in two's were a prominent part of the psychosis, e.g., one day she was afraid to face me because she remembered once having stolen 2 flowers from a garden belonging to some Americans.

Concluding Remarks

In conclusion, a few more questions raised by the data and some similarities to patterns isolated in the study of the families of schizophrenics in the United States can be briefly discussed. In the first respect, the occurrence of cousin marriage among South Italian schizophrenics furnishes a particularly challenging focus for further theoretical consideration. A high incidence of schizophrenia among offspring of consanguineous marriages has often been taken by biologically oriented theorists as evidence for the operation of hereditary factors. However, if such marriage occurs among the patients themselves rather than their parents, heredity cannot provide the explanation and the same phenomenon has a number of psychological and social ramifications. Both cases encountered are the type which Homans and Schneider [Ref. 3] predict for a society in which formal authority is held by the father on the grounds that sentimental ties more easily arise in kin relations counter to the authority ones, i.e., ego (male) married mother's brother's daughter.[9]

In the case of G. S. the cousin marriage was quite clearly bound up with a very strong attachment to the father, reciprocated by an equally strong one between husband and his mother and in a sense can be seen as an abrogation of the incest taboo in such a way as to accentuate the centripetal family tendency, i.e., the respective partners did not need to move outside to find mates as is generally the case. In both cases the consequence was a flying apart of the family equilibrium for lack of balancing ties, which did not often happen in other schizophrenic cases.[10]

Second, beyond the general differentiation of centripetal from centrifugal family systems discussed here, the data also point to some finer ways in which comparative analysis might be used to point out paths of potential breakdown in family systems which one might expect schizophrenic families to take. Initially, it was predicted that symbiotic relationships for female patients would most often involve the mother as a consequence of the sharp sex-role division which characterizes the Italian family. In fact, this expectation was not borne out. Five patients were very closely involved with the mother but four equally involved with the father and quite distant from the mother. However, this finding might simply indicate that the initial family model was inadequate rather than that the choice of intimate patients closely involved with the father were from Naples or its

9. One other Italian patient successfully rebelled against her mother's attempt to marry her to her brother's son.

10. Of course this does not mean that there is an inevitable relationship between cousin marriage and schizophrenia. In order to define better the relationship which these data indicate, it would be necessary to do considerable comparative work, utilizing societies in which some form of cousin marriage is more fully institutionalized than in Southern Italy.

immediate vicinity while four of those so involved with the mother were from peasant families or other areas. Most of the anthropological work which has been done on the South Italian family refers to the traditional rural pattern in which the father is apt to be a distant and authoritarian figure in the home [Ref. 14]. However, further consideration of the urban Neapolitan family indicates that a number of shifts have taken place in the direction of greater equality and communication between the sexes even though the double standard has been maintained. Given considerable seductiveness in the behavior of fathers to daughters even in the normal case, it is not surprising that for some schizophrenic cases breakdown took the direction of a very intense father-daughter involvement, or even actual incest.[11]

The mode of reasoning which we have followed here is to take a general model of the relevant family structure and isolate points of potential weakness, then looking to see whether or not the predicted breakdowns actually occur among schizophrenic patients. It is in this way that we believe comparative analysis of family structure could be very profitably adopted in the study of pathological family constellations. If it were possible to study schizophrenics in the Trobriand Islands, the classic case of the matrilineal society analyzed by Malinowski, one might look for breakdowns of the elaborate taboos surrounding brother-sister relationships, an area which his work points to as an anxiety focus [Ref. 13]. In a more practical perspective, one can consider some of the patterns characteristic of American middle-class patients. In an equivalent American sample of schizophrenic

11. For example, the low-status father in Neapolitan drama appears consistently over the last several centuries as a nice guy, lacking in effective authority because of his chronic lack of money, but nevertheless able to compensate his weaknesses with humor and affectionate qualities. Two non-psychotic informants in a control study interpreted the father-daughter card on the TAT as involving overt incest, quite expectable "because the daughter is attractive," and most of the others saw a quality of embarrassment as inherent to relations between father and adolescent daughter. That this form of incest should be the most threatening one follows from the fact that adolescent daughters are kept close to home while adolescent sons are outside to a considerable extent.

women studied by the writer, several patients were noted to have something approaching symbiotic dependency relationships in marriage. This can be related to the extent to which American society encourages a sharp discontinuity in parent-child ties, but at the same time idealizes marriage as a focus of a wide range of affective needs. The same pattern did not occur among the Italian patients, who tended to return to the natal family when frightened or in difficulties.

Finally, although up to this point we have been principally concerned with the isolation of patterns characteristic of South Italian schizophrenics as related to the cultural context, there are also instances in which the relevant patterns are quite similar to those which have been uncovered in the study of middle-class American patients. The work of Dr. Theodore Lidz and his associates [Refs. 2, 7, 9] stands out particularly for the extent to which a structural analysis of the family has been utilized in the United States. Among the patterns which have been isolated are that of a radical reversal of authority relations in the family, so that children rule parents rather than the reverse, marital schism and marital skew, in which either each of the parents goes his separate ways or one defines the family subculture at radical cost to the personal integrity of the other, and incestuous or homosexual seductiveness in the behavior of parents and children or between siblings. But all of these patterns could also be isolated in the Italian cases studied; e.g., in the case of G. S. described earlier in this paper, the exclusive dyad between father and daughter implies a marital skew as seen in the mother's statement that her husband and daughter were in league to get rid of her. In the case of D. P., another exclusive dyad where the relevant parent was the mother, a homosexual component was almost certainly involved: The two interacted on the hospital ward like lovers setting themselves apart by their private meanings. Other patients, where pathology was perhaps acted out in the family to a lesser extent, had dreams or psychotic experiences such as the fear that the mother had become a monster with bared teeth which very easily lend themselves to incestuous or homosexual interpretation.

Thus, it may be that if family determinants of schizophrenia are ever conclusively isolated, they will fall within the range of a violation of taboos such as that on incest within the elementary family which now appears to be a universal of social structure. However, before any of the many currently available formulations of intrafamilial behavior patterns can be taken as generally valid, a number of subtle problems in the differentiation of pathological from normal patterns must be resolved. Many of the fathers of schizophrenics in Naples manifested a passive relation to the environment, but how do they differ from others in a city in which a sizable percentage of the adult male population spends the day in the streets waiting for nonexistent work? Several of the patients markedly idealized the mother, but what is unique about this in the land of the Madonna and *mamma mia?* Some of the patients seemed to make little distinction between their own identities and that of the family collectivity, but how do they differ from others in a society in which one is dependent on a family for one's very existence from day to day? We would doubt that these problems can ever be resolved in a framework in which any particular set of social values or conditions is considered as inherently schizogenetic.

BIBLIOGRAPHY

1. EATON, J. W., & WEIL, R. J., *Culture and Mental Disorders.* New York: The Free Press, 1956.
2. FLECK, S., LIDZ, T., CORNELISON, A., SCHAFER, S., & TERRY, D., "The Intra-Familial Environment of the Schizophrenic Patient: Incestuous and Homosexual Problems," in *Individual and Family Dynamics*, ed. by Jules H. Masserman. New York: Grune & Stratton, Inc., 1959.
3. HOMANS, G. C., & SCHNEIDER, D. M., *Marriage Authority, Authority, and Final Causes: A Study of Unilateral Cross-Cousin Marriage.* New York: The Free Press, 1955.
4. JACKSON, D. D., "The Question of Family Homeostasis," *Psychiat. Quart.* (Supp.), *31*: 79–89 (Pt. 1) 1957.
5. KOHN, M. L., & CLAUSEN, J. A., "Parental Authority Behavior and Schizophrenia," *Amer. J. Orthopsychiat., 26*: 297–313, 1956.
6. LAMBO, T. A., "The Role of Cultural Factors in Paranoid Psychoses among the Yoruba Tribe," *J. Ment. Sc., 161*: 239–266, 1955.
7. LIDZ, T., CORNELISON, A. R., FLECK, S., & TERRY, D., "The Intrafamilial Environment of the Schizophrenic Patient: I. The Father," *Psychiatry, 20*: 329–342, 1957.
8. LIDZ, T., FLECK, S., CORNELISON, A., & TERRY, D., "The Intrafamilial Environment of the Schizophrenic Patient: II. Marital Schism and Marital Skew," *Amer. J. Psychiat., 114*: 241–248, 1957.
9. LIDZ, T., FLECK, S., CORNELISON, A., & TERRY, D., "The Intrafamilial Environment of the Schizophrenic Patient: IV. Parental Personalities and Family Interaction," *Amer. J. Orthopsychiat., 28*: 764–776, 1958.
10. LIMENTANI, D., "Symbiotic Identification in Schizophrenia," *Psychiatry 19*: 231–326, 1956.
11. LYKETSOS, G., "On the Formation of the Mother-Daughter Symbiotic Relationship Patterns in Schizophrenia," *Psychiatry, 22*: 161–166, 1959.
12. MAHLER, M. S., "On Child Psychosis and Schizophrenia: Autistic and Symbiotic Infantile Psychoses," in *Psycho-*

analytic Study of the Child. Vol. 7, New York: International Universities Press, 1952.

13. MALINOWSKI, B., *The Sexual Life of Savages.* London: Routledge & Kegan Paul, 1929.

14. MOSS, L. W., & THOMPSON, W. H., "The South Italian Family: Literature and Observations," *Human Organiz. 18*: 35–41, 1959.

15. MYERS, J. K., & ROBERTS, B. H., *Family and Class Dynamics in Mental Illness.* New York: John Wiley & Sons, Inc., 1959.

16. OPLER, M., & SINGER, J. K., "Ethnic Behavior and Psychopathology: Italian and Irish," *Internat. J. Soc. Psychiat., 2*: 11–23, 1956.

17. PARSONS, A., "A Schizophrenic Episode in a Neapolitan Slum" [this book, Chapter 9].

part two

Social Aspects
of Mental Illness

In this part Anne Parsons continues to explore the
theme begun in the last chapter: the relation between
adaptibility to social life and the structure of the
family.

Through an ingenious use of data, the author
shows in Chapter 4 that today in the United States
schizophrenia occurs primarily in those second-
generation Italians who have not been able to adjust
to the occupational mobility of their fellow Italians.
Typically, their lack of integration in the occupational
community tends to be associated with single marital
status.

As the rural Italian family struggles to adapt itself
to the alien values of an urban setting, the effects of
specific vulnerabilities inherent in the family structure
may be considerably magnified. The family's "resistance to infection," that is, to psychopathology, appears
to be lowered by conflicts in expectations which young

people must face between their family norms and the values of the surrounding world. Two cases are described in Chapter 5 in which a daughter expresses her family's conflicts regarding sexual norms, by rebelliousness in one instance and obedience in the other, followed in both instances by a schizophrenic episode.

A "familistic" culture is associated with personalized relationships in nonfamily settings as well. In Chapter 6, Anne Parsons shows that in the Italian setting relationships in the hospital approximate the "primary" type, with a de-emphasis on the functionally specific and affectively neutral aspects that govern relationships in American organizations. She does not limit herself to a mere description of these differences. As in all of her other work, she is acutely aware of the multiple linkages between the facts she observes and the socioeconomic context in which they are embedded.

chapter 4

Psychiatric Hospitalization, Social Class, and Immigrant Status

In a recent study which has had considerable impact on the psychiatric profession, Hollingshead and Redlich have demonstrated that there are some important class differences in treatment opportunities, as well as in the incidence of mental illness.[1] Their findings point to the possibility that specific factors associated with social class may have etiological significance for some syndromes. It is to this second point that this paper is addressed. It deals with the question whether patients of the lowest class (class V) at the present time come from a

1. A. B. Hollingshead & F. C. Redlich, *Social Class and Mental Illness: A Community Study* (New York: John Wiley & Sons, Inc., 1958).

This research was supported by a grant from the National Institute of Mental Health, Bethesda, Maryland (M-4449) and carried out while the investigator was the holder of an interdisciplinary training fellowship from the Foundations' Fund for Research in Psychiatry.

pathogenic subculture or whether they are deviants within an otherwise adapted or adaptable subculture.

Hollingshead and Redlich imply that there is something about the class V environment that is pathogenic.

. . . Class V respondents are individualistic, self-centered, sus-picious, and hostile to formal institutional controls. These character traits lead to further isolation and discrimination. In their social relations with one another, their feelings of distrust and suspicion hold sway when tensions develop between them. Consequently their social relations are brittle, often transitory, and emotionally unsatisfactory . . .

An implicit assumption that there is a kind of social disorgani-zation peculiar to the lower class also characterizes the work of Myers and Roberts, which was based on intensive case studies.[2]

We know that much of the urban working class through-out American history has consisted of recent immigrants and their immediate descendants. In the 1951 New Haven studies, by far the greatest number of persons characterized as class V consisted of immigrants from Southern or Eastern Europe and their immediate descendants, with the most important contin-gent from Southern Italy.[3]

The position of immigrants in the class structure has changed, especially for the second generation, through a process by which each wave of immigrants tended to move upward by being replaced below by more recent arrivals. Mobility in our society is not only part of the value system but is inherent, in spite of its being at the same time limited, in an open-class society. It is a structural feature in a society that admits suc-cessive waves of immigrants.

In this paper I shall argue that lack of mobility can be

2. J. K. Myers & B. H. Roberts, *Family and Class Dynamics in Mental Illness* (New York: John Wiley & Sons, Inc., 1959).

3. Immigrants from Southern Italy made up 48 per cent. in Class V, Poles about 12 per cent., other Slavic groups 6 per cent., French-Canadians 4 per cent. Twenty-five per cent. consisted in persons of Northern European or Yankee ancestry (Hollingshead & Redlich, *op. cit.*, p. 122).

"pathogenic" in a society based on collective social mobility. This is in contrast to cases of individual mobility, through achievement or otherwise, where it is the upward-mobile person who is likely to sever or loosen his ties with relatives and other former associates. Where members of a whole ethnic collectivity are given a chance to "better themselves" relative to new immigrants who are given bottom position, it is those who cannot move along with them, for whatever reasons, who experience a loosening of social bonds.

Mobility among Patients and Normals

It seems probable that second-generation immigrants who have remained in class V have failed to move up with others in their generation. Some supporting evidence for this hypothesis comes from data concerning Italo-American psychiatric admissions to a state hospital in 1939 and 1961 in Boston, where Italo-Americans constitute the most important segment of the urban working class today. In this respect, the city is similar to New Haven, the site of Hollingshead and Redlich's study of the relation between social class and mental illness.

I abstracted psychiatric and social information for 1938 and 1961 from the records of all patients admited to the Boston State Hospital, under the age of sixty, who were born in Italy or whose parents or grandparents were born there.[4] The first year was chosen because it was a depression year and because it was close enough to the period of mass immigration to find a substantially higher proportion of immigrants than today.

My focus in analyzing this material has been on three questions: (1) In what respects has the Italo-American patient population in the state hospital changed over time? (2) To what extent does the Italo-American patient population in the state

4. Only cases with both parents or all four grandparents born in Italy were included. Since cases were selected from admission lists by name, it is possible that some persons who had anglicized their names or some women of Italian descent married to non-Italians were missed; however, for 1961 a periodic check of all records was used for locating such cases.

hospital differ from the comparable normal population with respect to class status and occupation? (3) To what extent can relevant differences be related to factors in family organization? The purpose of comparison will be served by a study which I did of twenty second-generation Italian couples living in an undistinguished but solidly working-class and predominantly Italian area of Boston. They were selected through local leaders of a lower-class Italian neighborhood who were asked to give names of "typical" persons who could be interviewed; three different leaders were called upon independently for their judgment. None of the families approached refused to cooperate.

Socioeconomic Characteristics

As is to be expected, Italo-Americans admitted to the state hospital in 1961 are predominantly American born. This is in contrast to 1938, when more than one-half of the admissions were Italian born (Table 1).

Table 1—Italo-Americans Admitted to State Hospital in 1938 and 1961, by Place of Birth

	1938	1961
Born in Italy	52%	15%
Born in U.S.	48	85
N	52	96

In line with the change in the place of birth, the 1961 patients tend to be higher in class affiliation (Tables 2 and 2a).

Table 2—Patients Admitted to State Hospital in 1938 and 1961, by Social Class

	1938	1961
Class I and II	0%	2.1%
Class III	3.8	2.1
Class IV	13.5	28.0
Class V	82.7	67.8
N	52	96

Table 2a—Patients Admitted to State Hospital in 1938 and 1961, for Two Class Categories

	1938	1961
Classes I through IV	17.3%	32.2
Class V	82.7	67.8

However, the difference in social class between the two periods does not seem as important as the difference in education would lead us to expect (Table 3).

Table 3—Admissions to State Hospital in 1938 and 1961, by Level of Education

Education		1938	1961
Eighth Grade or Less		92%	59%
High School or Beyond		8	41
	N	52	96

To be sure, an absolute rise in education may still keep people on the lowest educational level relative to the rest of the population. This may explain in part the fact that the rise in occupational level for the admitted patients was minimal between these two periods (Table 4).[5]

5. The age composition has hardly changed between these two points in time:

		1938	1961
Under Age 35		36.5%	40.5%
35 or Over		63.5	59.5
	N	52	96

In addition, the age distribution by social class also remains approximately the same, the majority of class IV patients being younger in both years:

		Class IV		Class V	
		1938	1961	1938	1961
Under Age 35		55.5%	53.5%	32.5%	35.5%
35 or Over		44.5	46.5	67.5	64.5
	N	9	31	43	65

Table 4—Admissions to State Hospital in 1938 and 1961 by Level of Occupation

Occupational Level		1938	1961
I-II		0%	2%
III		0	1
IV		6	13
V		13	15
VI		8	10
VII		71	61
	N	**52**	**96**

The small occupational difference between the two years is nevertheless surprising, especially considering the great contrast between the American economy of 1938 and that of 1961. It would seem that the second-generation patients were not assimilated into the present-day working class.

Comparison between the patients and the normal respondents consisting of twenty second-generation couples who were interviewed in the community shows that, with three exceptions, the life style of the normal families was predominantly that of class IV, while a majority of patients represented class V (Table 5).

Table 5—Class Composition of Recently Admitted Patients and of Normal Families

		1961 Patients	Normal Families
Classes I-III		4.2%	5.0%
Class IV		28.0	85.0
Class V		67.8	10.0
	N	**96**	**20**

The normal informants were not selected on the basis of socioeconomic status, but rather as being typical of the working-class neighborhood in which they resided, according to the opinion of three local leaders.

In regard to the occupational pattern of these normal families, two features stand out: the family's dependence on a network of friends and acquaintances, and its attitude toward marital responsibility.

Much importance was attributed by the respondents to "connections" with the local political hierarchy or to a wide friendship network either for getting jobs or relocating in the event of job difficulty. About one-fourth of the informants made it clear that their jobs were acquired through political influence. Typical occupations were the following: TV repairman, depending on neighborhood contacts; plumbing inspector for the city, a politically acquired, secure job; longshoreman, pugilist, bartender, bookmaker, and such, the varied careers of particularly active and aggressive grammar-school graduates; cutter in the garment district; sales representative. About one-fourth worked in industries or small shops related to the artisan traditions which directed the occupational choices of many immigrants: shoes, garment work, furniture. Two men were studying to acquire technical positions, one of them full time; the remainder were working in a variety of semiskilled occupations.* Although some periods of unemployment had occurred, none of the men had worked only in very low prestige positions, as for example doing laundry or hospital work, or had held only odd jobs. For the most part the jobs were local ones and depended more on knowledgeability in manipulating the local system than on the fulfillment of standardized requirements.

A second factor related to occupational stability has to do with the life cycle. Almost all the male respondents referred to a period in adolescence or young manhood when they were not particularly interested in occupation or achievement as such, but

* *Editor's note:* In regard to the educational level of these "normal" families, the available data make a comparison difficult. Anne Parsons' material shows that in her normal sample nine out of twenty men, i.e., 45 per cent, had not completed high school. This would seem to compare with 78 per cent of the patients admitted in 1961. However, the figures given for patients include the women, while those given for normals are for men only. Anne Parsons notes about her interviews with normals: "Educational levels averaged higher for men reporting themselves than for reports by wives. It is possible that the men upped their own educational status when facing the woman interviewer."

in "enjoying life while you can." The expectation, however, is that this has to change with marriage, when one becomes responsible for a family, and the indications were that most of the informants had managed to cope with this responsibility.

This raises the question whether there is an association between marital and occupational status. Among the patients, of the forty-five men admitted in 1961, one-half were "drifters," in that they had never held any regular occupation. It turns out that whether or not an individual patient was a drifter was closely related to his marital status.

Table 6—Relation Between Marital Status and Occupation for 1961, Male Patients Only (N=45)

Occupation		Single or Divorced	Married
Drifters		65.5%	12.5%
Workers		20.5	81.2
Middle Class		14.0	6.3
	N	29	16

In contrast to the 1961 patients, there were fewer chronic drifters among the 1938 patients. Among them were a large number of patients who were on a regular working-class occupation listing, but with some specific reference to job loss, going on WPA, being unable to find work, and so forth.

Table 7—Occupational Distribution of Male Patients, 1938

Drifters	4
Occupation, job loss	20
Occupation	4
Total	**28**

In spite of relatively high rates of unemployment in 1938, the pattern of chronic marginality appears to have been less marked at that time.[6] It appears that the patients admitted in

6. As for female patients, those in 1961 who worked had occupations

1961 showed significantly different occupational histories from the nonhospitalized members of the same community. It would seem that this was probably not as apparent in 1938, when job interruptions tended to be common in the population at large.

It also seems that a smaller proportion of the patients admitted in 1961 were married, compared to those admitted in 1938.

Table 8—Patients Admitted to State Hospital in 1938 and 1961 by Marital Status *

Marital Status		1938	1961
Single		38.5%	53.1%
Married		28.8	28.1
Not Known		32.7	18.8
	N	**52**	**96**

One way of accounting for the low level of occupational attainment among the 1961 patients and for the high proportion of them who remained single lies in the lack of adaptability to immigrant life in the United States. It turns out that it is among the American-born rather than among the Italian-born that we find the single men (Table 9).

Table 9—Marital Status by Place of Birth for Men Admitted in 1961 (N=45)

	Italian Born	American Born
Married	83.3%	30.8%
Single or Divorced	16.7	69.2
N	**6**	**39**

---

of about the same prestige level as the normal respondents. Single status is not associated with drifting to quite the same extent as it is among males, though a few drifters appear, such as promiscuous women with children who live on welfare.

* *Editor's note*: This table has been computed from an available composite table that shows the distribution of diagnostic categories by year and marital status. Since the diagnosis is missing for seventeen of the 1938 patients and eighteen of the 1961 patients, information about their marital status is missing also.

If second-generation status is associated with a relatively high probability of remaining single, this should also be true for 1938 when, it will be remembered (Table 1), a much higher proportion of those admitted to the hospital were Italian-born. This is, indeed, the case (Table 10).

Table 10—Marital Status by Place of Birth for Men and Women Admitted in 1938 and and 1961 *

	1938		1961	
	Italian Born	American Born	Italian Born	American Born
Married	48.0%	8.0%	50.0%	24.5%
Single-Divorced	7.5	72.0	4.5	61.0
Not Known	44.5	20.0	45.5	14.5
N	**27**	**25**	**14**	**82**

The most important findings so far are that the present-day occupational level of the patients is significantly lower than that of typical second-generation immigrants in a working-class section of the city; that among the patients there is a disproportionately high number of single persons, and that single status seems to be associated with lack of occupational status. It also appears that among the 1938 patients, making allowance for the effects of the depression, there tend to be fewer drifters than among present-day patients.

As the undifferentiated and uneducated immigrant body of manual workers has become less significant with respect to the total population, it appears that a certain number of persons have been left behind or outside of the normal mobility pattern of the working class. I would be in agreement with Hollingshead and Redlich that there is today a social group (class V) ranking below the integrated working class (class IV) and that the former group is contributing disproportionately to the population of hospitalized psychiatric patients.

* *Editor's note*: Just as in Table 8, these figures have been computed from a table showing the distribution of diagnosed patients only, and not reporting the patients for whom diagnosis is missing.

It does not necessarily follow, however, that there exists a "class V" milieu which in itself produces pathology. To see a particular milieu as pathogenic, particularly to the extent that one considers early experience as a feature in the development of psychopathology, is to make some presupposition about the constancy of this milieu over time. I would rather be inclined to say that, starting from an initially less differentiated immigrant culture, some people make it into the contemporary working class and others do not, and that state hospital patients of immigrant background largely tend to come from the second category.

It will be remembered that the occupational level of the 1961 patients studied tends to be distinctly lower than that of members of the control group. Hollingshead and Redlich[7] as well as Faris and Dunham[8] have shown that one cannot explain the higher rates at the bottom level on the basis of "downward drift" from the higher class levels. Eighty-nine per cent of the class V patients in the New Haven study also had class V parents. Moreover, there are a great many persons in class IV, of immigrant parentage, whose parents came from class V backgrounds. In my own normal control sample, 70 per cent of the predominantly class IV informants had class V parents. "Normal" persons accordingly seem to have been more mobile than the patients.

In view of these considerations, research directed to the supposed pathogenic qualities of the "class V" milieu itself is unlikely to be fruitful. Rather, a refocusing of research concerning lower-class pathology is suggested, which can take two directions. First, considering the class system as a dynamic one, we may want to know why it is that some individuals move within it and others do not (or fall out of it). Second, with respect to the more specific question of ethnicity, we can ask what are the characteristics of a particular ethnic milieu which

7. Hollingshead & Redlich, *op. cit.*, pp. 244–248.
8. Robert E. L. Faris & H. Warren Dunham, *Mental Disorders in Urban Areas* (Chicago, Univ. of Chicago Press, 1939).

have made change and adaptability possible, and conversely, what strains and contradictions can account for the fact that some individuals, or some families, do not manage to adapt. To obtain answers to these questions it will be necessary to analyze certain characteristics of Italian culture that bear specifically on individuals' adaptation to life in the United States.

chapter *5*

Specific Patterns of Italian-American Life

It will be remembered that in the Italian working-class community, marriage and having family responsibilities are seen as the main source of motivation for work. This accounts for the observation made in the previous paper that most of the patients who are drifters, occupationally speaking, are also single. The fact that this tends to be true primarily for second-generation Italian patients in the United States today and not for those hospitalized thirty years ago who were primarily first-generation points to the factor of adaptability to American culture as a possible explanation. One source of failure among Italo-Americans of the young generations to marry and gain occupational status is to be sought in forces present within the Italian family that encourage prolonged dependency on parents.

What stands out among the patients is the extent to which

the family has become an exclusive and restrictive environment, rather than a point of leverage for movement into the outside world. In many cases one finds that the family itself has been reduced to an exclusive nuclear or parent-child unit, with the wider range of kin ties having been lost or abandoned. The strong maternal figure is endogenous to the Italian family. But among the pathological cases one often finds a patient who is the exclusive and continuous focus of forced feeding. Frequently a patient's attempts to form heterosexual relationships have been given up, or continue to be systematically frustrated by members of his family. Among male schizophrenics and defectives, peer-group ties are almost always lacking; this is in contrast to the normal adult Italian working-class male who may visit his mother faithfully every Sunday but who also spends many evenings at the bar with his friends, who teach him how to get along in the occupational world. The centripetal tendency of the Italian family may sometimes be so strong that it limits the possibilities of social mobility and change and thus directly contributes to the kinds of occupational and marital difficulties noted in the patients. Families may insulate their members from contacts with the wider community; alternatively, individuals may exert such strong centrifugal force in their efforts to achieve independence that serious conflicts are produced. These conflicts primarily revolve around submission to the father's authority, allegiance to the family of orientation, and continuing dependence on the mother for sustenance and support.

As might be expected, conflicts are often particularly acute during the period of adolescence. The young man faces the task of making his own way in the world, and of establishing himself as a man among men. At the same time he must refrain from rebelling too strongly. A delicate equilibrium between centrifugal and centripetal forces is necessary, and this can easily be upset by deviant features, either of the family itself or of its cultural milieu. When, as a result of immigration, these two sources of disequilibrium have a combined impact, it would seem that pathology is indeed likely to ensue.

For Italian young women the conflicts of adolescence are

fully as stressful as they are for young men, though the content and patterning of their struggles to achieve mature womanhood are of course quite different. The father's authority focuses on the maintenance of his daughter's virginity, and children of both sexes are taught to regard their mother as a wholly nonsexual being. Once again, a fine balance must be maintained within the family, and between the family and its surroundings, if the young woman is to free herself from family pressures enough to achieve successful adult status, without freeing herself too much. The case of Betty T illustrates the pathological results of centripetal forces that proved too strong for an immigrant family to contain, within an alien cultural setting. By contrast, Phyllis M failed to resist family pressures strongly enough, and on this basis succumbed to pathology in her turn.

Betty T: A Family Scapegoat

Betty T is the fifth of eight siblings born into a family that immigrated from a poor mountain area south of Naples. Her mother was orphaned at an early age and brought up by relatives of the patient's father. The two married when the mother was thirteen, and they came to this country after the birth of the first two children. The father operated a corner variety store in an undistinguished but solidly Italian working-class area where the family lived from the time of immigration. The mother helped in the store and was devotedly loyal to her family; in late middle age she appeared tired and worn from hardship but not beaten by it. Through most of her life, she lived with no blood relatives at all, a situation that is particularly difficult for the Southern Italian woman, who depends on her own kin for moral support far more than on her husband.[1]

Betty was always seen as an "I want, I want, I want" child:

1. F. Morrill, "The Influence of the Matrifocal Kinship Network on the Family Structure of the Italo-American," Manuscript, McLean Hospital, 1963.

When she was tiny her mouth was always wide open—wah, wah—then later it stopped and I never heard her tears but I remember her temper. The first words she knew must have been swear words.

The informant here is Julia, the oldest sister, who did much of the bringing up of the younger siblings while the mother worked in the store.[2]

Throughout childhood and adolescence Betty was considered particularly attractive and vivacious, more outgoing than her siblings, and musically talented. In a number of areas she was tacitly admired by her sisters because of what was considered an active and rebellious streak; this her older sister Rose reports laughingly: "She'd be doing the dishes and all of a sudden she'd throw the glass away saying it was much too hard to clean." The only abnormality noted prior to marriage was a series of convulsive episodes accompanied by rapid breathing which appeared in early adolescence in association with homosexual impulses:

Even as a child she was very sexy . . . in her sleep she'd get real close, begin to feel me up. I never told anybody this. I felt embarrassed to tell my mother. I don't even think she knew she was doing it half the time . . . it was mostly in her sleep. It was about the same time the breathing nervous business started [Mary].

In particular, she was known among her sisters for the way in which she was able to stand up against her father:

Boy, how that girl enjoyed a good time . . . even when she knew about the lickings she'd get, that didn't seem to stop her . . . Like I said before, many times we'd be out and I'd say to myself . . . 'My God, how can you have a good time when you know there's a licking waiting for you when you get home.' Everyone of us kids had our own share [of punishment]. In those days our father's word was the law . . . She resented him as far back as I can remember [Rose].

2. Cf. Myers & Roberts, *op. cit.*, who found that having been brought up by an older sibling was common among class V schizophrenic patients.

Parental strictness with respect to dating is characteristic in Southern Italy,[3] and conflict with the father on this issue is characteristic of second-generation girls. Betty was married at twenty-two in a rush ceremony after she let it be known at home that she had lost her virginity.

Betty herself, however, did not perceive her relationship with the father or siblings in terms of active competition or of success in gaining attention. Frequently expressing typical Italian family conflicts in paranoid language, she put the adolescent conflict in such a way as to suggest the appearance of psychotic, paranoid symptoms at that time:

He was either being with you or else you were being followed by him . . . he was always following, following, following, while teen-agers like to be left alone.

Her explanation of her difficulties was that his "ultra-strictness caused a persecution complex." Interestingly enough, she saw the hospital as a place where "you receive a sort of getting away from home conflicts."

Betty's illness as perceived by her family developed in two phases. In the first, they began to note that her life was following quite a different course from theirs and in the second, they began to define her as "mental." The first change in status took place a year or two after her marriage, when she began to have love affairs and to neglect her child; the second occurred on the death of the father when she was forty-three. It was only at the latter point that treatment was considered, and the first hospitalization took place on the initiative of her sister when she was forty-four.[4] From about twenty-four to forty-four she lived a somewhat deviant life, maintaining ties with her family but

3. Cf. A. Parsons, "Is the Oedipus Complex Universal? The Jones–Malinowski Debate Revisited," this book, Chapter 1.

4. She was admitted on a charge of assault and battery brought by her sister. However, with respect to the significance of the role of the police in working-class hospitalizations, it is interesting to note that the charge was invented by the sister and a neighborhood policeman to assure admission. In many instances the police are seen as a recourse for conflicts that cannot be resolved within the family.

not as closely as the mother and sisters, who formed a tightly knit group. Her husband deserted after a few years of marriage, and of her three sons, only the first was certainly fathered by him.

This man stuff started when she was about 26–27 years old. She'd say it right out loud. "I have to have men; one's not enough to put the sparkle in my eye." We [the rest of the sisters] led what you might call a conventional sort of life; . . . we always worked; to us it was a different kind of life . . . so different from what we'd call living . . . we used to get a kick out of her. My mother cried for days when we first knew what was going on [Mary].

When things went real bad for her with her husband, she moved in with this bad girl from around here who was living in X [a more disorganized neighborhood]. They say she was living with some Chinese fellow. . . . those days were rich days for Betty. She had fur coats, went to night clubs, didn't matter who she went with, Irish, Italian, didn't matter. . . . [Josephine].

For the point at which she was first defined as "mental," two different stories were given. According to Josephine, the crucial event was her reaction to hearing of the father's death. It was she who went to inform Betty, saying: "Betty, Papa died and I want you to come over and be one of us." At this point Betty broke into a stream of obscenity saying with "words of venom" that she had always hated the father and was glad he was dead. At the funeral she showed no grief. According to Mary, the break took place a few weeks before the father's death when he found her describing intimate details of her sexual experience to the mother; he told her to forget the number of his house. Both versions portray violations of key family norms, i.e. respect for the dead and the asexual image of the mother.

In this case the family does not appear to be significantly different in attitudes or way of life from other working-class Italian families, but the patient's own life history follows a course of progressive alienation from the family. It would seem that in this way they were helped by Betty, whose violations of norms were treated with humor and permissiveness if not encouragement. The development of Betty's illness seemed related to internal tensions in the family which could be vicariously dealt with through her. Though the mother and sisters all had "troubles" or neurotic symptoms, they seemed to be keeping their heads well above water and were closely linked together in the kind of matrifocal family pattern that is characteristic of the second-generation Italian family in this country as well as in Southern Italy.[5] One set of these tensions surrounds the role of the mother, who was herself an orphan. Though able to hold the family together, she was characterized by the others as often lacking in immediate affection or warmth, since she was always so busy. Other tensions surround the role of the father and the dating conflict, with Betty's fragile rebellion being magnified by her sisters; others again refer to the drabness of American working-class life with Betty representing the more glamorous if less moral alternative. Thus it appears that while family solidarity was maintained, this was at some internal cost to other members of the family as well. It was only when norms pertaining to family solidarity were violated that Betty was declared "mental" and expelled, other violations having been treated with humor that indicated vicarious participation.

Phyllis M: A Docile Daughter

Phyllis M is the third of six siblings born into a Sicilian family. The style of family life as remembered by her two older sisters was far duller than that of the T family.

Look, our life was like this. We'd go to school, eat, bed nine o'clock. We'd go to school, we'd come home, we'd eat, we'd go to bed at nine o'clock. That's all I remember. That's the way it was, day in and day out. Go to school, eat, bed nine o'clock, get up, go to work if we weren't going to school. We always had to go to bed early. My father was very strict about that [oldest sister, Roberta].

5. F. Morrill, *op. cit.*

The father had no relatives in the United States. Until two years before her death, the family lived with the maternal grandmother whose sister also lived nearby. Siblings of the mother were more prosperous and lived in other sections; a number of kin-group frictions were evident which finally culminated in a quarrel with the grandmother. On visits to aunts, uncles, and cousins, the patient and her siblings were taught to take the humble role of poor relatives. Both grandmother and father and, in later life, the mother, worked in laundries. The family income was adequate for survival but the life style never changed from that of the poor peasant.

Both parents appeared as seriously disturbed people. Their marriage was of the type that has been described by Lidz as "skew," [6] in which the tyranny of one partner is complemented by the abject submission of the other. The father, once briefly hospitalized with the diagnosis of paranoid schizophrenia, behaved almost like a caricature of the dominant, possessive, and emotional Italian male; the mother seems to have simply plodded through life making "pasta and beans, pasta and spinach, pasta and potatoes" and was severely depressed at the time I saw her. In this setting, Phyllis appeared as the favorite child primarily because of her simplicity and docility:

When Phyllis was a kid she was smart, she worked in the house, she washed the dishes, she'd go to the store for me, she'd do anything [Mother]. [Sister, Adele, interrupts:] Mama, you didn't like her just because she did all those things; it's because you loved her. [Mother:] Yes, I lika Phyl. Good girl, used to do everything I asked, go to store, wash dishes, clean the house . . . She was very clean. She took care of her clothes by herself, she'd iron, wash dishes, go to the store. Phyl was the best girl in the house.

In interviewing Phyllis it was difficult to gain an image of her adolescence beyond an impression of emptiness, though much of her psychotic behavior at the age of forty was appropriate

6. T. Lidz, A. Cornelison, S. Fleck, & D. Terry, "The Intrafamilial Environment of the Schizophrenic Patient. II: Marital Schism and Marital Skew," *Amer. J. Psychiat. 114*, 24:248, 1957.

to the period of American life when she was adolescent; e.g., "shimmying" to dance records.

Superficially much more conventional than Betty, in the early years of marriage Phyllis played the role of the devoted mother who remains close to her own mother. Not long after the general family disruption accompanying the break with the grandmother, when a divorced younger sister, Adele, took over the dominant role in the family, Phyllis moved to a housing project and the distance from her parents increased. In her mid-thirties, then mother of seven children, her first psychotic symptoms appeared in the form of paranoid delusions concerning a bad lady neighbor, an Irishwoman who gave her something to drink. When I first saw her at age forty-two, she was again living closer to her parents but actively resisting their influence in her life. The covert nature of the intrafamily conflicts can best be read from the content of her delusions which, in turn, correspond very closely to details appearing in family interviews.

In the first interview, the patient began by telling me she did not know where her husband worked, adding, "and I don't know much about him; he is never home." She then went right into a description of the psychotic experiences that led to her hospitalization:

Adele B[7] was right there on top of me—Joseph A [father] was jumping over the bed—I was really seeing him—they were drugging my coffee—trying to get information or something—right in my home—I never told them to stay with me. She wanted the money—is having trouble with mother's aid—the only other thing is that I seem to know when my family is near me.

The interview with the father turned into a kind of dramatization of his intense involvement with his daughter, as he emphasized and reemphasized all evening the tragedy of her marriage to such an "old man."

She met him when she was just sixteen. The guy that was going to

7. She always referred to members of her family with their full names while the common Italian usage is kin terms alone.

be her husband would drive her to work along with the other girls and because he made her pregnant, I had to get them married, but I never liked him ; he was no good. And what kind of man is it, an old man like that, to take out a young girl and make her pregnant?

It was clear that to him the event was still a contemporaneous one though nearly thirty years in the past.

In contrast to the other case where the family appeared to maintain an integrated surface by first encouraging and later expelling the patient, this family was characterized by the type of collective irrationality that has been described by Lidz:[8] there were very close correspondences between the patient's delusions and ideas held by other family members. Moreover, in some areas it was difficult to know exactly what had taken place: the most important of these being a complex question of whether or not the patient had had several children by a man other than her husband which in turn was connected with the father's leaving his male club because of the insults he received. The psychoses of the patient and her father seem closely intertwined, and her attitude of obedience during early years may actually have added to the family's pathological tendencies, rather than reducing them. The pathological nature of the family structure is clearly seen in those delusions in which Phyllis denied the existence of any physical or spatial barrier between herself and other members of the family. The earlier split from the maternal grandmother and the social distance between the mother and her siblings must certainly have been important for the development of this situation. Phyllis's parents in later life lived as an isolated couple to a degree that was unusual for families in such a setting. Thus in a certain sense there was no organized collectivity from which the patient could be expelled, for the siblings in this family had long since freed themselves from parental authority. It remained for the father's authority to be perpetuated, in schizophrenic caricature, by the daughter, whose docility may have eased her siblings' efforts to break away.

8. T. Lidz, A. Cornelison, S. Fleck, & D. Terry, "The Intrafamilial Environment of the Schizophrenic Patient. IV: The Transmission of Irrationality," *Arch. Neurol. & Psychiat.*, 79 : 305–316, 1958.

Discussion of Case Materials

While a number of studies indicate the existence of social and cultural variations in the incidence of schizophrenia, their exact patterning has yet to be unraveled.[9] Statistical distributions do not point to their own explanations, and there is a danger that they will lead to generalizations based on such global concepts as social disorganization, anomie, cultural breakdown, and so on.

One kind of methodological difficuty is illustrated by the hypothesis (to which Marie Bonaparte has called attention) that there is something tubercular-genic about Greek national character, since tuberculosis rates in Athens are unusually high. But tuberculosis is the result of a well-understood infectious process that is more likely to occur under conditions of urban economic deprivation which are indeed found in Athens, but also in Naples, Hong Kong, no doubt in Moscow, and in nineteenth-century London and New York as well. There is no need to add a sociocultural level of explanation since two processes are already clear: first, the bacillary infection which takes place within the biological organism; second, a range of environmental conditions that make the organism more susceptible to it or further its transmission, e.g. malnutrition, crowding of habitations, and so forth. In this instance we can say with assurance that the disease and its etiology are organic in nature, even though the conditioning factors show a determinate and statistically measurable social pattern.

In regard to schizophrenia, the question of causation and of the relation between statistical distribution and the internal structure of the disease becomes more complex, primarily because of the uncertainties surrounding the latter. This means that the weight given to indications of social variations is likely to vary according to the theoretical perspective of the interpreter.

9. For a summary of studies throughout the world, see M. Hammer & E. Leacock, "Appendix: Source Material on the Epidemiology of Mental Illness," in J. Zubin, ed., *Field Studies in the Mental Disorders* (New York: Grune & Stratton, Inc. 1961).

In regard to tuberculosis, no physician would consider the greater prevalence of the disease in slums as evidence against an organic theory of its etiology. It may also be the case that anyone who uses statistical studies in order to maintain that schizophrenia is socially determined is also on shaky ground. Statistical studies themselves show that schizophrenia occurs in a very wide variety of social conditions. Moreover, major advances in the understanding of this disease have come from intensive case studies that are usually acultural or asocial in that they focus on individuals, as such, abstracted from their social surroundings.

However, just as it is possible in the understanding of tuberculosis to link an organic infectious process to surrounding social conditions, it should also be possible to locate the social factors that serve either to condition the schizophrenic personality toward breakdown or to make the reintegration process more difficult once breakdown has occurred. Moreover, such an effort should take us beyond the implicit assumption of much psychoanalytic thinking that the postulated traumatic factors or structural defects which limit the adaptability of particular individuals are randomly distributed in space and time; we are far from certain that this is actually the case. The asocial assumption of randomness is very often maintained by the *ad hoc* postulation of a "basic" or "underlying" equivalence in the fact of observed variations either in the incidence or phenomenology of mental disease.

For each of the patients discussed in this chapter, it is quite possible to describe personality structures or mechanisms corresponding to those we would find among schizophrenics in quite different social milieux. Both showed gross failure with respect to the establishment of meaningful heterosexual relationships; both showed patterns of isolation and obsessive control coupled with indications of extreme dependency needs centered on primary objects; and both showed intensive aggressive feelings which were handled by means of projection and delusion. But in addition it also seemed possible to place these disorders in the specific context of conflicts that are characteristic of the Italo-

American adaptation to American urban life. Thus in various ways the two patients had made attempts to extend their individual values and life spaces beyond those of the family, and they showed personality attributes which they had picked up outside of the ethnic community. In certain respects an increased amount of visible personality disorganization can be related to the consequent potentiality for identity diffusion. Phyllis, for example, resembled many girls in Southern Italy in that as an adolescent she played the role of the docile good girl who becomes mother's favorite. However, in this country this role cut her off from the life around her to a much greater extent than it would have done in Italy. It appears that she picked up American adolescent models, even though unsuccessfully, and that they had considerable importance to her.[10] Much of the "inappropriateness" of her later psychotic behavior can be accounted for by her attempt to relive this period. One does not find this kind of juggling with the life cycle in a peasant environment.

When we try to relate the patient's personality to the family setting, we find that the same conflicts in the patient's personality can also be found within the family, though reacted to or resolved in different ways by other family members. Moreover, there seem to be certain structural features that account for inability to deal with acculturation conflicts. I should like to single out three of these for discussion: (1) the mother's loss of the tie to her own mother; (2) the size of the family; and (3) the failure of the father's authority to be effective.

The last is a factor which has already received considerable discussion as a common feature in the family of the schizophrenic. What can be added from a sociocultural standpoint is that processes of change may serve to weaken paternal authority.

10. A great deal of American adolescent life depends on school friendships rather than family or neighborhood belongingness. Many of Phyllis's psychotic fantasies centered on the space between home and school and when she described her prehospitalization life setting, she remarked plaintively that "there wasn't much people around—I looked in all the windows but there wasn't much people" (It. singular: *molto gente*).

The case of the European-born aristocrat, Mr. Dollfuss, described by Lidz *et al.*,[11] who withdrew into the study of Oriental mysticism all the while insisting that his family cater to his every whim, provides an example of a caricature of an original model remarkably similar to that seen in the second case discussed here. In both instances, one can see the caricature as a dramatization that deals with anxiety concomitant with the loss of the real role.[12]

The first and second factors, however, merit additional discussion in a way specifically relevant to the working-class Italo-American family. In such a family the link between mother and married daughters (and between sisters) is crucial to the entire structure, while men are much more loosely integrated.[13] In a structure of this sort one would not see a close mother-adult daughter tie as pathogenic in itself. However, what stands out in the two cases is that the mother of the patient did *not* have such links functioning in an effective way. Moreover, I saw several other second-generation cases where the mother expressed great pride in the competence and ability with which she had faced the new environment without the aid of consanguineal relatives, while at the same time she appeared to crush the patient, whose illness appeared crucial to her in maintaining her role in middle age.

Given the very common occurrence of matrifocal family structures in urban working-class groups, the investigation of the potential disruptions or complications in the ties between women and the consequent influence on pathological personality de-

11. T. Lidz, A. Cornelison, S. Fleck, & D. Terry, "The Intrafamilial Environment of the Schizophrenic Patient: I: The Father." *Psychiatry,* *20* : 329–342, 1942.

12. One similar case I saw involved the second-generation father of a patient who showed pseudo-American lower-middle-class patterns; actually living on disability, he kept a file cabinet close to his chair and talked insistently about his "papers" and bookkeeping. The close involvement of the father in the home in both these cases resulted from his failure to maintain roles in the peer-group setting which ordinarily symbolizes masculinity.

13. Cf. R. T. Smith, *The Negro Family in British Guiana* (London: Routledge & Kegan Paul, Ltd., 1956), for a description of the matrifocal family in British Guiana.

velopment seems important to the understanding of working-class psychopathology.[14] One such case observed was that of a young woman who became psychotic after delivering a child fathered by a paranoid-psychopath. She improved markedly, not through the establishment of any relationship to the father of the child, but after a reconciliation with her mother and the working out of mutually agreeable ways of supporting and bringing up the child. This illustrates the importance which solidarity among women has at this social level and the part that its presence or absence may play with respect to psychosis.

A final factor relevant to urban working-class psychosis concerns family size. The importance of large families for class V patients has been noted by Myers and Roberts,[15] who found a median of 6.5 siblings for twenty-five class V patients studied intensively (seventeen of these were of Italian origin) as opposed to a median of 3.5 for the class III patients. Since in Southern Italy families are very often large, socialization patterns are in many ways adapted to this fact (e.g., in the interest taken in children by relatives and often strangers), so that one cannot quite evaluate the results by reference to American middle-class norms. Although large families tend to be less adapted to urban than to rural conditions, nevertheless, under conditions of immigration, the family tends to become even larger (Table 1). Notably I found that the median family size for a sample of schizophrenic patients hospitalized in the United States was larger than for a comparable sample of schizophrenic patients hospitalized in Italy.

14. In studying perceptions of parental authority among schizophrenics and control subjects, Kohn and Clausen found that maternal authority generally appeared more important than paternal for the lowest SES, both for schizophrenics and controls (M. L. Kohn & J. A. Clausen, "Parental Authority Behaviour and Schizophrenia," *Amer. J. Orthopsychiat.*, 26, 2: 297–313, 1956.) However, one difficulty with this formulation is that the descriptive term "strong mother" refers primarily to a psychological trait rather than to features of social structure. The matrifocal family does not necessarily imply dominance of women, since women may, for example, band together over threats of desertion posed by men, or their authority may be restricted to specific aspects of intrafamilial operation.

15. *Op. cit.*

Table 1—Comparative Size of Family for Italian and Italo-American Patients[16]

Siblings Living Past 6 Yrs.	Italian Patients	Italo-American Patients
3 or less	60%	36%
4—5	24	20
6—7	16	28
8—9	0	12
10+	0	4
N	25	25

There is also a strong tendency for the schizophrenic patient to fall in the middle of large sibling groups. It appears that such families provide individualized relationships by a process of internal division into more tightly knit, partly overlapping groups of two or three siblings. In such families one finds either that the patient is an isolate or is locked in an incestuous or homosexual relation with a sibling. Thus there might well be structural factors inherent in the family as a small group that limit its effectiveness beyond a certain numerical point.

By way of summary, reference may be made again to the analogy with tuberculosis. Following this analogy, schizophrenia can be described as a disorder of intrapsychic structure which seems to be more likely to occur in the presence of particular kinds of social disorganization. Among the factors which I feel to be most important for members of the immigrant American urban working class are internal difficulties in the matrifocal family structure and problems of ego controls and identity formation relative to the expansion of the life space and the inclusion of a wider community. The adjustment of the large family to urban life is also a factor that particularly merits further investigation in the light of the rapid population growth that is taking place in many currently urbanizing areas of the world.

---

[16] These patients were primarily of the second generation. Four patients were third-generation, of whom three were small-family cases.

chapter 6

Some Comparative Observations on Ward Social Structure

Southern Italy, England, and the United States

   In the United States, a number of sociologists and social anthropologists have recently become interested in the field of psychiatry. One of the objects of their study has been the social structure of the mental hospital, i.e., the patterning of social relationships between patients, between patients and staff, or among the staff itself.[1] In such studies, the mental hospital is seen as a social system comparable to other social systems

   * This work was carried out on a research grant from the National Institute of Mental Health, Bethesda, Md., M-2105. I am particularly indebted to Prof. Vizioli for permission to carry out work at the Provincial Hospital of Naples.
   1. See A. H. Stanton & M. Schwartz, *The Mental Hospital* (New York: Basic Books, Inc., 1954) and W. Caudill, *The Mental Hospital as a Small Society* (Cambridge, Mass.: Harvard Univ. Press, 1958).

   Reprinted by permission from *L'Ospedale Psichiatrico* (Naples), April–June, 1959.

such as the factory, the community, or the family which have heretofore received the most attention from social scientists, being considered as a "small society" which has its own distinctive set of problems and social mechanisms for dealing with them. From this point of view, the study of the mental hospital is primarily of interest to the social sciences in that it provides a new field of data.

But in the United States such studies have not been the province of sociology alone: many have also been co-operative efforts in which psychiatrists have participated as well. For those psychiatrists who feel that psychological and social factors play important roles in the etiology of many forms of mental illness, it has become increasingly clear that the study of the social interaction of psychiatric patients is an effort which may further our understanding of its still mysterious aspects—in particular the mystery of schizophrenia which provides the largest contingent of chronic hospital patients, in Italy as well as the United States. One means by which it can be demonstrated whether or not there are social factors which are etiologically relevant to schizophrenia is by the increasingly detailed observations of correlations—or the lack of correlations—of changes in schizophrenic symptom patterns with changes in the social environment. In this paper, I shall present some comparative observations on social interaction on psychiatric wards in England, the United States and Southern Italy as a step in this direction. Since the majority of the studies of mental hospital social structure have been carried out in the Anglo-Saxon countries[2] they presuppose the constancy of certain social features of these countries. But precisely because they provide the possibility for the observation of further social variation, comparative studies in which radically different social conditions are taken into account are needed at present.

Concretely, I will summarize some observations of ward social life made in the Provincial Hospital of Naples, bringing out some of the principal points of contrast with public psychiatric hospitals in England and the Northeastern United States.

2. With the important exception of the studies of Caudill in Japan.

These observations have been made more or less accidentally as byproducts of a project to compare schizophrenic symptoms in these two societies on an individual case level: In Naples I spent three months as an observer on a mixed diagnosis female ward principally as a means for acquiring fluency with the language and some understanding of the situation of the psychiatric patient, and in the United States I spent some time at a state hospital for a similar case study project. Very briefly I visited a state hospital in England for the express purpose of receiving contrasting impressions to complement the Naples experience. The best way of presenting the contrasts is to describe my first experiences in the three respective hospitals.

In Naples, when I arrived on the ward that was to be intensively studied, I was immediately surrounded by a crowd of curious patients and nurses who in unison asked who I was, what I was doing in Italy, did I think Naples is beautiful and had I been to Capri, was I married or engaged and how old, did I have mother, father, brothers, sisters and wasn't it difficult to be away from them? did I know such and such a cousin Broocalin? etc. Exactly the same thing happened on every occasion I visited a new ward or a new hospital, and throughout one of the major difficulties in doing research was to succeed in talking to a single patient without interruption of this nature from other patients or nurses. At another hospital the rumor spread that my purpose was to tell fortunes and those who were not admitted for interview became quite resentful. And when I was taken to the female disturbed ward by the physician on duty in the absence of its administrator, both of us left soaked to the skin after a patient threw a bucket of water over us! The general laughter shared by patients and nurses prevented any resentment! Later via the patient grapevine I learned that the patients had feared replacement of their very popular physician on being introduced to the "dotoressa americana." Throughout a year of research, I maintained the feeling that whatever the unpleasant side of the wards, there was always movement and action: they never seemed like social vacuums, in which it was purely depressing or embarrassing to move.

In contrast, on my first day at the American state hospital, I had the feeling of being in a museum: the museum atmosphere of certain back wards has been well described by Von Mering and King.[3] Unaccompanied, I got lost in a maze of corridors and stood for several minutes bewildered before a patient noted my plight and gave directions. At that point, it first occurred to me that the statues could speak and that it would have been simpler had I asked in the first place. But in the course of a year's work, in spite of later forming a number of interesting relationships with staff members and patients, I was never able to enter without first fighting with a feeling of depression and uneasiness. In the English hospital, I was first struck by an atmosphere of ease and physical comfort in contrast to the starkness of the corridors of the American one: I arrived when small cafe tables were being set up for tea and coal grates provided a welcome contrast to the fog outside. But it took decided initiative, evoked by the memory of the not too distant Italian hospital, to break the social barrier which separated me from the patients, each of whom sat properly staring into her own solitude. Only one brave soul ventured to pressure the doctor who accompanied me concerning her possibilities for discharge, a pattern which would have been followed by 15 or 20 simultaneously had we been in Naples.

These incidents have been reported to bring out a very general contrast in the atmosphere of the ward. They should not be interpreted to mean that South Italian mental patients are always lovable and affectionate; obviously if they were, the hospital could shut down and send everyone home. On a finer level, we can now report some general groupings of types of disturbed behavior.

Aggressive Behavior

It may be that one reason Italian hospitals have been so slow in opening the doors is that in fact overtly aggressive behavior is more of a problem than in some other countries (e.g.,

3. Otto Von Mering, & Stanley H. King, *Remotivating the Mental Patient* (New York: Russell Sage Foundation, 1957).

in the English hospital there was a large mirror in the middle of the disturbed ward).[4] I saw a number of fights between patients, usually of a verbal nature but not infrequently ending in blows, hair-pulling, etc., so that patients had to be separated by nurses. In such cases, one or both patients are bound at the wrist and ankle so as to be held to one of the stone seats in the courtyard, which is the center of patient life. Thus punishment did not cut the patient off from social interaction, as does the seclusion more commonly used in the United States. Such fights appeared to give rise to line-ups between nurses and other patients. Each patient would try to defend her own honor, casting all of the insults, in which Neapolitan vocabulary is so rich, at the other. The casting of insults in turn became a means of lining up allies; and in contrast to what I have seen in an American private hospital, the nurses seemed to make very little effort to determine the objective situation, but rather were easily swayed by one patient or another so that one patient might be punished while another went free. Quarrels between nurses also sometimes result from quarrels between their favorites. On the disturbed ward obviously the frequency of patient quarreling is far higher so that the place is continually in an uproar: until 10 years ago a number of patients were kept continually bound but the present administrator has made considerable effort to free them. Although aggression is perhaps primarily of a reciprocal and transitory interpersonal nature, one also finds patients who alienate themselves permanently from others by continuous and intense aggression: isolation is sometimes used in such cases on the disturbed ward but not on others.

Repetitive Pleading

We emphasized the fact that the tone of the ward for one who enters is set partly by the crowd of patients who crowd around to plead for discharge. But on repeated contact, one is struck by the fact that this pleading often has a ritual character:

4. Although most experiments in this direction have shown that as freedom is given, patient aggression diminishes.

the same plea, "I wanna go home" is repeated over and over again, and it is not usually very easy to lead the patient into a consideration of some of the issues which may be involved in the particular situation. With varying structures depending on the patient's personality constellation or actual situation, the pleading usually seems defensive: thus patients who have entered with delusions of persecution relative to family members quickly come to express the other side of an ambivalent relationship by an obsessional plea to go home; depressed patients, who are not usually seen alone meditating on their sins, often take the center of the stage by pleading for attention to their unhappiness; manipulating or psychopathic patients assure the listener that everything is perfectly all right and they have never done anything they shouldn't but should only be allowed to leave. This pleading is also a major activity for patients who have little real chance of discharge or who have repeatedly been discharged with unsuccessful results.

From a sociological standpoint the plea to go home can be seen as a collectively supported ritual for the maintenance of contact with the outside world at the same time having the function of supporting denial of the problems which confront the patients in it. It is worth noting that although sometimes in individual cases it seemed that patients at least temporarily got considerable gratification out of the freedom from family pressures afforded by the hospital, this was not a belief which could be publicly expressed.

Physical Contact

In an American mental hospital, many patients set themselves aside as untouchables, and their fear of physical contact, often by persons of both sexes, gives confirmation to Freudian theories concerning the roles of heterosexual or homosexual panic in the genesis of psychosis. However, in the Italian setting the fear of being touched as such does not seem nearly as conspicuous. Patients are often seen in arm-and-arm promenades with each other on the ward courtyard and one of my primary means of making and maintaining contact with them was to adopt the same promenade pattern. Nor was it infrequent that I found myself hugged or kissed by women patients, in spite of injunctions from the nurses that such behavior was inappropriate towards a higher-status person.

However, there was a point at which patient behavior could transgress a norm implicitly established on the ward which separated socially acceptable affectionate behavior—even if mildly disapproved such as on grounds of status or insistence—from behavior of a more overtly sexual content which was tabooed. The existence of a line was made clear by reactions of nurses to one manic-depressive patient who in her usual hypomanic mode of existence was boisterously affectionate and a favorite of the nurses but who occasionally became more provocative, at which point aversion on their part became clear: they would repulse her with sharp remarks. Likewise two patients set up a relationship of mutual housekeeping in which they showed great affection and concern for each other during the day. However when it was discovered that at night they engaged in overt homosexual behavior, one was transferred, and both incurred considerable censure from other patients as well as nurses.

Closely related to the existence of untouchables is the fact that in mental hospitals one often sees patients who live in a purely private space in that their gestures appear to have no relation to those of others: psychiatrically, such patients may be characterized as posturing. Among the 150 patients of the ward observed, we noted only two who lived continuously in private spaces of this sort: one was not Italian and the other a university graduate. Moreover, the second, although she remained ill, went through a marked change in this respect after the observation period. The crowded and animated conditions of the ward made occupation of a private space extremely difficult and among very regressed or isolated patients, passive sitting on the sidelines seemed more common than active posturing.

Delusions and Hallucinations

A number of patients could be observed talking to delusions or hallucinations who generally on investigation turned out to be non-present neighbors or relatives. Gestures and verbal expression in such conversations usually had a very definitive quality and insulting language not very different from that of the actual interpersonal quarrels was common. Sometimes it was hard to tell if patients were talking to hallucinations or each other and occupation with a hallucinatory world did not necessarily preclude participation in the actual social one.

In comparison with the American state hospital, I felt that highly elaborate delusions and individual ways of expression were minimal. Those patients who do show an elaborate delusional system generally turn out to have a higher social and educational status than the others. Paranoid ideas, including feelings of persecution by family members and neighbors as well as magical and witchcraft ideas, are common also among the less educated schizophrenic patients but there seems to be less space to bridge between these and commonly held social ideas. In particular, there was far less of a tendency towards the elaboration of paranoid systems in which the hospital or doctors were held responsible for all of the patients' difficulties than in the American hospital. This goes with a lesser consciousness in either the positive or negative sense concerning the role of the hospital as a total social institution: for the majority of patients the hospital was simply a power which would release them or not, and not a significant social entity about which knowledge and concepts were to be acquired.

The term "hallucinated" had a special status in the ward vocabulary which expressed patient opposition to popular concepts of mental illness. The ability to reason was by doctors and nurses verbalized as the most crucial criterion of recovery and most patients had on admission been told they could not reason. Thus "hallucinated" became an insult—used often by patients with reference to other patients but never to themselves—parallel to the other insults in common use. Its extension was fairly large: for example I heard one patient call another hallucinating because she thought it was Tuesday and there should be movies when it fact it was Wednesday.

Treatment

Actually the ability to reason was by patients and often by nurses used as a criterion of recovery on a fairly superficial level, for elaborated observations on the rationality of conduct were not discovered. Rather treatment and recovery, and thus illness, were seen according to two principal norms: that one should eat and not worry. In fact mental illness often seemed to be defined as being thin and recovery as gaining weight: so that a patient might say "I was so thin when I came, now look how beautifully fat I am," etc. Forced feeding was seen, including the practice of holding patients' mouths open and shoving it in when food brought by relatives was refused. The bringing of food defined the symbolic ritual of visiting hour and a patient's relation to her family could be defined by her acceptance or refusal: families frequently mentioned failure to eat as the first sympton of illness they noted. It was also clear that value systems of both patients and nurses were not oriented to the synthesis or preservation of psychotic experience. Nurses saw electric shock, for example, as a means of knocking the remembrance of the disturbed period out of the head in association with the resulting memory loss, and were pleased with the results when patients showed amnesia. This relates to one of the most important characteristics of the intra-patient society, namely that it is present-oriented. In this it differs radically from the patient societies of American psychotherapeutically-oriented hospitals where patient discussions are a means by which therapeutic insights are discussed, tested, and consolidated.[5] Rather the patient society can be best seen as a perpetual interchange which is based on immediate feeling states and im-

5. See Caudill, *op. cit.*

mediate reactions to others rather than the exchange of biographical materials seen as distinct from the present context. It
could be proposed that in this sense there was considerable discontinuity between the patients' lives inside and outside the
hospital.

Social Isolation

Finally, in emphasizing the atmosphere of sociability and
motion on the wards, we do not wish to give the impression
that there are no socially isolated or extremely regressed patients.
Of the 150 patients on the intensively observed ward, there
were about 15 who habitually remained outside the flow of
ward life and made no efforts to contact others. Most of these
were schizophrenics and a number fit a particular pattern,
namely a regression to a primarily vegetative state where their
principal concern was with being fed. Such patients provoked
intensive mothering on the part of nurses or other patients and
some had parents as well who appeared regularly at visiting
hour to stuff food down their throats. Such patients were at
times sloppy or resistive to feeding but at others showed beatific
childlike expressions. The social interaction of some other
patients was somewhat marginal because of continual preoccupation with hallucinations or other phenomena such as borderline intelligence.

In sum, the ward society of the Naples provincial hospital
can be characterized as one in which there is perpetual motion
and activity and interpersonal interchange of a diffuse and
present-oriented nature. There does not appear to be a formation of stable groups such as cliques although a number of continuous two-person relationships exist. Not all patients are active
social participants and perhaps most show periods of withdrawal into their private worlds and some of the behavior is of
a not very highly integrated sort. However, the contrast between
the Naples hospital and the chronic wards of old-style American
and English hospitals is a very sharp one: the museum atmos-

phere or the quality of anomie, i.e., removal from the stream of social organization and events, is almost totally lacking in Naples. In conclusion we can attempt to relate this contrast to factors characteristic of the relevant societies and present some statistics concerning discharge patterns for schizophrenics as an index of the possible therapeutic value of patient society.

When one looks at the relationships between American and South Italian societies as a whole, at first it seems a paradox that the country which is by far the most advanced from the technological standpoint and most activist in values should appear to have the less active patient society. There are a number of fairly simple explanations for some aspects of this "paradox of progress." One of the most important facts is that the South Italian hospital is burdened with far fewer long-term patients with a bad prognosis both because higher death rates and other social factors limit the numbers of elderly patients and because the high death rate and general disruption of the hospital in the war years radically diminished the patient population: it has been noted that mental hospital population in Italy climbed upwards from the 1920's to 1940 but then radically declined and only since 1945 has begun to climb again.[6] But precisely because of more stable social conditions and advances in general medical care, the total population of American mental hospitals, but particularly the percentage of elderly patients, has increased steadily.

However, phenomena related to old age cannot wholly account for the phenomenon of lesser "anomie" or social inertia in the patient body, for our observations were principally of younger patients in both hospitals. Rather it seems possible that at all ages the greater the technological progress of a society the further behind do the mentally unfit seem to fall. Thus it may be that there is an inverse rather than direct correlation between the severity of potential personality and social disorganization and the state of industrial development of the society rather than a direct one; this is an assumption that has served many sociological studies. It was a great surprise to most of

6. See Lemkau & di Sanctis.

my Italian colleagues when I commented that in many ways American state mental hospitals can be worse than theirs. "How can this be in such a rich country?" Actually, from the material standpoint, there seems to be little difference between the American and Italian hospitals visited; both are overcrowded and understaffed with physicians.[7]

Turning to technical sociological concepts, we can try to explain the lesser anomie of the Italian hospital in terms of role differentiation and value systems. First, it is known that industrial societies are characterized by a very high degree of role differentiation, seen particularly in the amount of job specialization and the complexity of industrial or other bureaucratic organizations. But Southern Italy is not very extensively industrialized; thus the degree of role differentiation is low. In particular at the lower-class level, most jobs are fairly easily learned and can be taken over by almost anyone without special training. In addition, there is a lack of any very extensive development or commitment to social structures which include more persons than blood relatives or friends. As a cause or a consequence, it is the family which is the most important and extensive focus of social relationships, and the family in turn has greater extensivity and durability in time than is generally true in industrial societies.

These factors have a number of consequences for the mental hospital patient. First, because his activity in the outside world is far less specialized, it is more easily carried on within the mental hospital. Where work programs are carried out, they must in any mental hospital be of a highly diffuse nature. But

7. It is necessary to emphasize here that we are talking about the "typical" American state hospital "back wards" as they existed up to 1945 and continue to exist in complete or partial form today. In the post-war period, considerable attention has been given to the problem of the mental hospital and partly as the result of a self-conscious attempt at social reorganization, the same conditions have been wholly or partly modified in some hospitals. In addition, the differences between the private clinic and the public hospital is generally sharper in the United States than in Europe. The state of anomie cannot be said to be typical of the American private clinic which does have extensive resources in its hands.

although a hospital cannot hope to approach the degree of job specialization found in an industrial society, the occupation of a non-industrial one can much more easily be transplanted inside its walls. In fact it seemed that the work program of the Naples hospital, consisting principally in crafts and intra-hospital services is fairly successful, and given the generally very low economic rewards of the outside world, patients can be motivated to work even when paid exceedingly small sums.[8]

Second, the fact of greater family strength in itself provides a continual focus of social solidarity for hospital patients. It was our impression that there was far more visiting of even chronic patients in Naples than in the American state hospital by relatives, although this does not mean there are not patients whose families have abandoned them in the hospital. There seem to be two factors at work here. First, as a general rule family ties hold up better under situations of strain than social ties made in later life. However, given the greater extensivity and importance of the family relative to other social groupings in Southern Italy, the patient carries a greater part of his social world into the hospital by the fact of family visits. The South Italian family is an extremely permissive unit (outside of the area of sexual control of women) and there is little tendency to abandon a family member who does not live up to behavioral expectations. Thus the fact of mental illness as such does not seem to disrupt family ties although it may modify them. Of course, the family does not cease to exist in an industrial society although its functions are reduced. But the family itself is small in numbers and is more deeply imbedded in a context of extra-familial relationships, i.e., it is assumed that as soon as old enough to be independent, the individual will seek other social ties on his own. Thus the American mental hospital patient, who is likely to lose these "self-made" ties on hospitalization,

8. Sex-linked differences in occupations are also an important factor here. I observed only female wards, where many patients performed domestic duties. Beyond differences related to the degree of job specialization of the society, one would also expect women in general to be able to carry on customary activities better in a mental hospital because their activities are usually less specialized than those of men.

also is likely to have more difficulty in preserving relationships to the family if only because it is assumed that in the family one will have something to "talk about" i.e., activities centered in other social groups, and the patient does not. But this means that visiting hours may be extremely embarrassing and thus their frequency quickly diminishes: in comparison, South-Italian family conversation, like occupation, is less specialized. As a result, there is always something to happen at visiting hour, even if this consists only in the family's stuffing food down the throat of an unwilling patient.[9]

Third, it is well known that impersonal bureaucracy, in which the incumbent of a bureaucratic role is expected to follow the rules regardless of particularized personal ties, is a characteristic of industrial society. Impersonal bureaucracy is conspicuously missing in Southern Italy and even within the context of those formal organizations which do exist, the individual is very likely to by-pass the formal rules in order to do favors for friends or relatives. But this means that although the mental hospital is such a formal organization and by necessity has some rules, its spirit is not that of bureaucracy: rather it seems a giant network of informal ties. The importance of pleading and informal contacts in such a system is well supported by and can explain the continual plea of the patients "I wanna go home". But in many instances the informal spirit of the hospital may in itself be of therapeutic value; it has been shown that strict adherence to the norms of impersonal bureaucracy may have deleterious consequences for psychotic patients.[10]

Finally, the workings of the social class system play a role in determining the atmosphere of any mental hospital. Hollingshead and Redlich have recently shown that in the United

9. In this respect it is worth noting that most of the individual patients I interviewed in a rural hospital were far more "deteriorated" than those in Naples. But this hospital covers a very large district and distance and financial difficulties prevent most families from visiting.

10. Merton J. Kahne, "Bureaucratic Structure and Impersonal Experience in Mental Hospitals," *Psychiatry, 22* (November 1959), 363–375. See also Stanton & Schwartz, *op. cit.*, where it is shown that the patient favored by a nurse, who may put herself in a difficult position by giving special treatment, may often be the patient who gets better.

States a patient's class status is a primary determinant of the treatment received and that those patients who accumulate in the hospital as chronic cases are overwhelmingly from the bottom social groups.[11] Thus it appears that the mental hospital is comparable to the race problem as a blot on the face of American democracy. We do not know whether or not an equivalent social asymmetry would characterize chronic patients in Naples: the economically marginal groups are relatively so much larger than in the United States that it is difficult to make an estimate. However, in the United States, one may wonder if it is pure class prejudice which leads physicians to discriminate in treatment. It may also be that the situation of controlling state mental hospital patients is an extremely difficult one for physicians who assume a democratic ideology; thus they are left with a sense of embarrassment and lack of control which contributes to the intra-hospital anomie. The class system of Southern Italy is far less fluid than that of the United States and differences in education and economic status more extreme. But at least the differences are structured in a common value system (cf. the predominance of ethnic minorities in the American urban working class). In the mental hospital, this means that there are clear-cut channels of staff-patient relationships although they follow a superiority-inferiority axis. In other words, rather than a void, one finds that patients—in particular lower-status ones— tend to be put in the place of protected and guided children; the ethic is frankly paternalistic rather than ambiguously democratic.

The same factors which we have examined from the standpoint of social structure can also be examined from the standpoint of value systems. Max Weber had delineated some of the basic elements of the "Protestant ethic," a value system which in more general terms can be seen as characteristic of most industrial societies. According to Weber, the Protestant ethic is characterized by asceticism and constant rational discipline, i.e., the giving up of present-day pleasures in the interest of rationally conceived-of long-term ends. Some such value

11. A. B. Hollingshead & F. C. Redlich, *Social Class and Mental Illness* (New York: John Wiley & Sons, 1958).

system underlies all societies in which the degree of occupational specialization is such as to make long-term training and rational planning for future activities essential. Perhaps the United States has gone further than any European country in its emphasis on the "job" as the most meaningful focus of life.

However, in this respect Southern Italy provides again a sharp contrast. The lower-class value system is a variant of traditional Catholicism in which there are still magical residues; work is seen as an imposed necessity rather than a positive value. On the lower-status level a partial compensation for economic insecurity is provided by an emphasis on the immediate pleasures of dress, food, humor, gossip, etc. In the terms used by Talcott Parsons, the value system can be characterized as expressive and particularistic; the principal emphasis is placed on the expression of immediate feeling states and on the forming of and acting in social relationships in the immediate rather than on rational planning for long-term ends. Even at the professional level, job performance is a less crucial focus of self-esteem than in the United States.

However, whatever the deleterious consequences of such a value system for the economy, again we can find in it explanations of the lack of anomie in the mental hospital. Since the major value focus is on immediate expression, the transition a patient suffers on entering the mental hospital is not nearly as sharp a one as it is in a society in which the central meaning of life is derived from long-term plans or jobs which by necessity are disrupted by hospitalization. This in itself can account for much of the feeling that life within the hospital is not very different from life outside of it. In both, those at the bottom of the social scale can do very little to change their unfavorable position, but are quite successful in passing the time in conversation, laughter, the active expression of anger and resentment, and indulgence in those minor pleasures that the pocket-book permits. By contrast, an American who has committed his life to the "job" and the ideal of social advancement has far fewer defenses or ways of passing time when fate puts him behind the doors of a mental hospital. An important factor in the social inertia of the American hospital is the guilt and failure complex which the fact of hospitalization in itself entails. The patients in Naples I questioned on this certainly did not like being hospitalized, but it appeared to disrupt their self-esteem much less: in the words of one patient, "what destiny wills happens," but she did not see herself as dead to society.

These considerations can account for the lack of "freezing" in statues of the hospital patients. But if the hypothesis that chronicity in schizophrenics is due to the anomie of the hospital society as seen in industrialized countries, one should also find less chronicity in a hospital such as the one in Naples. In an attempt to check this hypothesis, we examined discharge statistics for schizophrenic patients and compared them with the findings of Wing, Denham and Munro for an English hospital at the time before an active treatment program was instituted. They found that 37 per cent of schizophrenic admissions for the years studied had not been discharged within two years, after which point most remaining patients stay much longer if they are ever discharged living.[12]

At the same hospital, G. W. Brown has found that there is a high correlation between having been visited in the first few months and the fact of eventually being discharged: it was those patients who did not receive visits who made up most of the 37 per cent who were not discharged.[13] But it was our impression that extremely few newly admitted patients failed to receive visits in the Naples hospital. Thus if Brown's hypothesis is valid, far fewer patients should remain two years or longer without discharge.

We tabulated a series of 130 female schizophrenic[14] first admissions to the Naples hospital of all ages in 1952-53 in order to determine their hospital status as of December 31, 1958.

12. Quoted in G. W. Brown, "Social Factors Influencing the Length of Hospital Stay in Schizophrenic Patients," unpublished manuscript.

13. G. W. Brown, *op. cit.*

14. Patients diagnosed as paranoid psychosis, schizophrenia; dissociative syndrome; or puerperal, confusional or acute hallucinatory psychosis if no precipitating agent such as fever or alcohol was noted. In this work, I was aided by Miss Aurora Ben Vignati.

Thirty-one per cent of these patients had remained two years or more without discharge, in comparison with the 37 per cent found in England, including 15 per cent who were still in the hospital as of the end of 1958. Twenty-two per cent were discharged in less than two years and have not returned to the provincial hospital and 5 per cent discharged after two years have not returned. By far the largest group, 40 per cent discharged in less than two years and 7 per cent discharged later, have returned to the hospital any number from one to six times in the period covered. The cases in this group averaged 3 years and 7 months in the hospital in 5-6 years, i.e., more than half-time.[15]

The study revealed that more patients are becoming chronic than we had expected from social structure considerations.[16] In addition the number of patients not returning after a single hospitalization is not exceptionally large, given a common assumption that a fourth to a third of schizophrenic first admissions recover or improve in any case. The most interesting finding was that such a large number of patients go in and out of the hospital; in other words, they become semi-chronics, having two sets of social roles, one within and one outside the hospital. This means that they are not wholly cut off from the

15. The detailed breakdown for 130 patients is as follows:

Discharged in less than two years:	69.2%	
Without readmission		21.5%
With readmissions		40.0
Transferred		4.6
Deceased		3.1
Discharged after more than two years:	15.4%	
Without readmission		4.6%
With readmission		7.0
Transferred		2.3
Deceased		1.5
Continuous hospitalization to December 31, 1958:	15.4%	

16. The continuous hospitalization group is smaller than was found in England. However, the figures are not strictly comparable because for technical reasons we were able to include only first admissions while the English authors took all admissions. If there is a difference, the percentage should be higher for all admissions.

outside world but at the same time are not successful in maintaining a continuous adaptation in it.

There are two directions in which it is possible to look for explanation of these findings, and their failure to wholly accord with our original expectations. First, having emphasized those factors of the hospital social structure which by contrast with some other hospitals seem to work against chronicity, we can turn to those social factors in the Naples hospital which appear to work in favor of it. Second, the figures can be seen as pointing to factors other than the social ones considered as working to keep the patient sick; it would probably be naive to consider schizophrenia as a purely socially determined phenomenon and the similarity in discharge patterns across social lines mitigates against it.

But there do seem to be a number of social factors in the Naples hospital which work in such a direction as to keep patients in the hospital or to return them once they have been discharged. The most important factor is probably the economic one. Actually there are a number of patients in the hospital who are clinically very much improved—and who contribute considerably to setting the tone of ward social life—but who cannot be discharged because there is no place for them to go.

However much family loyalty is emphasized by the value system, it may wear thin when the patient is an extra burden in an already crowded and undernourished household. Thus a patient may be maintained in the hospital even if somewhat improved because at least he is fed there and is out of the way. Thus visits may become a token apology for the failure on the part of the family to take concrete action towards discharge, or patients may be returned when things get hard at home or the family "needs a rest".[17] When patients do not have close relatives willing to take them, it is very difficult to discharge them even with medical encouragement; unemployment is so

17. We found a similar in-and-out pattern to characterize Italo-American patients in the United States and one family periodically brought the schizophrenic sister in during the summer quite frankly explaining that they "needed a rest."

high and the opportunities for living outside a family setting are so limited.

A second factor is the social attitude towards mental illness, which is no less severe than in industralized societies and far more so than among the middle classes in the United States. A mental patient is defined as crazy and his hospitalization becomes part of police records: mental illness is not popularly seen as a disease which can be treated like any other (and even for some serious medical diseases such as tuberculosis there is considerable fear which creates social prejudice rather than sympathy for the victim). Thus having once been hospitalized, a patient encounters many difficulties in getting along outside after discharge. We found that the immediate family tended to deny the fact of illness, at least at first, but this was not true of more distant relatives or neighbors in many cases. Thus a patient's chances of getting married or acquiring a job are sharply limited after the first hospitalization and this may account for many returns. One paranoid patient on readmission told me that all the neighbors said she was crazy and her boy-friend's family wouldn't accept her for the same reason where-upon a listening nurse commented: "She's not hallucinated; that's true for most patients who come back."

Two other closely related factors are the denial of mental illness built into patient society and the social distance between patients and physicians. We noted above that the patient's repetitive "I wanna go home" seemed to have a ritual quality: by repeating and mutually confirming the desire to go home, the patients deny the fact that they ever have been ill and so lift from themselves the burden of social censure. However, this denial results in a weakness of any commitment to the hospital as such or lack of co-operation in the treatment program; the patients do not want to feel associated with the hospital because such an association would mean that they must perceive themselves as crazy. It also results in a fragmenta-tion of patient society since most patients who are unwilling to admit that they themselves are crazy are less so to say that their neighbor is, and it leads patients to pressure their families to pressure the physician for premature discharge, putting him in a difficult position. This feature is not specific to Southern Italy but common to all environments where the mental patient is seen as a social outcast.[18]

Although it is structured in terms of a paternalistic ethic which lessens the communication barriers in some respects, the social distance between physicians and most of the patients can also be seen as a barrier to the achievement of patient commitment to treatment programs. In respect to education and some crucial values, the distance between physicians and lower-status patients is far greater than it is in the industralized countries, simply because physicians as educated professionals share the knowledge and scientific values of the rest of the western world (in fact several Italian psychiatrists have been innovators in organic treatment) while numerous patients are illiterate or semi-literate. This means that medical explanations of disease may not penetrate to either patients or families and they themselves may have quite different concepts of what needs to be treated and how. The physician may find that his advice is being neglected in favor of that of the *fattucchiere* (magical practitioner) and one patient encountered was strongly resistive to taking drugs because she felt her disease was one to be cured by a visit to the shrine of a saint, not by medicine.[19] It also means that sometimes physicians have to fight heroic battles of persuasion to convince the family when hospitalization is necessary on the ground of public danger. In addition, the factor of education makes for considerable social distance between physicians and

18. At a second hospital visited in Naples we found some changes in this patient attitude; they accepted hospitalization to the extent of conceiving transfer to an open ward as an earned privilege and some modified the "I wanna go home" to "I wanna go upstairs (to the open ward)." This change was associated with an active attempt on the part of the staff to change social attitudes concerning mental illness and made possible by the psychiatric unit's being part of a general hospital; thus it was not perceived as the "nut house."

19. Actually we found more favorable attitudes to modern medicine on the part of uneducated patients than we expected and this is a rapidly changing variable, particularly in the urban area.

nurses who thus do not have an active role in treatment, although there is a sufficient number of them.

And finally a factor which may have importance for the high rate of returns is the "forgetting" ideology of treatment as described above. We noted that the intra-patient society is present-oriented in that patient interaction consists in expressions and social exchanges relative to immediate feeling states. In addition it supports a collective denial of the fact of mental illness. Thus the patient society cannot reinforce the commitment of patients to the treatment program nor can it serve as a testing ground in which patients discuss and consolidate understanding which they gain concerning their past social difficulties, working out new adaptation patterns which may prove more effective. Rather the patient's own predispositions and those of their families coincide with factors built into the hospital value system to encourage a denial that anything has ever been wrong.[20] This we think may account for a number of quick recoveries; in a sense it was impressive to see how many patients who came in after severe anxious or aggressive episodes very quickly perked up and became socialized in the first few weeks of treatment. At the same time, this improvement must be seen as based on repression rather than integration of conflict: it entailed a simple putting out of the mind, whether because of social encouragement or the effects of the organic treatments extensively used. Unfortunately, it seems to be the case that what is put out of the mind comes back; thus when patients return to the original conflict-producing situations, there seems to be a high probability that symptoms will return.

To sum up, we think that it is clearly established that there are variations in the symptoms and personality characteristics of mental-hospital patients which are best understood in terms of specific factors of the social milieu. Such differences can be seen even within common diagnostic groups within which it is evident that there are also common symptoms, as for example the delusions and hallucinations characteristic of schizophrenia

20. This trend was usually countered by physicians, but often actively encouraged by nurses.

which appeared in both of the hospitals studied. That there are such social variations is not a new finding to most psychiatrists; they were noticed at least a century ago. However, only in the light of the recent movement of "milieu therapy" has the study of these variations been seen as having crucial importance for etiological research and the setting up of treatment programs. Between the "typical" old-style English or American hospital and the Naples provincial hospital we believe there is one crucial difference which has special implications for treatment programs whose goal is to modify the symptoms of schizophrenia by social means: namely that in the latter case there is far less inertia and disorganization of the normal channels of social communication than in the former. This can be explained in terms of certain general features of the relevant societies such as type of role differentiation and value system.

However, although it seems to produce fewer and less extreme forms of disorganization of the personality culminating in the bizarre, the non-industrial society of Naples nevertheless produces schizophrenia of sufficient severity as to necessitate long-term hospitalization for some patients. This means that the etiological explanations of schizophrenia advanced by several sociological or anthropological writers in the 1930's, according to which schizophrenia was seen as "caused by" industrialized and highly differentiated societies, cannot provide the whole story. Rather social factors must be seen as one among several which produce and channel the course of schizophrenia. When one examines the breakdown of a schizophrenic patient in detail, one generally finds some adverse social conditions; likewise, when one seeks to explain why one patient remains years in the hospital and another is quickly discharged. To know why one patient broke down when similar social difficulties might have left another person unscarred, it is necessary to turn to the consideration of the earliest bases of personality structure as laid down in the child. And in turn, to know why unfavorable conditions of early development have left personality weakness in one person while another has successfully compensated them, it may be necessary to turn to the neurological or biochemical substrata of personality.

part three

Cultural Themes in Expressive Symbolism

In the following chapters Anne Parsons addresses herself to problems of cultural and individual symbolism. Chapter 7 provides a theoretical analysis of the differences between magic and delusions: belief in magic ties the actors to a set of cultural prescriptions and to a collective conscience; by contrast, in paranoid delusions communication with the collectivity has broken down. Delusions differ from magic beliefs in that they do not follow the culturally prescribed principles of causality or goal-oriented action.

Yet, though elaborated through withdrawal from reality into a private world, delusions draw, for their formation, upon the resources of the culture. In Chapter 8 Anne Parsons shows that individual delusions draw their content from social structural arrangements. In a society where particularistic relationships are stressed, the maleficent delusional agents are personal ones, that is, concrete individuals who actually exist within the individual's life space. By contrast, in societies where universalistic norms pervade almost all but the private spheres of life, the deluded individual converts his interpersonal relations into an abstract delusional system of impersonal maleficent forces.

Chapter 9 examines, through a case study, the expressive mechanisms. The author concludes that expressiveness of affect cannot be simply explained in traditional psychoanalytic terms as the breakthrough of id impulses; in some cultures it is, on the contrary, a mechanism adaptive to social and cultural reality.

chapter 7

Expressive Symbolism in Witchcraft and Delusion

A Comparative Study*

Witchcraft beliefs and delusions of persecution are two extreme examples of types of symbolism which must be understood in function of their value as representations of internal psychic reactions rather than as empirically valid representations of the external world. Both express subjective motivation: they have in common the fact that they do so by means of a belief about the motives of a real or imaginary external

* This paper is based on research conducted under a grant given by the United States Public Health Service, Institutes of Mental Health, Bethesda, Md., to whom we are greatly indebted. We wish also to acknowledge Dr. Grete L. Bibring, Beth Israel Hospital, Boston, as sponsor of the project, and Dr. Harry C. Solomon, Superintendent of the Boston Psychopathic Hospital, for permission to publish data from the hospital files.

Reprinted by permission of the Société Internationale d'Ethnopsychologie Normale et Pathologique, from *Revue Internationale d'Ethnopsychologie Normale et Pathologique,* Vol. 1, No. 2, 99–119.

agent. Prior to the theoretical advances in understanding of non-rational symbolic processes which have taken place in the last half-century both in psychiatry, as represented by psychoanalytic theory, and in cultural anthropology, they were identified as "irrational" beliefs. But in spite of these advances, the tendency to assimilate the two forms has not disappeared. Within psychoanalytic theory the formation of delusions has been explained as a process of projection in which a threatening affect which has been denied by the conscious ego returns in the form of an external perception (11); by this means psychic equilibrium is re-established. Psychologically oriented anthropology has also had recourse to the concept of projection; consequently witchcraft beliefs have been considered as a mechanism which restores psychic equilibrium in the face of overwhelming anxieties or hostilities. Little detailed comparison has been made, but, since both distort empirical reality in function of motivation, a basic similarity has frequently been affirmed. Whether from the standpoint of the assumption implicit to psychoanalysis that all of the "primitive" symbolic processes in which motivation is primary have something in common, or whether from the standpoint of the conviction of a number of anthropologists that the symbolism of non-literate societies is subject to interpretation on the basis of psychological principles common to our own society, it is the movement towards assimilation rather than a search for distinctive features which has been most prominent in recent decades.

But, as Lévi-Strauss has stated (5), although there may be resemblances between the symbolic processes of the primitive, the abnormal (and the child), one should not lose sight of the fact that there are both children and abnormals in non-literate societies. In other words, we do not know whether or not these processes are equivalent, or if they are, in what specific respects, prior to a comparative analysis in which the variables are chosen from among all of the possible combinations provided by these three dimensions. The aim of this review is to further exchange between anthropologists and psychiatrists: our own interest lies in the area of symbolic content, and empirically, in that of the cross-cultural study of schizophrenia. Most important, we feel that comparative studies are lacking and badly needed at the present time. Consequently, we have decided to present a case history, chosen for the reason that the same manifest symbol can be viewed from either the psychoanalytic or the anthropological standpoint. The patient is a 37-year-old woman of Italian peasant origin hospitalized in the United States with a diagnosis of paranoid schizophrenia. Her symptoms include auditory hallucinations and withdrawal and passivity alternating with aggressive and self-destructive behavior, but of greatest interest to us is a delusion in which she sees herself as the victim of a spell effected by means of the evil eye, an idea which in itself is frequently found in Italian peasants even long after emigration to the United States. Focusing on a single symbolic construction which can be considered as either a delusion or a cultural belief, we hope by a sort of comparative analysis to be able to isolate some ways in which we think that the pathological specificity of the delusion is more striking than its resemblance to the same symbol as it might appear in a normal context.

More specifically, we have selected three more or less independent foci for organization of the case material. First, since it might be said that, given the correspondence in content with symbolism normal for the culture, it is impossible to characterize the case as pathological by the diagnostic criteria applicable to our own society, it is necessary to justify our initial assumption that the symbol is in fact delusional. However, on a rough empirical level the distinction appears to be less difficult to make than the assumptions of many anthropologists who have worked in the field of mental health would indicate. In this case, it requires nothing more than a conscious cross-cultural application of classical descriptive psychiatry; by stating the diagnostic indices used, the correspondence of the patient's behavior with that of other patients placed in the same category can be demonstrated. Reciprocally, we will also sum up the indices by which the patient's behavior differs from that of a normal person in her own milieu, thus justifying the appellation "pathological" in the latter as well as for the psychiatrist.

However, this first distinction is purely empirical and has to be made on the basis of the total behavior of the patient; it does not in itself provide any clues to a theoretical distinction between the psychic mechanisms involved in the formation of the respective beliefs. For this latter problem, we will have to restrict analysis to the symbol alone, comparing its structuring for the patient with that which would be found in a non-pathological believer in witchcraft. Here we have selected two foci of organization, namely the problem of relationships between symbol and the situation to which it refers, and, since both witchcraft beliefs and paranoid delusions (in some cases) involve personalized persecuting agents, the problem of agent choice.

The patient, Angelina Perella,[1] arrived in Boston, Massachusetts, with her husband and two of their eventual family of nine in 1921, toward the end of a wave of Italian immigration whose magnitude can be judged from the fact that in 1950 one out of every fifteen residents of the United States was born in Italy. The Perella family settled in a predominantly middle-class suburb, where Mr. Perella became a garage worker. Thus superficially, they were considerably closer to assimilation with American culture than the large majority of first-generation Italian-Americans among whom—or at least among the women— the phrase "going to America" was used to denote a trip from the Italian quarter to the central shopping district. Nevertheless, like most Italian women, Mrs. Perella showed little proficiency in English at the time of her hospitalization fourteen years after immigration, and was able to name three large cities in Italy but only one in the United States on the psychiatric examination.

She was born on June 19, 1898, in Piave, Province of Venice, as the second female child of nine live births. Her parents, both of whom were still living in Italy in 1935, were tenant farmers of marginal economic status. Angelina worked in a factory from the age of 14 to about 17, but did not work subsequently when the entire family was transported to Avellino, near Naples, where they lived for three years in a state barracks

1. Angelina Perella is a pseudonym.

during the First World War. Avellino has sent many immigrants to the Boston area: it was here that Angelina met the man whom she married after a two-year courtship and with whom she emigrated at the age of 23.

We know nothing beyond the bare facts of Mrs. Perella's early life, since our knowledge of the case comes solely from hospital records. However, the husband's anamnesis was unusually complete, for he, to the contrary of his wife, spoke English fluently, and, moreover, was willing to reveal many intimate details, among which we find the fact that, to his knowledge, his wife had never evidenced any pleasure in sexual relationships, giving as a reason (although she gave birth to nine children) her fear of pregnancy. In addition, he felt that she tended to take her responsibilities as a mother too seriously, that otherwise she was a sociable personality, less inclined to worry than he, "practical rather than imaginative," but that over the years she withdrew more and more from social relationships, explicitly in order to care for the children. She was a nominal Catholic, but during the years prior to admission attended Mass rarely, since she felt it impossible to take all of the children. He considered her "unusually superstitious."

About June 1934, at which time the patient was pregnant for the ninth time, she became even more "superstitious." Between June and the September delivery, Mr. Perella spent a considerable sum of money in gratifying her whims, including the purchase of a live pig which he killed so that she could drink its blood. Six days after being delivered in a general hospital, the patient was visited by three neighbor women, including a Mrs. J. Later the same evening, she complained to her husband that Mrs. J. had bewitched her and that she had come under the influence of the evil eye. It is at this point that we can place the beginning of an acute psychosis. She began to complain of being hot and cold alternately and of feeling generally sick; her breast milk and her lochia dried up. No medical basis for these complaints was discovered, and 12 days *post partum* Mrs. Perella was returned to her home, diagnosed as homesick by the hospital staff.

On return, she found four of her children ill and was further convinced that malign influences were at work, that both she and the family were in danger, and that had she not returned from the hospital all of the children would have died. This and subsequent happenings over the next nine months were attributed to the spell cast by Mrs. J. who, according to the patient, was extremely jealous because of the many friends who paid visits and brought presents on the birth of her various children. When Mrs. J. paid a few calls, the patient did not directly accuse her of witchcraft; however, she was extremely disagreeable.

One month after delivery, the patient went to a fortune teller to have the spell lifted. Subsequently, her condition seems to have improved, until December when she developed a marked swelling and pain in her left arm which a little later gave place to the same affliction of the right member. This too was evidence of the evil eye cast by Mrs. J. During one visit to the fortune teller, Mrs. Perella was asked if Mrs. J. had taken anything from the house. Mr. Perella related on request that Mrs. J. had taken and not yet returned two dresses belonging to one of the little girls. This was evidence that they had been used to work a charm on the little girl because she had become thin and did not seem to be in as good health as formerly. At the same time the patient began to talk about a dream that she had in the hospital following delivery in which the devil appeared, showed her a large knife, and told her that it was with this she would have to kill the child.

She was then informed by the fortune teller that there must be something blue in the house which caused her troubles. After considerable fretting and searching, she discovered an old American flag in the bottom of a trunk; she then rinsed the blue portion in cold water according to directions to obtain relief. Over this period she was extremely depressed, often telling her husband that somebody would eventually kill him because he did not believe she had been bewitched. Between January and May 18, she improved somewhat while following the fortune teller's prescriptions. The latter date is that of her last visit to the fortune teller who informed her that she would soon find a tin can filled with money which they were to share. Mrs. Perella then began to act very mysteriously towards her husband, telling him that there was a great deal of money in the house. The morning of May 19, she got up at five o'clock and spent the entire day prowling about the house, opening cans, and insisting when she found no money that someone else had taken it. She became afraid that people had found out about the treasure, and, believing she had already found it, were going to kidnap her children and hold them for ransom. She kept the windows and doors locked, stated that the watch-dog had been won over by thieves so that he would not bark, and showed an ever-increasing restlessness. Her husband called a doctor who saw the patient several times over the next ten days and finally advised commitment to a mental hospital. Over this period she slept little and ate almost nothing. On May 30, Mrs. Perella was admitted to the Boston Psychopathic Hospital.

Most of the psychiatric observation we have covers the week of May 30 to June 7. As to her condition at that time, we may abstract from the hospital records:

On admission, the patient was overactive, overtalkative, and very resistive—requiring to be kept in seclusion for several days. She slept poorly but attended to her vegetative functions without prompting. . . . She exhibited no stereotypies or ritualisms . . . (several days later) has quieted considerably and is a great deal more co-operative. Objectively, the patient seems to be bewildered and distressed . . . cries readily, is very suspicious of anything done for her in the hospital—physical and mental examinations, medications, etc. and constantly anticipates injury of some kind.

The psychiatrist qualified his mental status examination and felt himself unable to make more than a provisional estimate of the degree of cognitive disturbance due to the patient's difficulties with the English language. However, we can cite the following material as to thought content:

. . . it is quite clear that there has been inexplicable and sinister activity going on about her for some time. "People" call her crazy and say that many of the things in her house have been stolen (cf. information from husband), although actually they are prizes salvaged from the city dump by her children. Automobiles go round and round her house in the evening with their lights turned off apparently to prevent her from catching a glimpse of the occupant. Suspicious characters have been loitering around her grounds and flashing lights through the windows at night. "People" have been entering her house the past two or three weeks and turning everything upside down, disarranging her clothes, hiding one of a pair of shoes or a single stocking, so that she has great trouble in mating her wearing apparel. They have even gone so far as to heat her bed in some way, possibly by placing a fire under it so that she was unable to sleep and had to stay up most of the night. She at first denied ever having talked of the evil eye, but later stated that visitors at her home had repeatedly remarked that she had the evil eye . . . She at first denied searching for money about her house, saying that all her acquaintances did this but not she. Later she admitted that she looked for a cache but only in one room, while "other people" had ransacked her entire house. . . . During the course of the interview, she repeatedly twisted her hair into a knot at the back of her head, but had no hairpins with which to hold it in place. After a few moments of animated conversation, the chignon was loosened and the patient never tired of calling the examiner's attention to this as evidence that something was amiss.

Note vagueness of style and the use of the paranoid mechanism of denial and return in the form of a positive statement (to be discussed below) on occasions when the patient is confronted with her past behavior; she denies having talked of the evil eye, then states that "visitors in her house" accused her of having it. Likewise, she denies having searched for money, later states that she did in a particular instance, and that "other people" had done so. Note also the image of fire under the bed as a probable non-technological equivalent for the electricity image frequently found in paranoids.

The examining psychiatrist was not certain as to the presence of auditory hallucinations; however, on one occasion the patient stated that she was unable to answer a question because "head no feel a good, talk a talk a talk." This is a phrase frequently used by Italian patients to describe auditory hallucinations. In sum, although there may be some inaccuracies of detail due to the language barrier, the mental status information generally checks with that given by the husband and clearly substantiates the diagnosis of paranoid schizophrenia.

On June 7, the patient was withdrawn from the hospital by her husband against medical advice, as frequently happens in the case of first-generation Italian patients for whom the value of family solidarity outweighs the commitment to specialized professional care. On June 12, she was readmitted in the following circumstances as described by Mr. Perella. She was considerably improved after the hospital stay, but a neighbor woman was called in during the day as a precautionary measure. On this date, the neighbor did not arrive on time and the patient was left alone with her three youngest children. As the patient later recounted to her husband, someone came to the door to ask the time, and as the kitchen clock was not working, she went upstairs to look for a timepiece. Once upstairs, she forgot the errand and (probably commanded by hallucinatory voices) took off all her clothes, rubbed her body with bathing alcohol and ignited it. She was next seen by the landlord, walking down the stairs in flames with a child under each arm. On June 22, she died in the hospital of severe burns.

The circumstances of her death are sufficient to place the patient outside the norms of her own culture. From the psychiatric standpoint, the following signs which determined the diagnosis can be briefly summarized; a) after the birth of her ninth child (with some forewarnings during pregnancy) the patient went through a distinct *personality change* in function of which: b) her behavior and ability to perform her normal role began to *disintegrate,* terminating in a state of *acute confusion* (from May 18 on); c) in the confused phase, rapid and apparently inconsistent *alternation of affects* (from co-operation to extreme suspicion, from passive withdrawal to overt aggression) were observed (as far as can be determined, the patient did not possess a consistently aggressive or suspicious personality before the change); d) it is highly probable that *auditory hallucinations* were present; e) in the confused state, the patient describes herself as the victim of a series of mysterious and indeterminate events in the *vague style* characteristic of paranoids; f) after a period of improvement, the confusion returned suddenly and terminated in a *self-destructive act,* committed without determinable motive. All of these symptoms could be found in any psychiatric text as characteristic of paranoid schizophrenics.

From a biographical standpoint, three phases can be roughly delineated in the patient's married life (for lack of information, we exclude early life). The first extends up to the ninth pregnancy; it is characterized by a number of symptons which can be called neurotic, i.e., frigidity and compulsiveness as indicated both by overconscientiousness in care of the children and by her "unusually superstitious" nature.[2] But no gross pathology is observable in this period, and, although the presence of severe anxiety is indicated, the patient was able to function in her social role. By sharpest contrast, in the third period which follows failure of the magical attempts at self-cure, complete ego breakdown occurs; the patient is no longer able to function in her role and eventually destroys herself. Moreover, this period is characterized by total breakdown in symbolic functioning. To others, the patient is able to communicate only the impression of confusion—of vague mysterious events whose referents are undiscoverable to the non-specialist. That the cognitive structure of normal effective communication, as indicated by the use of language, was disrupted is probable.

However, the second and intermediate period which extends from the announcement that she has come under the influence of the evil eye until the breakdown of attempts at cure structured via this same symbol is more difficult to characterize; it is this period which will be the focus of our intensive analysis.

2. Of course since the source we possess is secondary, such a value-loaded assertion has to be qualified. It may be that the patient actually was "more superstitious" than other Italian peasant women of the first generation, and consequently the presence of neurotic anxiety can be assumed. It may also be that she is simply "more superstitious" than her husband, who is a non-believer, would wish.

After the fact, it is easy to spot indices of pathology during this period and presumably a skilled psychiatrist would have been able to spot them had he seen the patient at that time. But at first glance, it appears that the anthropological observer or the believer in the evil eye might not have found the means of distinguishing the belief from the normal for the very reason that the patient defines her situation in culturally formulated terms. Given her definition of the situation, she acts appropriately in seeking the fortune teller's aid in lifting the spell. Moreover, up to a point these means of cure are effective. It is only when they themselves are put in doubt, i.e., when the patient constructs further paranoid agents who stole the money that she was to give to the fortune teller, that pathological thinking extends beyond all bounds.[3] But given the *post-facto* evidences of pathology, at least an attempt to isolate the pathological specificity of the thinking of this second period is legitimate; it is to this task that we can now turn.

To restate the question briefly, given that the symbols of this period correspond in content to the general cultural pattern, in what ways can they be distinguished both from the standpoint of their structuring in this case and from the theoretical point of view? In this formulation we will refer to Freud's Schreber case (2) and to other articles in psychoanalysis and anthropology on the formation of the two types of belief. Throughout the discussion, we will make extensive reference to the works of Kluckhohn (4) and Evans-Pritchard (1) on witchcraft in Navaho and Zande societies respectively, while on delusion formation we will refer to Freud's Schreber case (2)

---

3. At this point, the case resembles one which has been collected by Benjamin and Lois Paul (unpublished field notes) in an Indian village in Guatemala. The patient maintained that an illness which had been intended for another person by witchcraft had been mistakenly given to her. Her *denial* of her own situation as culturally defined (others saw her illness as the direct result of witchcraft) is exactly equivalent to that found in the Western paranoid who feels he has been "railroaded" into the mental hospital by mistake since he is "really" not ill. Moreover, the Pauls' case felt that her persecutors were accusing her of having too much money; in the culture involved, possession of too much makes one susceptible to witchcraft.

and to articles by Waelder (11) and Tausk (10). In addition it will be necessary to intersperse some empirical material on normal witchcraft beliefs in Italian society. Our foci of discussion are the following: first, what is the relationship between symbol and situation in each case; and second, how is the persecuting agent chosen?

Both Kluckhohn and Evans-Pritchard emphasize the function of witchcraft beliefs as an explanation of and as a means of channelling anxiety which results from random misfortunes which could not have been prevented by ordinary means of empirical or normative control. That the actually observed distribution of witchcraft beliefs according to evoking situation follows the pattern that would be expected from this assumption is clear in the data that they present: death and illness are by far the most prominent foci, while certain other categories of events seem outside the range of witchcraft. Among the latter, Evans-Pritchard presents the examples of the adulterer and the incompetent apprentice carpenter who breaks the wood; the actions of both are considered within the realm of human control, whether technological or moral, while death and illness are not. Rather it is the witchcraft belief itself which provides the means of control whether in the form of preventive measures —amulets, incantations, etc.—or of *post-facto* rituals of exorcism or acts of vengeance against real agents supposed to be witches.

Not only does the distribution of witchcraft beliefs follow a predictable pattern, but also the anxiety sources behind them can be discovered rather easily by the observer. When the Zande takes an anthropologist to visit a sick relative, the latter will agree as to the description of the symptoms and will understand the Zande's concern, although he will differ on explanation or prescription and although his greater understanding of illness may make the event seem less mysterious. Thus *although the witch herself is a non-empirical symbol, the situation in which she is evoked can be empirically located*. From this standpoint, witchcraft beliefs appear as elaborations which depart from commonly defined situations and whose result is *cognitive-*

ly to explain the situation by construction of a causal agent and by relating a number of discrete situations under a general category, and *expressively*, to alleviate the anxiety, concomitant to the situation in channelling it through a set of expectations and in furnishing the means for symbolic counter-action. Secondly, there is a *reversible relationship between symbol and situation* in that the possessor of the symbol can himself return to the situation to which it refers, i.e. explain it to an outsider.

But for the observer, the location of the source of anxiety behind paranoid symbols has proved much more difficult, and although considerable effort has been devoted to the problem, there is still some disagreement as to the interpretation of delusional symbols. The most striking characteristics of paranoid thinking are its vagueness and looseness of structure. If a Zande happened to say that his family was under a spell, one might ask him what he meant and receive the reply that his brother had just died suddenly; this event could only have been caused by witches. But the paranoid's situational referent would never be so clear; his circumlocutions might include some situational justification (as a secondary process) of the belief that he was being persecuted, but unless a "translation" from paranoid language can be obtained, one is never sure of the referent. Theoretically, this fact can be formulated in two ways: first, paranoid thinking is *irreversible*, i.e., one cannot ask a paranoid what he meant; and two, paranoid symbolism lacks the dual character (*à deux faces*) of normal expressive symbolism which in fact is always partially cognitive, i.e., refers simultaneously to an objective situation (cognitive referent) and to its effect on the subject (expressive referent).[4]

Given this lack of cognitive referents, only two possibilities are open in the interpretation of the delusional symbols: one can say that they refer to an abnormal subjective experience which is outside of the limits structured by normal communicative devices, or one can say that they express "unconscious"

4. See Parsons, Shils, *et. al.* (9) for the theoretical distinction between cognitive and expressive assumed here.

motivations and attempt to interpret them by genetic reconstruction as has been done by psychoanalysis.

Thus in summary fashion two provisional oppositions between witchcraft and paranoid symbolism can be stated: a) witchcraft symbolism refers to socially defined (and/or conscious) situations, while paranoid symbolism relates to purely subjective situations (or unconscious factors); and b) the relationship between symbol and situation is reversible and structured in the case of witchcraft beliefs and irreversible and unstructured in the case of paranoid delusions. Since the relationship is structured for witchcraft beliefs, it follows that there are "appropriate" situations in which they can be evoked; this point will serve as a basis for further discussion.

But some anthropologists may consider the assumption that witchcraft beliefs relate only to conscious anxieties as somewhat arbitrary; Kluckhohn in particular has emphasized their function as a means of expression for unconscious hostility. Nadel (8) and Evans-Pritchard as well as Kluckhohn have demonstrated that there is a cross-cultural variation in the pattern of choice for those considered as witches and that the actual choices in a particular society can be explained in terms of the tensions inherent to the social structure. Witchcraft beliefs from this standpoint can be seen as expressing these tensions in a displaced form; in this sense one might speak of an unconscious determinant. However, this problem is more relevant to our second problem, that of agent choice, than to the first and can be left aside for the moment.

Actually if one attempts to evaluate the role of the unconscious in witchcraft beliefs from the standpoint of evoking situations, several questions to which presently available research does not furnish answers are raised: e.g., to what extent does the believer himself independently perceive a specific anxiety source relative to a given evocation of witches; second, can an anxiety source external to the subject (whether social or natural) always be located by the observer; third, what is the relationship between primary witchcraft belief as related to external situations and secondary anxiety due to fear of the witches themselves or anticipated consequences of witchcraft? In order to answer them, an isolation of levels of meaning would be necessary since the witchcraft symbol is presumably over-determined. For example, the Italian mother who fears when her child is praised too highly by a stranger that the evil eye may make him ill may on one level be channelling a conscious fear of illness and on another, expressing unconscious resent-ment of the praise; thus even if an external referent is present in all cases, the presence of additional unconscious elements is not excluded. However, for several reasons it seems best to leave aside this problem for the present paper, even at the risk of the accusation that we are eliminating the essential. Al-though other relationships are by no means excluded, the avail-able data indicate a primary relationship between witchcraft beliefs and specific external anxiety-provoking events; it is this relationship that has been most clearly formulated in anthro-pological theory. It is also in this respect that the contrast with paranoid symbolism is most obvious; it thus serves as the best starting point in clarification of the differences. Secondly, start-ing from a theory of motivation in the cross-cultural interpre-tation of symbols always creates a certain risk that a culture-bound view will be imposed upon the data; starting from situa-tions may eliminate some of this risk.

When we first examine the situation in which Mrs. Perella sees herself as the victim of the charm cast by Mrs. J., as she herself defines it, it is the similarities to culturally-structured belief which are most apparent. An informant in Boston's Italian quarter has described the symptoms of the evil eye in much the same terms which, according to the description we possess, Mrs. Perella used: she felt generally sick, and alternately hot and cold, and had difficulties in nursing. Secondly, she attributed the children's illnesses to the charm; children are considered the most frequent victims of the evil eye in Italian culture. But we would nevertheless hesitate before overestimating the coinci-dence: although, since the data are limited, it is necessary to use a certain amount of hypothetical reconstruction based on the assumption that the patient's thinking resembles that of other schizophrenics, some lines of distinction can be proposed which could be tested on other cases. First, it appears as if Mrs. Perella *first* complained that she was being bewitched and *then* began to complain of the physical symptoms usually attributed to the evil eye; moreover, no intermediate signs which indicate to her that she is in fact under a spell are evident. There is an apparent discrepancy in timing which means that the concept of witchcraft symbolism as an explanatory framework applicable to a specific category of events has to be discarded at the outset, for *an explanation must follow and be appropriate to the event which it explains.* Actually in most witchcraft cases, rites of divination are performed to find out *whether or not* witchcraft is involved and if so, who is responsible. Thus witchcraft is conceived of as a possible explanation and one which may be appropriate depending on an agreed-upon definition of the situation, while Mrs. Perella herself defines the situation before the application of any conventional means of interpretation.

In fact, of course, the sequence of events of a psychotic breakdown is not so simple, and a secondary report is bound to be highly selective in the direction of normal experience. From the literature on paranoid symbol formation (2, 10, 11), we can suppose that Mrs. J's visit to the hospital provoked an impulse on the part of Mrs. Perella which was then rejected from consciousness. Subsequently, she must have felt a sense of estrangement and a series of bizarre subjective symptoms inexplicable on the basis of existing expectations (i.e., not corresponding to the normal *post-partum* condition with which Mrs. Perella as the mother of nine would presumably have been familiar). The formation of the belief *both* explains and to the patient "is" the disease since she does not believe that she is ill independently of the charm.

But there is a common sense in which a belief can be maintained against opposition which has to be discarded in this case. Given the cultural difference, it is likely that Mrs. Perella might not understand the psychiatrist's definition of the situation as one of emotional conflict, or if she did, consider her own, that she was a victim of a charm, as superior in the light of her own cultural identification. However, it is the factor of timing which makes it possible to discard this interpretation; but we have first to state more clearly the psychoanalytic theory of the mechanism of projection in psychosis. According to Freud and Waelder (2, 11) a delusion of persecution (when an agent is involved) is the return, in the form of the belief that the agent is a persecutor, of feelings formerly attached to the latter. Thus Freud states that the proposition "I (a man) love x (a man)," one which is unacceptable to the ego, may be denied by reversal of subject-object relations and by *a transformation of affect into belief,* to give "x hates me." According to this formulation, it would appear that Mrs. Perella's belief about the charm is actually a *transformation of* an impulse felt towards Mrs. J. rather than a *belief about* the situation of illness. To the observer, this is seen in that the belief was formed at the moment when Mrs. J. paid her visit to the hospital and before the patient discusses her physical symptoms. These latter would have to be explained as further manifestations of the psychosis, either in the form of a description of actual sensations or in the form of a rationalization (secondary elaboration of the delusion) for the belief that she was being bewitched.

Thus although the communicable content of the symbol which the patient adopted does correspond to the normal precisely because she took over a common cultural representation (rather than a bizarre invention such as the influencing machine described by Victor Tausk), its subjective content differs and is incommunicable except to those familiar with schizophrenic symptomatology. It is in this sense that Mrs. Perella's belief is culturally inappropriate. She does not interpret the situation as would normally be done; for example, by pouring oil upon water to determine from its spreading or failure to spread whether or not the evil eye is involved. Rather, she assumes immediately, and with a type of absolute conviction characteristic of paranoids, that it is.[5] In fact, the symbol refers to a different situation

5. Paranoids may call upon conventional means of verification for their assertions, but only as part of a process of secondary elaboration which rests on a prior conviction. In this paper, we refer only to the

from the normal, and, as seen by the lack of the intermediate signs by which a social definition of the situation would be reached, the relationship between symbol and situation is unstructured (or better, structured by means of principles other than those of cultural belief systems whose laws must be sought in personality theory). Had she used such interpretative signs, she would have been able to communicate her belief to others, assuming they were of the same culture, who would have accepted (or rejected for predictable reasons) her definition of the situation. As it is, although these others recognized the words, they did not understand their meaning and called her "crazy." [6]

But it is precisely this communicability which characterizes cultural belief systems. A cultural belief system from one standpoint is a set of general categories, with fixed cognitive referents, possessed by all of the members of the community; specific and individual experiences can be referred to them and thus, via the return route from the general and communicable to the specific and individual, similar experiences are evoked on the part of others and "understanding" is reached. But in order that the categories remain stable—and consequently common to the community—specific steps by which one proceeds from a particular situation to the category are necessary.[7] Experiences

initial delusion formation which accompanies an acute state, not to such systematizations more characteristic of chronic cases. Mrs. Perella's discovery that Mrs. J. had taken her child's dress as a means of effecting the charm falls in the latter category and as such both indicates a degree of systematization and is more closely integrated with cultural symbolism.

6. Of course the data from the second period do indicate that the content correspondence with cultural symbolism enabled the patient to "fool" others for a time and even to act effectively. But the husband's report indicates that he felt that "something was not quite right" although part of her behavior was understood. As a non-believer, he would have rejected the witchcraft explanation in any case, but had its utilization been normal, as a bi-cultural individual he would have understood it through his knowledge of the situations in which witchcraft beliefs are evoked.

7. Of course these criteria need not all be explicit. Although to the anthropologist, the events which a Zande explains as due to witchcraft may belong to the category "anxiety due to unpredictable causes," the Zande does not see it that way. Rather he will relate them on the basis of a particular feeling tone: the symbolized relation exists only in the witchcraft imagery.

can be referred to them and thus, via the return route, from the general and communicable to the specific and individual. Thus in the case of witchcraft, it is necessary that a set of criteria by which a particular event can be attributed to witchcraft be utilized; if this were not so, any event whatsoever could be so explained and the distinguishing capacity would vanish. A nonpathological deviant might change the meaning of the categories, but in most circumstances (where culture change is not involved), social correction mechanisms would operate against him: e.g., a Zande might for personal reasons say that witches had induced him to commit adultery, but he would be laughed at because everybody knows "witches don't do that." Such correction mechanisms are notably inefficacious in the case of delusions. In fact to say that such categories are both culturally and situationally appropriate is to state the same relationship in two ways, since cultural categories themselves carry with them some means of determining the range of situations to which they belong.[8] As such they contain a cognitive element by necessity and cannot be considered as pure expressive symbols as those of a schizophrenic might.

Another way of defining the lack of situational appropriateness of schizophrenic belief would be in terms of the "spread of meaning" by which psychiatrists have long characterized it. This can be seen in the case of Mrs. Perella when she attributes a series of apparently unrelated events to the charm cast by Mrs. J. without using independent criteria of relevance; it is as if the charm gave meaning to her entire life. The fact that she considers a single agent responsible for a series of events does not in itself place her beyond the limits of cultural symbolism: in all societies in which the witch exists as a stable social object, and in the case of certain stereotypes in our own society which have been explained in terms similar to witchcraft, the agent once defined as responsible may be evoked again with little reality

8. In slightly different terms, cultural categories are reversible, i.e., if they are not understood, the speaker can either return to the situation to which they refer or substitute equivalent terms for those which did not communicate. A schizophrenic cannot substitute other terms at will; his delusion is both fixed and irreversible.

testing. But again, we can isolate the difference by regarding the discrepancy of timing between the emergence of anxiety and the attribution of responsibility. Mrs. Perella does not, once she has blamed Mrs. J. for symptoms which she herself felt while in the hospital, forget the matter and *then* re-evoke Mrs. J. as agent after she discovers her children ill and again finds herself in an anxiety-provoking situation to which the same symbol might be appropriate. Rather the affect has spread to the point of eliminating distinctions between situations; the latter simply justify it secondarily. The selections inherent to a secondary report are in this case revealing; as her husband sees the situation, the patient felt herself continually under the spell and consequently found nothing unexpected in the further, and situationally unrelated, misfortunes. Moreover, she does not, as a neurotic might, simply exaggerate a given situation by fearing that the children might die of what was probably a minor illness. Rather she states it as a positive fact, via the paranoid mechanism of transformation of affect into belief, that the children *would have died* had she not returned from the hospital.

Secondly, in this particular case the delusion is not internally consistent, for she holds herself rather than Mrs. J. responsible. Rather the affective meaning of events has "spread" beyond the cognitive framework so that it is hostility or anxiety rather than situations which might provoke them which is constant; the malign influence of Mrs. J. reappears when one child is observed to have lost weight, but when Mr. Perella reveals his skepticism, the patient again shows inconsistency and states that "they" may kill him because he does not believe, not that Mrs. J. will react in some fashion. The constant element is that she sees her anxiety *as* reality via the mechanism of projection. In a sense it is for this reason that cognitive consistency lacks.

In concluding discussion of the first question, the following propositions can be stated as provisionally differentiating the two types of symbolism in regard to the structuring of relationships between symbol and situation. 1) Culturally defined witchcraft belief both provides an expressive form and fulfills a need for explanation by attributing a number of causally distinct (from the scientific standpoint) situations to a common agent; by this means consistency of action is assured in spite of the random arrival of misfortune and the resultant affects which might otherwise disorganize behavior; 2) in schizophrenic symbolism, on the other hand, the relationship to the immediate anxiety-provoking situation is secondary; rather it is the presence of a negative affect which is constant and which itself creates the symbolic framework while the cognitive aspect of the latter may vary. Thus in the second case, the symbol is no longer a *link* between the individual and a given external reality, but rather *creates* a new and purely subjective reality by transformation of affect. One might speak of a reversal of relations between cognitive (and culturally-structured) categories and affective processes as another way of stating the Freudian definition of psychosis as a dominance of id over ego processes.[9]

The second problem which we have to consider is that of the choice of agent. Anthropologists have made a number of hypotheses as to the bases of choice for witches (in those cases where they actually exist as social objects; in those where they do not, the same principles may be applied to the qualities which are attributed to them). As stated above, empirical observations indicate that the choice is predictable in function of tensions within the social structure; as a general rule one can say that witches are most frequently those persons against whom hostility is commonly felt, or representatives of these persons. Thus if the obligation to support the old is enforced but at the same time this obligation creates considerable economic strain, it is likely that old people will be frequently accused of witchcraft. But if the real object of hostility is one whose position within the social structure is such as to make direct expression of hostility too disruptive, another object may be substituted by

9. On the assumption that neurosis does not involve such a reversal of relations between affective and cognitive, one might question the current usage of the term "projection" as a neurotic mechanism; the latter is based on *selection* in function of affective factors rather than transformation and is not dissociated from cultural (or ego) symbolism. Neurotic perceptual distortion may be equivalent to witchcraft belief as discussed here.

displacement; thus a man may accuse another in the next tribe of witchcraft when his own brother is the real source of tension. In other cases, it seems that witchcraft accusations act as a balancing mechanism which counteracts real power relations; e.g., the rich are accused of witchcraft in a number of societies. This has a number of effects both in relieving some of the psychological pressure on the poor, in depreciating the value of wealth in a certain measure and consequently insuring against too great disparity, and in certain cases, it acts as a real sanction in that the rich know that if they do not donate sufficient sums to specified ceremonial occasions, they themselves may become victims of witchcraft (the assumed agent is frequently a potential victim). Although it will not fit all cases, the assumption has also been made and confirmed in some that those who deviate from the given social norms are among the most suspect. Thus in the concrete social structure, witchcraft accusations may act either negatively as a mechanism for the resolution of tension created by a given set of norms or positively as a sanction which reinforces these same norms.

However, on the level of symbolic processes which most concerns us here, it is the characteristics by which the witch is defined which is most important rather than the choice of real objects or the real effects of the belief on the psycho-social situation. In fact, witches are more often heard about than seen; anthropological research has had considerable difficulty in gathering accounts from the victims of witchcraft or from those actually so accused, although such do exist. It seems possible to account for a large percentage of witchcraft belief on a purely symbolic level; consequently it can be best analyzed not in the perspective of the choice of real object, but, like the images of Russians held by Americans who have never seen one, and vice versa, in terms of the composite characteristics of the image. Kluckhohn's data for the Navaho list a number of defining characteristics: witches are associated with night (they are feared only at night); with incest (it is necessary to commit incest to be initiated into a witch society); with animals (for the Navaho and many other societies, witches possess the capacity of taking animal guise), with death and with illegitimate possession of wealth (witches rob graves); and with out-groups (the neighboring Zuni are frequently accused of witchcraft). In sum, the witch is everything which the good Navaho who fears him is not. The latter identifies himself as a Navaho rather than a Zuni, as a man and not an animal, as one who works by day and sleeps by night, with his wife and not his sister, who obtains wealth by sheep-herding and cultivation and not by robbing, and finally, as someone who is alive and very much afraid of corpses. Each characteristic of the witch has its reciprocal in the positive characteristics by which the group (or individual) identifies itself.

A similar process of polarization has been described and analyzed by Moscovici (7) for the formation of representations in propaganda. In this research, pairs of qualities of which the negative is attributed to the rejected opinion while the positive defines the group's own values were isolated: e.g., Communist believers in dialectical materialism characterize psychoanalysis as idealistic, while for integrist Catholics it is mechanistic, in contexts in which it is opposed. In both cases, the rejected view is represented in terms contrary to the group's values. On the basis of the foregoing data on witchcraft imagery, we should like to apply the same principle: namely, that a series of negative qualities are structured around the witch in a relationship of reciprocal opposition to group identification. A further assumption which can be made is that the structuring of negative qualities in itself—because they are seen as oppositions—provides the basis for a structuring of positive qualities and consequently reinforces identification: it structures both external world and the subject's relation to it. In this sense, one can speak of "projection" but the process is quite different from that involved in the psychoanalytic theory of delusion formation; in delusions neither reciprocity nor the independence of subject and object is present.

Moreover, it follows that the witch must have a certain degree of stability as a social representation, for he is an element of a total symbolic structure, i.e., the negative.

Our choice of the term "representation" rather than agent or object is intentional, but it raises a problem of levels of analysis which has been left implicit up to this point. For the witch-object is not necessarily constant; a person may be accused of witchcraft on one occasion and then forgotten, or, as is true in the case of the Italian evil eye belief, he is not always held morally responsible for his acts and is sometimes chosen on the basis of a randomly distributed characteristic, namely, the possession of heavy eyebrows. In considering witchcraft as a cultural belief system, we have isolated it from what in terms of the general theory of action (9) would be called action processes in social or personality systems. Cultural forms, precisely because they are categories abstracted from concrete experience and exist only in consciousness, cut across the boundaries of personality and social structures. Thus with some justification, the Navaho definition of the witch can be interpreted in terms of a generalized representation of Navaho consciousness and in terms of the characteristics of the symbol alone. But pathological processes occur only in concrete personalities; consequently for the psychotic agent the problem is one of a real relationship to the object who becomes the persecutor (which may be formulated by a general theory of personality dynamics) or of particular associations which determined the substitution of a symbolic object for the real one. Holding this distinction in mind, we can turn to an analysis of Mrs. Perella's choice of persecutor.

Psychoanalytic theory furnishes several possibilities as to the basis of choice of agent. From Freud's paradigm of paranoid projection (stated above) we would assume that Mrs. Perella's delusion is a form of denial of homosexual wishes: consequently Mrs. J. was chosen because of a former homosexual attraction to her. In line with the increasing emphasis on the mother-child relationship in schizophrenia, one could equally well say that Mrs. J. represents the patient's mother: that in maintaining that Mrs. J. is a witch, she is denying a previously stable attachment to the latter, and perhaps her own feminine identification as well. The interesting fact that Mrs. J's surname is one that may also serve as a Christian name and is actually that of the patient's mother would support this interpretation; such associative bases of choice have been discovered in other cases. Moreover, Mrs. Perella's mother gave birth to nine children and she herself became ill during the ninth pregnancy. We do not posses sufficient information to make a valid dynamic interpretation, nor is it necessary for the present problem. The essential is that in spite of the theoretical indeterminacy which characterizes the present state of psychoanalytic research on schizophrenia, it is a generally recognized principle that the *persecuting agent in a paranoid delusion is either a formerly loved object or a representative of such an object* (see Freud, 3).

But in this respect the basis of choice is clearly different from that of the witch. In the case of either witchcraft symbolism or of the representations used in propaganda, the qualities of the object are those which for a given set of values are constantly negative; it is precisely this constancy which gives them the potentiality of structuring the world for a given culture and consequently of serving as expressive forms. But in the case of schizophrenia, which involves a breakdown of ego-functioning, i.e., of cultural forms, the persecutor is or represents a formerly loved object. A transformation of love into hate is inherent to the mechanism of projection as it operates in psychosis; this transformation differentiates it from the ego-mechanisms which regulate the relationship between the two by structuring them in relation to the external world in a consistent fashion, although both may involve distortion of empirical reality. The difference between witchcraft beliefs and delusions could be summed up from both standpoints, that of choice of agent and that of relations between symbol and situation, in stating that the first structures relationships between subject and object by a process of polarization which divides the characteristics attributed to the self from those attributed to the (real or symbolic) object, while the delusion operates by a more direct *transformation* of subjective feeling into objective conviction which eliminates this very degree of independence.

However, the case for complete differentiation of the two forms cannot be considered conclusive in all respects even in the light of presently available material. Several striking facts need more detailed consideration, among which are the similarity between the causal language of paranoids and that found in some of the descriptions of self-defined victims of witchcraft which have been collected. Both say frequently "they are doing such and such to me" in a form in which effects are directly and often impersonally seen to follow from the actions of external agents; in both the victim is unqualifiedly passive. In the area of means by which witches are thought to cause diseases, i.e., the injection of objects into the victim, spraying of poisonous gases in the atmosphere or the more general use of poison, there are crucial resemblances to paranoid symbolism. It might be possible to base research on the assumption that there is a progressive differentiation of function such that witchcraft beliefs have both a cultural-ego function in identification and serve as a more "primitive" means of expression, while in our own society the two functions are separated in propaganda (and other types of selective perception on the level of values) and mental illness respectively. Moreover, presumably a number of the self-defined victims of witchcraft must by our standards be mentally ill. A psychoanalyst has recently remarked to us that the first person to believe in witches might well have been a paranoid. If this statement were taken metaphorically rather than literally, it might serve to deepen our psychological understanding of witchcraft phenomena.

BIBLIOGRAPHY

(1) EVANS-PRITCHARD, E. E., *Witchcraft, Oracles, and Magic among the Azande.* New York: Oxford Univ. Press, 1937.

(2) FREUD, S., "Le Président Schreber," in *Cinq Psychoanalyses.* Paris: Presses Universitaires de France, 1954.

(3) FREUD, S., "A Case of Paranoia running counter to the Psycho-analytical Theory of the Disease," in *Collected Papers,* Vol. II. London: Hogarth Press, 1949.

(4) KLUCKHOHN, C. K. *Navaho Witchcraft.* Papers of the Peabody Museum of American Archaeology and Ethnology. Cambridge, Mass.: Harvard Univ.: XXII, 2, 1944.

(5) LEVI-STRAUSS, C., "Introduction à l'œuvre de Marcel Mauss," in Mauss, *Sociologie et Anthropologie.* Paris: Presses Universitaires de France, 1950.

(6) LEVI-STRAUSS, C., "L'Efficacité symbolique,' *Revue de l'Histoire des Religions,* 1951.

(7) MOSCOVICI, S., "Logique et langage dans la propagande: quelques résultats," *Bulletin de Psychologie,* VIII, 7-8.

(8) NADEL, S. F., "Witchcraft in Four African Societies: An Essay in Comparison," *Amer. Anthropolog. 54*:1, 1952.

(9) PARSONS, T., SHILS, E., et al., *Towards a General Theory of Action.* Cambridge, Mass.: Harvard Univ. Press, 1951.

(10) TAUSK, V., "On the Origin of the Influencing Machine in Schizophrenia," in *The Psychoanalytic Reader,* Fliess, R., ed., Vol. I. New York: International Universities Press, 1948.

(11) WAELDER, R., "On the Structure of Paranoid Ideas; Critical Survey of Various Theories," *Internat. J. of Psychoanal., 32,* 1951.

chapter 8

Abstract and Concrete Images in Paranoid Delusions

A Comparison of American and South Italian Patients

There seem to be very marked differences between delusional perceptions of patients in an American private hospital and one in Southern Italy. In American delusions there is a very strong tendency toward abstraction. Actors in these delusions include, in addition to concrete individuals, such abstract social entities as Communists, an advertising agency, or the hospital perceived as a unitary whole. This tendency to think of the enemy in ideological or institutional terms is almost completely lacking in the delusions of Southern Italian patients. These, in contrast, although showing plentiful evidence of projection and dissociation, are centered almost completely on concrete persons and events within the patient's immediate context of family and neighborhood. Although one might say that

Presented before the round-table meeting on cultural factors in delusional systems, American Psychiatric Association, May 1961.

there was far more "reason" for these patients to construct delusions about the hospital, given the close restrictions on patients' behavior that were imposed by the locked ward system and by hospital personnel, I found that most patients merely considered the hospital as an external restrictive force that did not arouse enough concern to enter into their psychotic ideation. The lack of abstractness in the thought processes of Southern Italian patients no doubt reflects the fact that in their cultural setting primary group membership alone is socially meaningful, while for middle-class Americans secondary institutions are crucial to the formation of an individual's sense of identity.

Among twenty-five American cases studied, fifteen showed institutional and ideological delusions in a conspicuous form, while a like number of Italian patients showed none at all.[1]

Three patients in a private mental hospital may be considered first. Patient A was a college graduate from an intellectually inclined and cosmopolitan upper-class family. Her father, a lawyer, held rather conservative views, while the relatives of her deceased artistic mother were socialistically inclined. Just before hospitalization the patient had spent some time discussing politics with her father. An earlier psychotic breakdown had taken place just after a visit to her maternal aunt and uncle. The patient herself, in several problems of choice with which she was faced, was uncertain as to whether to identify herself with the legal profession, as represented by her father, or with various wandering artistic friends, more closely linked to the image of her mother, whom she had encountered in college and on trips to Europe. Talking about an immediate past phase of muteness, patient A explained:

I thought I would be a good weapon in the struggle between Communist and Western powers—my aunt and her husband are Socialists, I thought they might be Communistic. I read the *Look* article about the radio-active family—that's how I felt, spreading

1. The closest approximation to an abstract type of delusion occurred in one Italian patient who said that the nurses on the ward were in collusion against her. She quickly abandoned the hospital theme, however, by adding, "like daughters in a family."

radioactivity. I had a lot of information on me—anything I did would mean that all the Americans would be swept off the earth and I thought the hospital was a big factory that observed guinea pigs—everything was arranged. You never can tell who the doctors are, they keep records and know all about you.

Patient B's father was a Madison Avenue man. The family, a rather badly disorganized one, with a psychotic mother and a heavily drinking father, had early in its history become addicted to psychotherapy; both the patient and her father tended to see the world through psychodynamic eyeglasses, and she quickly became involved with other patients and the hospital society, albeit perceiving them psychotically. Patient B talked about her life in the hospital:

What is it that the people on the ward know about me that I don't know? I just feel so degraded. It's getting more complicated every day—the books, the TV, they're all written for me, it's one big advertising campaign at my expense. They are redoing the hospital —switching the male and female wards—it's all planned by an advertising agency for my benefit. I feel as if I'm losing all my individuality, trying to conform to a norm.

Patient C was a small-town girl; her father, a physician, was Protestant, while her Scandinavian husband was Catholic. Her psychotic breakdown involved conflicts surrounding the areas of medicine and religion. The parents had objected to the marriage both on religious grounds and because the father was very seductively attached to the patient. Father and husband came into acute conflict over the issue of whether he, as a physician, should treat his own grandson, the father declining on the grounds of medical ethics and the husband insisting on grounds of finance. The resulting conflict of loyalties provided the onset for the patient's withdrawal into psychosis. This is how she spoke right after admission:

I have made images out of people on the ward. My family was in danger. Now I am killing all the people on the ward—it's my fault because I made images out of them [i.e., equated them with persons at home]. They have turned against me—Mrs. R [a Jewish patient] thinks I am condemning the Jews—The Catholics think I'm condemning the Catholics—Dr. X is the Pope, I'm trying to glug up his medicine.

In all three cases there is a very close relation between the content of delusional thinking and the actual social situations in which the patients are involved. Moreover, all three of these patients show a common characteristic. They tend to juxtapose personal details and ideas about ideologies or institutions, such as the conflict between Russia and the United States, or the hospital seen as an entity which is coordinated or planned with exclusive reference to the patient. This kind of juxtaposition has been noted very often by psychiatrists, and in fact might be conceived of as one of the qualities that makes paranoid thinking often seem so chaotic. It is a characteristic that Norman Cameron has described, and to which he has applied the concept of "interpretation of themes."

Although it now seems pretty well determined that schizophrenia and paranoid thinking are not limited to any particular cultural environment, this specific characteristic may very well be so limited. A number of observers, such as Louis Mars in Haiti and T. Adeoye Lambo in Africa, have noted that in these non-Western societies technological concepts or sophisticated paranoid "systems" only appear in patients who have had superior education; the delusions of less highly educated patients are instead likely to be based on concepts of magic and witchcraft shared by other persons of the same cultural background. I should like to furnish added support to this view by presenting two further case excerpts, both concerning patients hospitalized in Southern Italy. Patient D, the illiterate daughter of an ambulatory fruit vendor on the outskirts of Naples, described how she got to the hospital in the following terms:

I was afraid—I was afraid—I had a fight in the middle of the night and while I was fighting in the middle of the night I said, "No mama." Then mama was dead next to the cupboard where the pictures of the dead people and saints are. Then I got scared and

I began to cry because I thought, I thought that mama was dead and after I began to cry, I grabbed my mother's medal and my brother stayed in the bed. Then I began to fight all of them, then I was wearing a nightgown, and then it was very long. Afterwards my brother held mama's shoulders from behind but it was mama who held me—then she [mother] said, "Come, come we are going to make a visit up to the City Hall," I went up to the City Hall and she took me where the doctor was and the doctor didn't want to see me, his face fell, he didn't want to look at me, this is what he said: "No, there's nothing wrong with this kid; it's not my business, it's in her head, you have to go somewhere else," and he wrote out the slip and gave it to me and put it on my hand and I came here, first to the observation ward, then to this one.

Since the father's death, the family had been supported by the mother's work as a maid, and the patient did most of the housework. Her first psychotic episode at the age of seventeen followed immediately on the father's death and involved similar frightening perceptions of the mother, then seen as a monster. The excerpt above refers to her third admission at age twenty-one. The patient, an adult brother and sister, and three younger siblings all shared one room and three beds. I learned from the family that a fight did indeed take place in the middle of the night and that the patient was usually hospitalized when she had her rare but very intensive aggressive outbursts. These were in contrast to her usual behavior, which was more restrained than that of any other family member. The mother was not actually hurt; the pictures of the saints and the family dead are those found in the place of honor in any lower-class Neapolitan home.

About patient E, the most educated of the sample of twenty-five schizophrenic women I observed in Southern Italy, I find the following in my field notes:

The charge, made by the S. family, was that the patient had thrown a shoe at their daughter on two occasions. The patient became extremely hostile when a policeman tried to intervene. She went into a tirade about the evils done to her by the S. family: they tried to penetrate her house and she will certainly not sign any paper permitting that woman to get back in; who knows what poison was in the coffee they have offered her; the daughter of the S. family is a public disgrace for her carrying on with men; they have invited her cordially to their house only to beat her and throw her under the bed, and if she were not in the hospital she would certainly bring a countercharge. The policeman finally gave up and left, concluding that she could not reason well enough to sign the papers anyway.

An inhabitant of Ischia, with a moderately well-off artisan father, this patient had nearly completed her training as an elementary school teacher. The fight with a neighboring family, in which the other party as well as the patient were actively involved, represents a very common reason for hospitalization in this setting. The patient actually had shown psychotic symptoms over many years but had remained at home up to the time of the described episode.

As the case of patient E shows, educational level is not the only social factor that has an influence upon delusions. The immediate involvement of the patient in reciprocal interaction accompanied by strong love or hate relates to general characteristics of the society, as does the concern with the sexual behavior of others and the meaning of social invitation.

While a sense of vagueness and depersonalization accompanied the juxtaposed abstractions expressed by the American patients, as if they were desperately trying to organize an over-complex world, the Neapolitan patients vividly communicated terror, anger, and all the details of immediate experience, using language with remarkably concrete and explosive forcefulness. None of the latter patients complained of depersonalization.

The implications of these and other findings concerning cultural differences in the content of delusions are difficult to evaluate, given our current lack of a coherent theoretical explanation of schizophrenia. There are two perspectives in which one can look at such data. The first is that adopted by most organic theorists and also by most psychoanalysts, namely, that the differences are superficial or incidental and that what is essential to schizophrenia is invariant. The second perspective is that adopted by Dr. Weinstein,* namely, that we can build on those works of Sapir and others that show the very crucial ways in which culture affects the perceptions of all of us. This viewpoint can be extended to include the perceptions of schizophrenia and to show how delusions are dependent on cultural conceptualizations. From this perspective, I would say that in a certain sense the delusions of the schizophrenic present a microscopic model of the social structure. Thus in our own society, where the individual life course involves choices between religious or ideological values and relatedness to large-scale institutions, we find conflicts among these institutions and ideologies represented in the delusions of schizophrenics. In the simpler society of Southern Italy, which is family- and neighborhood-centered, delusions focus instead on family members or neighbors. Even when patients are in a large hospital, this has so little intimate importance to them that it is not perceived delusionally.

Other cultural influences also are evident in the delusions of women patients from Southern Italy. For example, fears of gossip or of being called a bad woman are characteristic of most single patients, and fears of infidelity on the part of husbands are characteristic of those who are married. Such delusions reflect the strains of a culture in which premarital virginity and monogamous marriage are strongly upheld, while at the same time attitudes toward sexuality are far from being puritanical. This is in marked contrast to Dr. Weinstein's data from the Virgin Islands, in which fears about sexual behavior appear far less frequently. In that society, illegitimacy and casual sexual relationships are not condemned.

I should like to stress that the cultural perspective alone is not sufficient for the understanding of psychotic delusions. Certain delusional ideas seem to occur and reoccur quite remarkably across a wide variety of cultural settings, for example: fears of poisoning, change in sexual identity, or being influenced by highly charged forces, whether technological or magical in

* *Editor's note:* Reference is to Dr. Edwin A. Weinstein, moderator of the round-table meeting at which this paper was delivered.

origin. This content was present in both my American and Italian samples. Moreover, many images pointed to the importance of homosexual drives in both groups, although the explicit content differed. Many of the Italian patients feared women who drilled holes, penetrated their houses, offered terrifying phallic objects while threatening bewitchment, and so forth, while the Americans more often explicitly referred to homosexual fears or to homosexuals being interested in them—again showing more willingness to abstract when expressing their delusions.

In ending I should like to raise the question whether there is a necessary incompatibility between seeing delusions as expressions of primary instinctual drives and seeing them as products of a particular cultural environment. Although these approaches seem hard to reconcile at the present time, they are not mutually incompatible. A patient cannot express an instinctual wish without using language and cultural symbols. Moreover, the form in which such a wish is expressed is highly dependent on the particular social constellation in which the patient lives. I would not wish to think of either the culturally derived symbolic form or the instinct as having such pre-eminent importance that the other must be relegated to the realm of the incidental or superficial. Rather I wonder if by the further comparative study of schizophrenic patients in different settings we might not arrive at better formulations than we have as yet achieved of the relationships between instinct and culture and between early development and adult life, as well as attaining greater understanding of the process of symbolization itself.

chapter 9

A Schizophrenic
Episode in a
Neapolitan Slum*

During the last ten years, a few case histories
have been published of schizophrenics originating in cultural
settings quite different from those which usually provide the
clientele of psychodynamic psychiatry. Cross-cultural examination of such clinical material can provide a useful research

* This paper is based on work carried out at three hospitals in
Naples and its vicinity under a research grant from the National Institute
of Mental Health (M-2105), Bethesda, Md. I should particularly like to
acknowledge the cooperation of Professor Vizioli, Director of the Naples
Psychiatric Hospital; Professor Cristini, Director of the Psychiatric
Emergency Ward at the Morvilla Hospital, Naples; the late Professor
Ventra, Director of the Psychiatric Hospital of Nocera Inferiora; other
staff members of these hospitals; and Aurora Benvignati, graduate of
the UNSAS School of Social Work in Naples, who made an invaluable
contribution in interviewing patients' relatives.

method for psychiatry in that it takes advantage of the natural laboratory setting offered by the wide range of variability among human societies for testing assumptions about the determinants of psychopathology. At the same time, if the anthropologist working in a field setting can learn to deal with his material on an individual case level, his method will be brought closer to that of the psychiatrist, so that a more meaningful exchange of materials becomes possible.[1] This paper, which presents the case history of a young psychotic woman hospitalized in Naples, Italy, is intended as a contribution of this sort.

In the reciprocal confrontation of psychoanalysis and cultural anthropology, a host of questions has been raised concerning the respective roles played by instinct and culture in the development of both normal and abnormal personality patterns. The contributions of Edward Sapir, Ruth Benedict, Margaret Mead, and others have brought two propositions increasingly into the awareness of psychiatrists: First, that personality constellations depend to a considerable extent upon features of culture—such as family structure, child-training practices, and possibilities and limitations in the expression of affects—which vary among human societies; and second, that perceptions of abnormality, including those of the psychiatrist, are to a considerable extent dependent upon the observer's particular view of what is normal.

However, neither of these two propositions in itself provides the answer to a third question: Can one nevertheless describe specific pathological reaction types in a way that is at least partially independent of cultural variation? The realization that varying norms may determine pathological behavior and perceptions of it does not necessarily preclude the possibility of

1. See especially: Melford E. Spiro, "A Psychotic Personality in the South Seas," *Psychiatry* (1950), *13* : 189–204. Melford E. Spiro, "Cultural Heritage, Personal Tensions, and Mental Illness in a South Sea Culture," pp. 141–171; in *Culture and Mental Health,* ed. by Marvin K. Opler; New York (The Macmillan Company, 1959). Benjamin Paul, "Mental Disorder and Self-Regulating Processes in Culture: A Guatemalan Illustration," *Interrelations between the Social Environment and Psychiatric Disorders* (Millbank Memorial Fund, New York, 1953). T. Adeoye Lambo, "The Role of Cultural Factors in Paranoid Psychosis among the Yoruba Tribe," *J. Mental Sc.* (1955), *101* : 239–266.

culturally invariant features of psychopathology, but rather should stimulate the investigator to a more rigorous isolation of constant elements from the wider symptom complexes often taken for granted in everyday psychiatric practice, in which there may be considerable normative bias.

In other words, I believe that the method used by some research workers of describing personality and its potential disorders *solely* with respect to a normative context is insufficient, among other reasons because, carried to its logical extreme, it leaves no room for a scientific theory of personality independent of the normative biases of particular observers.[2] For this reason it seems important to initiate a series of comparative studies searching for *both* variations relative to the cultural context *and* invariant features. The case of Giuseppina M will be presented with these two distinct questions in mind: (1) Which aspects of a complex of symptoms and behavior can best be understood by reference to the general knowledge of schizophrenia, independent of the cultural context in which it occurs? That is, in which ways does Giuseppina M very much resemble schizophrenic women seen in the United States? (2) Which aspects of the same complex can be better understood by reference to the specific cultural setting in which they are located? That is, what differentiates Giuseppina M from schizophrenic patients commonly seen in American psychiatric practice?

Case Material

Naples is a preindustrial city with a standard of living closer to that found in the Orient than to that of any other Western city. Living under foreign domination for much of its

2. Compare Sapir's example, "Two Crows denies this," given in support of the view that the anthropologist as well as the psychiatrist can go wrong if he expects all of the members of a culture to conform to a particular view of its norms. Sapir's definition of a psychiatric approach in anthropology was one which would isolate individual variations in cultural perception. See Edward Sapir, "Why Cultural Anthropology Needs the Psychiatrist," *Psychiatry* (1938), *1*:7–12.

long history, it has never created a successful urban economy, and its present population of over a million seems squeezed into a grotesquely overgrown town. A large proportion of the poorer population lives by various uncertain expedients known as "arranging oneself"—begging, the sale of contraband goods, parasitism on foreign tourists, and so on. The economic situation acts against much faith in rationally planned individual advancement. The family system, which involves chaperonage of women and close postmarital parent-child ties, in many ways resembles a peasant one, and magical beliefs are still found among the lower classes. Much of the lower-class ethic is based on a concept of honor according to which one is obligated to respond to an offense—to oneself or one's intimates—with an affirmative rebuttal. The crowded living conditions and the habitual poverty have combined with a considerable urban sophistication to give rise to a distinctive expressive animation which permeates the city, the legendary home of love and laughter.

Giuseppina M was born on November 20, 1932, in the San Lorenzo quarter, a particularly crowded section, which includes the central railroad section and a black-market district. Her father was formerly an artisan, skilled in the making of tortoise-shell goods, but he now for the most part holds only temporary unskilled jobs because of increased competition from industrial goods. The one-room home which he and his wife inherited from his artisan father is a *basso,* a ground-floor dwelling typical of the Neapolitan slums; when the door is left open, the family's entire living accommodations can be viewed from the street.

The parents were married about 1930 after a stormy courtship in which the father disfigured his reluctant beloved so that no other man would take her from him; she has a faintly visible scar from the razor cut on her still attractive face. At the time, *lo sfregio* (disfigurement) was an accepted means of expressing jealousy. As the father has grown older, he has become more easygoing, but also more indifferent; during the war, he was interned for a while in a local German labor camp, and the indifference has been particularly conspicuous since then. He nevertheless appears to be a person with a certain amount of warmth, and to occupy himself during unemployment spends many hours chatting with his numerous friends in the quarter.

The mother, born in the same quarter, is the daughter of a chauffeur who until his death was an old and trusted servant in a wealthy professional family. Her conscious values owe much to her father's upper-status connections, and a long-cherished dream of hers is an improvement in social status—at least to the point of moving from the *basso* to an upper-floor apartment. She sees her marriage as decidedly unhappy, principally because of her perception of herself as having status aspirations in contrast to her husband's "vulgarity," and because she feels that the social pressure resulting from *lo sfregio* forced her to marry before she could make up her mind. Like her husband, she has numerous friends in the quarter but proudly speaks of them as among the most "civilized" of the women. Small, attractively dressed, and quiet, she appears to have been quite successful in learning higher-status speech and mannerisms, but she expresses many depressive feelings.

The patient is the youngest of three siblings. A sister born about 1931 is currently living at the parents' home with her son and working as a salesgirl; she married about 1948 but is partially separated from her husband—he lives across the street with his own parents, and they visit frequently, but she treats him like a small boy unable to live up to a man's responsibilities. A brother, born in January, 1932, died of tuberculosis in 1954. His memory is very much idolized by the mother, who is still heavily involved in a grief reaction for him.

The patient's delivery was a difficult one, after which her mother suffered from hemorrhages and was unable to nurse her; as a result she was sent away to a colony of wet nurses near Rome. On her return, she appeared to be a bouncing baby in the best of health, but her mother states that "from the time she began to reason," Giuseppina accused the mother of neglect for not having nursed her as she had the other two siblings.

From this developed what her family sees as a consistent personality pattern—a tendency toward "jealousy." "Jealousy" is a frequently used word in Naples, meaning quickness to show emotional reaction, such as having temper tantrums when affection and material tokens of it are perceived as offered in a discriminatory manner. Throughout childhood the jealousy pattern was revealed in Giuseppina's constant complaints that the mother made better clothes for the sister, although the mother maintains that in order to resolve the situation she made identical dresses for the two.

In mannerisms and personal appearance, the patient is far more like her father than her mother; she is a small, somewhat plump girl, 'cute' but not strikingly beautiful, rather typical of the milieu and less carefully put together than her mother. She has always managed to secure prestige and friendships in the neighborhood, being particularly admired for her success in securing compensation payments after she was laid off from a job. In the hospital, she did not present herself as having status aspirations and did not express snobbish attitudes concerning other patients. Nevertheless, when she wants to, she is as capable of speaking refined Italian as her mother is, and went to considerable effort to secure an elementary school certificate, returning to night school after the war, which had interrupted her studies; neither the ability to speak Italian as well as the Neapolitan dialect, nor the educational achievement can be taken for granted at this social level in Naples. She did well in school and in the two jobs, ironing in laundries, which she held before marriage. At the same time—and the significance of this in the family setting became clear when her nine-year-old nephew, returning home dirty and using the language of the streets was severely reprimanded by his grandmother—she learned some of the less refined mannerisms of the neighborhood, as shown in the abusive rhetoric she used with quite a flair in the hospital.

Thus in a sense the patient's personality and history can be seen as a series of alternations between identifications with maternal and paternal social reference groups. The same conflict is seen in the courtship period, which also marks the beginning of the difficulties that culminated in the psychotic break. First, although her mother had an up-and-coming neighborhood man, who has since achieved white-collar status, all picked out, the patient rebelled against this choice. In the hospital, she fantasied leaving her present husband and marrying her mother's choice. The man whom she eventually did marry is similar to her father in social status; he also is a partially employed artisan, well regarded for his *savoir-faire*. The contrast between Giuseppina's noisy and obviously lower-class mother-in-law and her more refined and quiet mother is very striking. Second, the courtship situation was such as to produce a considerable alienation from her family, in particular a disruption of a previously close, affectionate relationship with the father. Further, during the courtship the brother died, and this event probably aggravated the mother's depressive tendencies.

The patient met her future husband when she was about eighteen, and they were officially engaged for four or five years. Like that of the parents, the courtship was stormy throughout, to such a point that no one in the family wished to take the role of chaperone for fear of the couple's constant quarrels. These also had "jealousy" as their basis, a fear shared by both partners that the other would desert in favor of a third person. Giuseppina's jealousy convinced her fiancé that she was very much in love; others saw the relationship as of the intense sort that can "drive you crazy." Because of the frequency of quarreling, both families were opposed to the marriage, and in order to force the issue the patient's father stated that he would no longer allow her to eat at home until the engagement was broken. The result was an elopement and immediate marriage. The husband reports that there had been premarital sex relations. Female premarital chastity is highly valued throughout Southern Italy, but in this case, as far as I know the matter did not become public, and they were not married in disgrace.[3]

The rather sharp break that the marriage produced in

3. Elopement creates some social censure, but in the city this usually abates after the couple is safely married.

Giuseppina's ties to her family was accentuated by the fact that her mother was at the time in a "particularly nervous" period (at the time of interviewing she felt much improved as a result of a thyroid operation). Either just before or soon after the wedding, the two had a fight in which the mother threw a pair of scissors at her daughter; but somewhat contradictorily she also refers to having cut a photograph of the patient and her husband in half, preserving only Giuseppina's photo, thus symbolizing her wish to keep her close at home. However, in order to accentuate the separation, the couple took a room at a considerable distance from either family.

Giuseppina almost immediately became pregnant; sometime before she delivered, her mother went to the hospital for the thyroid operation. Psychotic symptoms first became evident during the early months of marriage and pregnancy. Her mother's vagueness about the onset confirms her distance at the time; she reports only that her daughter thought that there were spirits in the house, and she believes that some sexual difficulties arose in the marriage, Giuseppina's husband, Mr. M, reports that she had hallucinations of water running and that she began to see shadow women coming toward her at night, whereupon she screamed and began to fight back at them. He also felt that her jealousy took a pathological turn when she began to accuse him of sexual involvement with her mother and sister.

The patient herself reports the onset in terms of a sudden and intense terror experienced on hearing voices:

. . . I kept hearing a lot of noises, the noises, so that I was very frightened, so much so that I was always praying, praying, praying, because I was so afraid. I heard noises of all sorts, noises and also voices, if that is what you mean. One morning I had a fright, Madonna, I had really a voice so that suddenly I ran to the priest who said to me, "Maybe it could be—" because it was an acquaintance this voice, it could be a dead person, "Don't you want to have a mass said or something?"

The voice was that of a woman characterized by the mother as her friend rather than her daughter's, who died before

Giuseppina's engagement as a result of an abortion for illegitimate pregnancy.

Perhaps because Mr. M felt incompetent to deal with the situation alone, the couple then moved in with his mother, where they remained until after delivery of a healthy girl. However, after delivery the symptoms worsened; unable to tolerate Giuseppina's behavior, the mother-in-law expelled the couple, and the husband decided to take her to the psychiatric emergency clinic. Just before admission, her paranoia expanded into the feeling that everyone was against her, and she interpreted random movements made by the child as expressing aggressive intentions toward her.

The month spent in the emergency clinic was a particularly traumatic one:

. . . I only went to the emergency clinic for a declaration of the nervous system [to have a physician's report filled out], but they made me go inside, then they attacked me every day for going next to the window . . . there were all the nurses that did this . . . they were all daughters of a family, perhaps, who knows, things between them. . . .

From her reports it emerged that the nurses (there are only two on the ward, as there are two daughters in her family) had restrained her, telling her she was crazy, from standing by a window through which she believed she saw her dead brother outside. Also she was particularly afraid of being held down on the bed by the nurses during electroshock treatment, and mentioned that earlier girl friends might have "done bad things" to her. Feeling that she was rapidly becoming worse in the hospital, her husband decided, against medical advice, to withdraw her. But in the street outside she went into such a temper tantrum—saying that if she had remained in the hospital she would have inherited a large sum of money from a woman who was dead—that he decided to call the police, and from the police station she was admitted to the provincial hospital.

It was at this point that my contact with her began. In the first interview she appeared well-ordered, was somewhat hyperverbal, and indicated her anxiety only by indirect statements —for example, she said that someone might be sending Americans to the hospital to find out who was crazy. During the first three weeks, she retained an elaborate delusional belief concerning impregnation by means of the soul of a bird belonging to a woman friend:

. . . I really felt the conditions of an interesting state [delicate, upper-status expression for pregnancy] although I have menstruated. It has been a little bit of a new thing, it's a new thing because when someone is in an interesting state that business never happens. . . . [*Interviewer*: The first day you told me something about a bird.] Oh, yes, yes, from the bird on the ground, no? On that moment seeing in that moment the breath of the bird it happened to me . . . two days passed and I felt movements. Feeling some movements from fear, then what did I do, I have a glance at the lady that had the bird, no? Giving a glance I didn't want to say it was her fault because who knows if she had something to do with it, something shall we say to make me hear this noise, because I was afraid, that it was really like a destiny, as if she had resuscitated the bird and I couldn't think about it. . . .

. . . who knows, maybe it walked in from behind, it made my spine twisted here so that when I went to the hospital giving me electroshock after I felt a pain. . . . I think maybe it was the soul of the bird that walked, who knows, in any case it happened to me that I, my behind here, you know, it didn't go straight any more, but it went twisted this way and that's the truth.

The pregnancy belief is thus associated both with the experience of hearing voices and with a sense of body deformation.

During these first three weeks, she was quite confidential in interviews. The principal themes were the delusional pregnancy, her fear and hostility vis-à-vis the nurses at the emergency clinic (which did not spread to those at the provincial hospital although she received more electroshock there), the initially frightening voice, hallucinations of her brother, and a fear of having tuberculosis. She frequently referred to women in an indeterminate way, and presumably the voice and the woman referred to as the agent of the pregnancy are various aspects of a single significant female object. This object is very closely identified with herself:

[*Interviewer:* What did the voice say?] What did it say? It said that I—she—had suffered because I was engaged and all through the engagement we were, we were married, and so on. It was almost like her—like her, shall we say, her behavior. Then she had suffered . . . She had many sufferings, many things, they couldn't have her, she died. . . . Yes, and this, shall we say, I was engaged, and then I had almost, identical, her personality.

A sense of guilt is also centered on the same person, which presumably is at least partly explained by the fact, implicitly confessed above, that like her mother's friend she had premarital sexual relations:

. . . she said to me when she died I cried a lot. Why did I cry so much, she asked me? . . . he [a male cousin whose voice reassured her in the hospital] says that when someone cries a lot for a dead person, it means that he feels guilty about something. . . . I was crying because—she was a friend, I was over there all the time, shall we say inside her house and we went to the movies with her boy friend. . . . I cried from the bottom of my heart, but how I cried! I also was guilty about something.

She also reveals intense feelings of terror, and a belief that she can play the savior role toward the woman and at the same time achieve salvation:

Do you know that a photo came out in the newspapers . . . a photo with all the teeth sticking out . . . all of her lineaments from when she was alive, no, only that she had the teeth that way, sticking out. It came out right in the newspapers so that I was scared, and then she told me that I was the boss of her life and then she would have left me that little book [savings account book], but I never took anything. Then one day I read in the newspapers that at the Pediatric Clinic there, where she was when she died . . . there was a clinic for children and they were remodeling it. I heard right in my ears what she said—that she would be very pleased if her money—it pleased her that a hospital would be remodeled with her money and that I would take the rest.

During the same three-week period, she also began to bring up some of her difficulties in maintaining close relationships within the family. However, after an interview in which I began to sound her out, American fashion, about her conflicts with her mother, our relationship suddenly changed in that she became markedly less confidential. This change coincided with a clear-cut social improvement; she became far more coherent in verbal expression, and for the first time her real child emerged into conscious consideration and displaced the delusional pregnancy. For the remainder of a three-months' hospitalization, she wanted immediate discharge on the grounds that a small child should not be home without its mother. Some events which took place during the second and third months of hospitalization are illustrative of the way in which social recovery was effected.

First, when visited by her relatives, she tended to show exaggerated emotional reactions. For example, one day when her husband and child visited, accompanied by the in-laws, she conspicuously took the child from her sister-in-law and promenaded around the ward mothering her—the nurses watching carefully lest she throw the child on the ground. Likewise, she conspicuously demonstrated both affection for her husband and hostility against him, the latter with an elaborate verbal and gestural rhetoric which was coherent if not very polite. When her father and husband came to see her, after a visit to the ward physician to ask if discharge could be considered soon, she perceived that they were afraid to tell her what the physician had said—that a few more weeks of hospitalization would be advisable—and threw a temper tantrum which sent both off the ward looking sheepish.[4] She consistently greeted her father with far

4. At this point I intervened and, as I had been taught to do with paranoid patients in an American hospital, tried to clarify the facts concerning the physician's recommendation. The nurses, who supported the husband's and father's failure to tell her she would have to stay, bodily carried me from the scene. They informed me that one does not communicate unpleasant facts to the sick, and told the patient that she would leave the hospital in a few moments.

more genuine affection than her husband, and toward the end of her hospitalization, following a successful visit from her mother, she began to show increasing affectionate concern for both parents, referring constantly to herself and her family as "we" rather than to herself as a misunderstood "I."

A second illustrative event occurred not long before her discharge, when I happened to encounter her in the ward courtyard in the company of a depressed patient. When the latter suggested that mental illness can make you lose interest in your children, Giuseppina began to show an intense anger reaction, exploding principally against me for failure to secure her discharge (at her request I had brought the matter up with the physician, but he still did not believe that the moment was opportune), and emphasizing her respectable position in society as a mother and married woman. She also implied that the other patient might not be so respectable. But here, as at other points, she appeared to be using a highly elaborate rhetoric as a defense mechanism; this rhetoric was both internally coherent and highly communicative, which had not been true for the more intimate earlier statements about herself.

In the period immediately following her discharge, she spent the days with her mother, with whom she was at this time on particularly good terms, and the nights with her husband. The mother and daughter identified with each other as afflicted by destiny with "nervousness." Almost immediately she became pregnant again, and she began to look for a room close to her mother's home. At this time, she claimed complete amnesia for the acute phase, saying she had been "out of her head" and would not otherwise have said and done what she did. Eighteen months after her discharge, conflict with her mother had reappeared, and she and her husband were now living at a greater distance from her family. She was keeping house adequately and had not been rehospitalized, but she showed considerable aggression against both her husband and her children, and her delusional fears had returned concerning sexual relationships between her husband and her mother and sister.

The Selection of Cases for Study

This case is one of 25 young schizophrenic women whom I saw in Southern Italy, a sample gathered for comparison with a sample of 25 female schizophrenics of comparable age and length of hospitalization seen in a private, psychotherapeutically oriented hospital in the United States. The aim of the project was to isolate both similarities and cultural differences with respect to a variety of features of schizophrenic symptoms and personality. However, such an aim presupposes that diagnosis is carefully controlled; if there are no reliable diagnostic indices, it would, of course, be impossible to select such a sample. For this reason, for the Italian sample, whenever any questions arose concerning the diagnosis, the case data were reviewed by a senior consulting psychiatrist in the United States and one in England.

The 25 final cases were chosen from an initial sample of 30, five being discarded at the stage of consultation because of disagreements or other complexities—for instance, cases classified as "borderline," "schizo-affective," and the like were not included. For the final sample, there was agreement with the official Italian hospital diagnosis in 20 cases. No attempt was made to distinguish subtypes, and several differentiations currently made in Italy—such as schizophrenia, paranoid psychosis, dissociative syndrome, catatonic state, and so on—were lumped together as equivalent to the broader American conception of schizophrenic reactions.[5] Most of the five disagreements can be explained as resulting from administrative mistakes such as may happen in any hospital; for example, one patient initially diagnosed as "depressive state" was clearly paranoid when seen on her third admission, but the official diagnosis had not been changed. The high level of agreement is particularly significant

5. It is important that the diagnosis is usually made by the director of the hospital in Naples. The term schizophrenia is placed on records only in the most severe or chronic cases because of the prejudicial consequences it carries, and some of these other terms may be preferred for this reason.

in the light of the fact that both consulting psychiatrists were psychoanalytic in orientation, while the predominant current of psychiatric thought in Naples is organic.

Features of the Schizophrenic Episode Shared by American Patients

For a diagnosis to be used cross-culturally, the illness diagnosed must have at least some invariant features; and, as was noted above, one of the tasks of the comparative study of psychopathology might be to isolate them from larger symptom complexes which are dependent on the cultural context. The term most commonly used for schizophrenic reaction in Naples at present is dissociative syndrome, a term which sums up the global dissociation of behavior and representational processes considered characteristic by many descriptive psychiatrists.[6] The schizophrenic reaction may also be characterized in terms of the presence of delusions and hallucinations or in terms of a disturbance of affect; these features can be discussed as they appear in the psychosis of Giuseppina M.

First, there is no doubt that Giuseppina showed both delusions and hallucinations. She herself dates the onset of psychosis to the time when she felt terrified by hearing voices. Subsequently she developed a number of delusional ideas, some of which have a classical paranoid form: that shadow women were attacking her; that her husband was sexually involved with her mother or her sister; that her child had aggressive impulses toward her, as interpreted from random gestures; and that the nurses at the emergency clinic wished to harm her. In addition, she expressed

6. See the article by Carlo Felice Coppola, Staff Physician, Naples Psychiatric Hospital, "I Limiti della Schizofrenia e la sua Indipendenza dalle altre Psicosi," *L'Ospedale Psichiatrico* [Naples] (1957) 3 fasc., July–September: 259–314. The distinguishing features of schizophrenia are discussed, and among those isolated are: dissociation (of representations); disturbance of affect (prolonged latency in response, abnormal persistence, lability, incompatibility with surrounding events, and so on); autism (confusion of fantasy and reality); and hallucinations (including delusions in the American sense).

fear of bodily deformation, denied the death of her brother, and fantasied a purely narcissistic resolution of her difficulties —that she would become rich by a large inheritance, part of which she would donate to a pediatric clinic. All these beliefs involve a breakdown of the boundaries between internal and external reality.

However, if delusions are simply considered to be non-rational beliefs, one must raise the question of whether they appear as pathological only to the psychiatrist, whose concept of rationality derives from his scientific training, or whether they appear so also to the people who make up the social setting— and who may accept beliefs which would be regarded by an observer from another social setting as projections of fears or desires into reality. The concept of the believable, for Giuseppina's intimates, does not preclude spirits' haunting houses, the dead reappearing in dreams, a pregnancy's going wrong if the mother's food cravings are not gratified, or one's best hope for success in life lying in an unexpected inheritance rather than in work. Thus all of these elements of Giuseppina's psychosis reflect beliefs common in the relevant social environment; for example, the mother herself at one point thought that there were spirits in the house and for this reason encouraged the couple to move. However, by this same token it is unlikely that Giuseppina's holding these beliefs caused her relatives to take her to the hospital and to agree with the hospital personnel that she could not "reason."

In other words, since the relatives, rather than rejecting the psychiatric definition of the illness, emphatically affirmed that the patient was "crazy," they must have possessed some criterion according to which they also saw a difference between schizophrenic and normal thinking. Actually, when the material is examined, it is not difficult to find evidence that Giuseppina herself perceived the psychotic delusions as deviant from the social standard of credibility; for example, she was quite aware that "when one is in an interesting state that business never happens," and so had to provide secondary rationalizations for her conviction of pregnancy. Likewise, her mother was particularly troubled by her direct affirmation that she *had seen* her dead brother, for although in Neapolitan popular lore the dead may appear in dreams, or their spiritual presence may be felt, one is not permitted to deny death by affirming the actual presence of the dead person. The same is true of the affirmation that she would have received an inheritance if she had stayed at the emergency clinic. Again, fantasies of such an acquisition of wealth are common among poor Neapolitans, but normal persons do not have public temper tantrums because an expectation of this kind is not fulfilled. In general, one might say that the common cultural beliefs in magic and the supernatural differ from delusions in that the person holding the former is able to relate belief and situational reality with a fluidity which is lacking in the person suffering from a delusion.[7]

The second relevant criterion concerns affect. In the classical textbooks, schizophrenia is defined in terms of lack of affect or "inappropriate" affect. However, the latter term implies a normative standard as to what affect is appropriative, and such standards are known to fluctuate widely. Many forms of affective reaction which would be inappropriate for the professional psychiatrist may be far less so by the more tolerant conventions of the Neapolitan slum. Thus the patient's father was not judged crazy when he sliced the mother with a razor, for the gesture

7. See Carlo Felice Coppola, "Diagnosi Differenziale fra sintomo del Mutamento Pauroso e Stato d'Allarme nevrastenico," *L'Ospedale Psichiatrico* [Naples] (1960) 1 fasc., January–March: 1–38. In attempting to differentiate neurotic from schizophrenic anxiety, the author observes (p. 28) that ". . . as long as it is not explained, as long as it appears as irrational panic, fear is an intolerable suffering for the individual; so it has an inherent need of explanation by laws of causality, just as a chemical body needs to saturate its own valences. But in the case of neurosis, it gives rise to a fluid link (that is, a reasonable, logical, or representative explanation that can be discussed) while in the case of schizophrenia, it gives rise to a stable link—that is, a delusion." A similar comparison might be made between delusions and culturally appropriate beliefs in magic or witchcraft—the latter, because they are socially shared and exchanged in communication, could be seen as closer to neurotic mechanisms for dealing with anxiety. See "Expressive Symbolism in Witchcraft and Delusion," [this book, Chapter 7.]

has a commonly understood social meaning, which in this case influenced the mother to marry him.

But again it is more difficult to give a commonly understood social meaning to the patient's affects; in fact, her relatives indicated that they found her feelings impossible to understand, and she herself said that she felt badly misunderstood. Two phenomena of the acute phase are relevant in this respect. First, although her husband found the jealousy she expressed during courtship to be quite comprehensible, he began to think of her as crazy when she expressed the idea that he was sexually involved with her mother; for although jealousy is freely expressed by Neapolitan wives and girl friends, it usually concerns more obvious threats of infidelity and is not likely to involve older persons within the family. Second, the patient herself talked of terror—not jealousy—at the point of onset, when she began to fight with shadow women. Thus intense panic, giving rise to delusion formation, and alienation from any appropriate social object—which the shadow women revealed—would seem to be the most important features of the schizophrenic reaction in Naples, as in the United States.

Further similarities can be found by going beyond description and into dynamics. First, Giuseppina's delusions can be seen as based on the mechanism of projection, as is true of paranoid delusions in American culture, even though the content of delusions in the two cultures varies considerably. Second, homosexual impulses related to a primitive oral attachment to the mother—which, according to psychoanalytic theory, projection is a defense against—can be seen as important dynamic determinants in the case of Giuseppina. This is shown by her concern with girl friends who had "done bad things" to her, by her choice of a female agent for the delusional pregnancy, and by her intense hostility toward the nurses who had placed her on the bed in a passive position. Moreover, the pregenital nature of the impulses is shown by her feeling of bodily deformation in the anal area and the terror evoked by the image of teeth. The intensity of her need for her mother is revealed at many points—in her childhood jealousy, in the coincidence of the breakdown with a period of alienation from her mother and the coincidence of reconciliation with improvement, and in the half-carried-through attempt to identify with her mother by learning higher-status social patterns. Giuseppina's accentuation of her independence in courtship and marriage shows the other side of an ambivalent relationship.

Features of the Schizophrenic Episode Specific to the Cultural Context

Certain other features of Giuseppina's illness do not correspond to common assumptions about schizophrenia in the United States. At various times in the history of American psychiatry, generalized inhibition of affect and continuous social insecurity have been considered to be the essence of the schizophrenic personality, so that schizoid has come to mean cold, withdrawn, and tending to live more in ideas or fantasy than in the immediate social reality. But these traits are not characteristic, to any marked degree, of most Neapolitan schizophrenic women.

In the case of Giuseppina, although one can meaningfully speak of withdrawal from reality into fantasy in describing her symptoms, one cannot characterize her as a globally withdrawn or inhibited personality, either before the onset of psychosis, during the acute phase, or in the postpsychotic period. On the contrary, she seemed almost a polar opposite of the classical "schizoid" personality—even in the acute phase of psychosis, the outward expression of her emotional reactions was like a continuous explosive force. And she was characterized by her relatives as "jealous and capricious"—personality traits which are fairly common in her environment,[8] as was her tendency to dramatize by rhetoric and gesture.

8. About one-third of the 25 patients in the Italian sample could be characterized as jealous and capricious, like Giuseppina. The other two-thirds appeared "quiet and good," inhibited in the expression of aggression but not in the manifestation of childlike affection. See "Family Dynamics in South Italian Schizophrenics" [this book, Chapter 3].

A second feature closely related to the cultural context is the fact that the period of courtship and the beginning of marriage was the time of particular stress during which the psychotic episode was precipitated. A difficult and traumatic courtship such as Giuseppina's is not at all unusual in the cultural setting, and the only difference between her and many others who violate chaperonage norms and overthrow parental vetoes is that the situation really did drive her crazy, while others might use such a phrase merely to dramatize their difficulties. It was also true of Giuseppina and of almost all the schizophrenic patients I saw in Naples that they retained an elementary facility in handling conventional social situations, and perhaps for this reason the problem of 'making contact' was not too difficult in most instances.[9]

These contrasts can be related to the nature of the family system and its relations to the surrounding social world. First, Southern Italy, unlike American middle-class society, does not require, as maturity is reached, a progressively increasing independence from the natal family. Rather, for women, at least, too much independence leaves one open to the suspicion of being a bad woman. Actually, in the city young girls are not wholly bound by the home role—for example, Giuseppina attended school and held outside jobs. However, growing up in a Neapolitan *basso* provides little in the way of solitude or physical isolation from others, so that the process of social exchange is a constant one, and the gestural and verbal components of this exchange are a direct continuation of those learned in the initial family attachments. This can be compared with the situation of

9. The informality of the hospital and elaboration of nonverbal communication were important in this respect. A lesser social withdrawal among schizophrenics has also been observed in Japan by Caudill and among South American Indians by Stainbrook; the latter reports a conversation, with an acute catatonic terrified by spirits but not afraid of people, "because they are human beings." William Caudill, "Observations on the Cultural Context of Japanese Psychiatry," pp. 213–242; in *Culture and Mental Health,* ed. Marvin K. Opler (New York, The Macmillan Company, 1959); see especially p. 233. Edward Stainbrook, "Some Characteristics of the Psychopathology of Schizophrenic Behavior in Bahian Society," *Amer. J. Psychiat.* (1952) *109* : 330–335; p. 333.

the American child or adolescent who must venture out into a wide and empty social space on his own. The very common social ineffectiveness and gross affective inhibition of the American preschizophrenic might be seen as the result of a failure to make the leap from the family world into a discontinuous outside society.

This failure has usually been related to intense anxiety and dependency needs. However, given a centripetal family system such as the Southern Italian one, it is the dependency which is the most obvious phenomenon. The very widespread occurrence of acute conflicts associated with courtship—the rebellion which appears in patterns such as violating chaperonage rules and marrying after elopement—may be necessary so that a dependent attachment to the natal family can be broken. This appears in the psychotic sample in that, for all of those patients who broke down either before or soon after marriage, some association with courtship problems could be discerned. And like Giuseppina, most of the married patients showed some retreat from the marital situation back to the shelter of the natal family in conjunction with psychosis.

In the sample of American schizophrenics studied, two very common personality trends were often badly juxtaposed in a single patient: a conspicuous infantilism and a precise and controlled but unenthusiastic adulthood. Many southern Italian schizophrenic women also have childlike personalities, but with less distortion or unpleasantness. The difference may be the result of a social structure which in demanding less individually also provides mechanisms which limit gyration into the bizarre.

Finally, the apparent ease with which the patient was able to recover from acute psychosis in an impersonal hospital situation provides a convenient focus for considering the relations between individual psychodynamics and cultural expressive mechanisms. One might attribute Giuseppina's social recovery to the continued presence of the dependency objects—that is, the frequent visits of her family. However, during the acute phase she was 'out of contact' with her family, and its members, by calling her crazy, excluded her from social participation. Thus there must have been some internal change which modified the overt psychotic symptomatology to the point where readmission to the family became possible. As a beginning, one could point to the emotional and exaggerated behavior of the patient in the hospital as cathartic and say that she was able to 'express' her conflicts, the process of expression being abetted by her membership in a society which demands far less rational control than many others require.

A further clue to the recovery mechanism can be found in her vehement response to the patient who suggested that mental illness might make one lose affect for one's children. Her response was a rhetorically elaborated self-defense against the implication that she did not really care about her child, which served simultaneously to vanquish the attacker and to express the rage which she then felt. The continuing unconscious operation of the psychotogenic problems is indicated by her defensive quickness to respond, but the response itself, including the derogation of others, is not qualitatively different from the response which any Neapolitan of her milieu makes to an offense. It can be taken as an example of the honor ethic: Rather than dutifully admitting one's faults and weaknesses, as in Anglo-Saxon culture, one denies them, throwing the offense back on to the offender in the best possible style while setting up oneself as a paragon of all possible virtues.

In a sense this is an ethic based on denial; certainly the patient's improvement cannot be attributed to her acquiring a rational understanding of her emotional problems. Had I at that moment reminded her that she was not actually a respectable woman, by her own standard, because of the premarital sex relations, or suggested that she 'really' had aggressive feelings toward her child, I would no doubt have received a good blow for my pains, or at least have had several generations of my ancestors roundly cursed. Nevertheless, there is a crucial difference between this response and the more revealing but less coherent ones of the acute phase; the patient had regained the ability to use conventional expressive mechanisms and thus to make others respond to her. None of her intimates would have taken her self-defense as evidence that she was crazy.

However, one must be extremely cautious about assuming that the patient has expressed *rather than inhibited* her conflicts. If one assumes that all intimate conflicts are openly expressed in an emotive culture such as the South Italian one, it becomes extremely difficult to see why mental illness should occur at all—that is, why did not Giuseppina express her conflicts earlier and save herself the trouble of a psychosis? That she did not indicates that some conflicts were repressed; moreover, the continual operation of repression can be seen not only in the above episode, but also throughout the postpsychotic period, in which, for example, she seemed to repeatedly emphasize her intense interest in the child, as if to squelch the aggressive impulses which were revealed by projection earlier. It might be better to see her outburst against the other patient as reinforcing rather than eliminating repression—that is, as hysterical. The difference between Giuseppina and the patients commonly seen in American hospitals who recover from acute psychotic episodes by means of inhibition and affective constriction, then, would lie principally in the mechanism by which repression is reinstated, not in the presence or absence of repression as such.

In other words, although repression is reinstated, it seems that the improvement took place by means of expressive mechanisms—that is, a conscious dramatic emphasis of emotionality—rather than by means either of an avoidance of affect and constriction or the achievement of insight. This raises a seeming paradox: Psychosis may be seen as the break-through of conflicts from repression, and social recovery as a process of re-repression, in an expressively oriented culture as well as in one which emphasizes rationality and self-control. But like most seeming paradoxes, this calls for a closer analysis of the concepts involved, since it is by no means established that the anthropologist who makes the distinction between rationally and expressively oriented cultures means the same thing as the psychoanalyst who distinguishes between repression and break-through into consciousness of unconscious conflicts. For the patient under discussion, the terrifyingly intense affects of the psychotic period seem to be very clearly different from those of the postpsychotic period, which are held fairly well under ego control. In the latter the elements of coherent style and communicability are highly significant; in the former they appear to be threatened with disruption. Moreover, those affects which tended to disappear with social improvement are condemned in her own culture as well as in many others—for example, homosexual impulses and intense destructive wishes toward an infant —and they reappeared later on when she again became somewhat disturbed.

Thus it might be useful to make a distinction between uninhibited instinct, seen as terrifying in any culture, and socialized affect, expressible in many different ways and within different limits depending on the cultural value system. It is the threat of the first which drove the patient into psychosis, and it is the use of socialized mechanisms of expression to which recovery can be attributed. Socially acceptable affect is in any culture limited to certain tones in the total human spectrum which psychoanalysis is attempting to analyze. But given the requirement that affect in any culture characteristically must be socialized to some extent, one no longer has any basis for saying with certainty that instinctual drives are more openly expressed in Southern Italy than anywhere else; the difference between this culture and a puritanic one may lie principally in the channeling of affect by means of dramatization rather than by a deliberate attempt at consistency, control, or self-understanding.

In this respect, the work of an Italian anthropologist, de Martino, is of particular interest.[10] In interpreting the funeral laments still used by Lucanian peasants, he comes to the conclusion that the highly dramatic re-evoking of memories of the deceased on which they are based—which an Anglo-Saxon could easily see as evidence that there is far less inhibition of grief than he is accustomed to—can be conceived of as a mechanism for isolating the participant from the destructive potenti-

10. Ernesto de Martino, *Morte e Pianto Rituale nel Mondo antico* (Turin: Einaudi, 1958); see especially Chapter 2, pp. 57–110.

alities of the immediate and most poignant grief reaction; the repetition stereotypes the affect so that it is depersonalized and mastered and given meaning in a wider cultural framework. In her improvement, Giuseppina appeared to be using just such a detachment mechanism; by repeating, formalizing, and exaggerating certain affects she was enabled to repress others, to isolate herself from the destructive consequences of the psychotic break-through, and to reachieve a role in culture.

Thus rather than appearing as evidence for the greater acceptability of id impulses, the highly dramatic expressivity of South Italian culture might be given a particular place among the ego mechanisms, different from, but in this respect fulfilling the same function as, an emphasis on rational self-control. Expressive ego mechanisms are, of course, not lacking in scientific and professional cultures, but with a few notable exceptions[11] they have been grossly underemphasized by psychoanalytic theory, in which Freud's rationalist definition of the ego still holds sway. When one looks at unconscious impulses as expressed in the delusions of the psychotic patient, Freud's theories seem far less culture-bound than some anthropologists have believed. However, before it is possible to work out a unified model of personality which can be successfully used cross-culturally, it will be necessary to amplify the definition of the ego to include the honor ethic of the Neapolitan slum resident as well as the rationalist and introspective ethic of the psychoanalyst.

11. Including Freud's "Wit in Its Relation to the Unconscious," pp. 663–803; in *The Basic Writings of Sigmund Freud,* ed. A. A. Brill (New York, Modern Library, 1938).

The recent work of Bateson and his associates points the way to a much more precise attempt to deal with expressive difficulties in schizophrenia than has yet been accomplished. See Gregory Bateson, Don D. Jackson, Jay Haley, and John Weakland, "Toward a Theory of Schizophrenia," *Behavioral Science* (1956) 1 : 251–264; and Jay Haley, "Paradoxes in Play, Fantasy, and Psychotherapy," *Psychiatric Research Reports,* No. 2, Amer. Psychiatric Assn., December, 1955, pp. 52–58.

part four

Religion and Social Change

These three chapters deal with the relation between religion and social interaction, under conditions of radical change. Anne Parsons' sensitivity to the variant symbolic meanings implicit in all ceremony, and her appreciation of the subtle fit between ritual form and personality content, are used to advantage here.

All three contributions are concerned with the pathological accompaniments and strains of religious conversion; all interpret the significance of the mixing of old cultural elements and new; all deal with Catholics who have become—at least in some doctrinal regards—Protestants. But the findings demonstrate that these transformations are not so much incomplete as they are complex. "Religion" is not an abstract category, but an interpretable body of acts and their accompanying understandings, given life through the social maneuvers, both concrete and symbolic, of the participants.

237

In all three cases, the author is dealing with the adjustments of those who must find their faith in what is, for them, a different world. Her insights are particularly telling in the sphere of sexual and generational differences, and familial relationships— those between husbands and wives, and between parents and children. She shown that contradictory elements may be bound up within a single personality, rather than counterposed in terms of different groups; that individual personalities are very differentially integrated; and that both "personality" and "culture" must be abstracted from concrete behavior, if we are to understand either personality *in* culture, or culture *in* personality.

Two chapters deal with a Pentecostal congregation composed primarily of first-generation South Italian immigrants to the United States; the third paper, a brief book review, discusses a quasi-Protestant cult leader. All reveal Anne Parsons' attempt to escape the limitations of disciplinary parochialism.

chapter 10

The Pentecostal Immigrants, I

A Study of an Ethnic Central City Church*

In a recent particularly thought-provoking book, *The Suburban Captivity of the Churches*,[1] Gibson Winter has raised a challenge for contemporary American Protestantism. His major thesis is that the denominational churches in the suburbs have lost the sense of mission and ministry, and along with it the sense of the church as a community based on faith, as a consequence of a number of complex processes character-

* I am indebted to John Boyles for critical comments on this paper; to many other students at the Yale Divinity School for the discussions which have inspired it; and to the Foundations' Fund for Research in Psychiatry for support during the period in which my observations of the Pentecostal immigrants were made.

1. Gibson Winter, *The Suburban Captivity of the Churches:* An Analysis of Protestant Responsibility in the Expanding Metropolis (New York: The Macmillan Company, 1962).

Reprinted by permission of the Society for the Scientific Study of Religion, from *J. for the Scientific Study of Religion*, 4 (1964), 183–222.

izing the development of modern metropolitan areas. Tracing the changing ecological pattern of church distribution and membership over the past few decades, Dr. Winter shows how the suburban church has become progressively more isolated from central city areas, having to devote more and more efforts simply to maintaining its own community consisting in the highly mobile populations of the suburbs. The congregation thus becomes a social grouping which is subtly distinguished from significant other congregations in terms of similarity of socio-economic status and consumption styles. At the present time, middle-class Protestantism has little or no relation to the working-class Protestantism embodied in the very different ethnic churches and small store-front sects. In this respect, the organization of Protestant churches parallels the structure of American society as a whole in which geographical distance and the isolation of residence from place of work make for a much greater degree of segregation along class lines than is found in many other societies.

However, the loss of the sense of mission and ministry is more than a simple consequence of geographical insulation from the working-class. The suburban churches are seen not only as using socio-economic criteria as the primary basis for membership, but also as being introverted in the sense that their multitudinous "organizational" activities have as their primary end their own perpetuation. Thus the church is not usually in the forefront of social change, as it has been in many past epochs. This introversion is in turn related to an excessive privatization of the religious life: just as the suburban residence is separated from the place of work of the breadwinner, so is religion separated from the social responsibility that goes with public life. The danger is that it can increasingly become simply another variant of psychotherapy. Winter comments that the suburban minister does come into contact with human suffering in the form of illness, death, and intra-family turmoil among his parishioners, but having little or no contact with their public lives, he may be at a loss when it comes to creating standards for moral action and choice in the wider community. But if the

Christian minister truly means it when he tells his parishioners to "love thy neighbor," he should refer not only to his wife and children and his neighbor of like socio-economic status in the split-level ranch house next door, but also to all of his neighbors in the metropolis, the nation, and the world: Christianity is a religion based on universal principles of brotherly love. Both Winter and other writers have pointed to the kinds of depression or lack of a sense of faith and community that can underlie the frenetic and introverted "organizational" activities of the suburbs. It is as if the morally responsible being cannot live without some representation going beyond the immediate present in social relationships of that to which he is responsible. Thus it is evident that leading an exodus from the suburban captivity would be a very worthwhile contemporary mission for the church.

But to think about such an exodus is far easier than to actually accomplish it. One of Winter's suggestions is for new forms of church organization which would link up the suburbs with the central city area in a wider metropolis. However, such organization cannot be created without some knowledge and understanding of the religious groups which already exist in the central city area, which is far from being the spiritual void it is often thought to be. One need only take a walk through a crowded slum section and count the "Jesus Saves" signs, either in neon or the more modest hand-done lettering characterizing the store-front churches, in order to see this fact. The problem is not one of a total lack of religious organization, but rather of the existence of religious groups whose belief systems and style of worship can be quite different from those of the denominational churches.

In other words, the great difficulty lying in the way of the creation of a unified metropolitan religious community lies in the fact that there are great schisms between social groups in the metropolis. To a great extent of course, this is a consequence of the role played by immigration in American history. By and large, the urban working-class is made up of immigrants and their descendants, and the original Anglo-Saxon settlers have been pushed or repulsed outwards into the suburbs as new arrivals have taken over their former homes. In the early part of the century, the most important groups were from Roman or Orthodox Catholic areas of Southern and Eastern Europe; today the urban slums are being filled by Negro migrants from the South or the West Indies and by Puerto Ricans. The cultures of these people are quite different from those of England and Northern Europe and this diversity is certainly a factor underlying the tendency of white Protestant Americans to band together with others of like socio-economic status in religion as well as other spheres.

However, it is also a fact that the defensiveness inherent to contacts with people of other cultures may disappear when their life-ways come to be understood. It is in this respect that the religious specialist may call upon the anthropologist. Anthropology as a discipline has had a particularly rapid growth in the United States in part just because of the great variety of life-ways that can be observed within the metropolitan area. As a specialist, the anthropologist tries to understand social groups which differ from his own: usually through the method of participant observation, or simply by attending functions at which he would not be present were it not for his profession, he tries to find out what these activities are like—how they work and what kind of standards and beliefs govern those who do participate as true members. The minister on the other hand is quite a different kind of specialist. Living within the community to which he definitely does belong, he tries in some way to provide answers to the questions of meaning asked by his congregation and to point the way towards moral action. Thus the anthropologist is an outsider while the minister is an insider, and the perspectives of the two differ in relation to this fact. But given the very great internal complexity of American society, it may be necessary to add a new dimension to the role of the minister if he is to deal successfully with relationships in the broader society, rather than simply with the private conflicts of members of a homogeneous congregation. Among other things, he needs to know something about religious organizations other than his own, and in this respect anthropology may be able to provide a great deal of descriptive material.

In the recent past, the various forms of sect religion which are found both in American central city areas and in the newly developing countries of Latin America, Africa, and the Far East have been a special focus of anthropological study. One thing which has become apparent is that there is a great variety of possible religious syncretisms, each of which occurs in some group which, while in contact with one of the major religions possessing a highly developed literary tradition, also is still anchored in tribal, proletarian, or peasant life. Many of these are closely related to culture change, such as the African sect described by Messenger[2] which re-interpreted the teachings of missionaries so as to fit the model of its own kinship structure according to which God had to have elder brothers as well as a son.

While few of the immigrant residents of American urban slums were born in tribal cultures, many did come from Roman Catholic peasant areas where the popular religion is far more animistic than that of Catholic theologians. Not all of them have remained within the Catholic fold. While few working-class immigrants have been attracted to the more traditional Protestant denominations, a great many have converted to the Church of God, the Jehovah's Witnesses, the Pentecostal churches, and the great host of small and more or less independent small sects which are generally ranked at the bottom of the religious prestige hierarchy. Such sects are an important part of Puerto Rican life in New York City today; they also occur in Puerto Rico itself[3] and throughout Latin America. In a certain sense they can be seen as present-day re-enactments of the Reformation, a fact that makes them of particular significance for any attempt to apply contemporary social science methods to questions concerning the history of religious institutions. In this

2. John C. Messenger, Jr., "Reinterpretations of Christian and Indigenous Belief in a Nigerian Nativist Church," *The Amer. Anthropolog., 62,* 268–78 (1960).

3. Sidney Mintz, *Worker in the Cane: A Puerto Rican Life History* (New Haven: Yale Univ. Press, 1960).

paper, I should like to describe an Italian immigrant sect, calling itself the *Chiesa Evangelica Italiana* or the Italian Evangelical Church. Located in the central city, it would fall into the group of ethnic churches as delineated by Winter (*op. cit.* pp. 123–32) in that a major function was certainly to preserve a traditional community based on an interlocking of cultural, social, and family ties. At the same time, there is no doubt but that it acted as a dynamic force in social change. I will attempt to present the data in a double perspective which brings out both conservative and dynamic elements.

The Italian Evangelical Church
An Interpretation

The largest body of the congregation and the one which held the dominant position consisted in a group of middle-aged and elderly immigrants from rural areas in Southern Italy who had converted somewhere around the time of arrival in the United States. Important sub-groups consisted in their American-born children and grandchildren, and a smaller group of post World-War II arrivals, many of whom had converted in Italy and come to the United States with the aid of fellow Protestants. There was considerable open conflict between the immigrants and the American-born generations, resulting in a separate but subsidiary set of English-language activities whose religious style was much more directly inspired by the contemporary American revivalism of the Billy Graham type than that of the Italian-born membership. My own observations center primarily on the latter group: for a period of about 18 months I attended Italian-language services and Bible class on Sunday mornings and on weekday evenings.

Calling itself Pentecostal in theology, for full membership the church required an adult conversion experience, symbolized by water baptism, and a revelation from the Holy Spirit manifested by speaking in tongues. Beyond the constant elements of Christian theology such as faith in Jesus Christ as the Son of

God, articles of faith referred to the Bible as the revealed source of all doctrine, to the literal existence of the devil and of evil spirits as his agents, and to the eventual resurrection of the body. The church would thus in contemporary American terms fall into the category of fundamentalism or evangelicism. However, as I shall try to show, the meaning of fundamentalism is quite different when it is a question of recently converted Protestants than when it is a question of a conservative attempt to preserve traditional beliefs against inroads made by modern intellectual criticism. In addition, the church should be considered as revivalist in that emotional expression in services was open and often vehement rather than quiet and restrained, and it had many of the characteristics of the sect in that it saw itself as a distinctive religious community isolated from the world.

However, by the time I observed it, the congregation had made many steps from sect status to that of the more substantial church. Thirty years earlier, a small group of converts had rented an upstairs room from a storeowner, but with increasing membership and increasing prosperity among the members, a fairly substantial edifice was constructed which, moreover, then ceased to coincide with the residences of members. Bordering on a slum section torn down by Urban Redevelopment, it was peopled by a congregation of either upper-level working-class or lower-middle-class semi-suburbians, who commuted in by car. Average Sunday attendance was about 200, which is well above the level of store-front churches. However, it remained a sect in that religious activities were so extensive as to take up most of the non-working time of the members (with three-hour services on Sunday morning), and in that it maintained a number of strict taboos over daily life, notably in prohibiting drinking and smoking.[4]

The new church building was a symbolic expression of the

4. However, the taboo on alcohol conflicted with certain ingrained Italian cultural patterns, and the latter did not easily give way. At the home of one member who was very strict, I was served cherry soda in a bottle shaped like a wine bottle along with the spaghetti, but at the home of a family close to the pastor, I was given both wine and liquor. A public wedding I attended was completely dry.

values of ascetic Protestantism as epitomized in the simplicity of New England architecture. But the significance of this only stands out when we make the comparison with the over-elaborate Baroque of the Catholic churches in which most of the members had been brought up. Lacking even the simplest of crucifixes, the front of the church was adorned only with the lectern, a large cut-out Bible, and "Thou shalt not make unto thee any graven image, or any likeness of any thing that is in heaven above, or that is in the earth beneath, or that is in the water under the earth" (Exodus 20:4) in gold lettering around the choir. The significance of this again only stands out by reference to the past. At least in its peasant variants, South Italian Catholicism is far from being a monotheistic religion in that quasi-magical cults of local saints and the all-important Madonna make up a vital part of the religious life. Thus for many of these people a very literal throwing out of the graven images, or the candle-lit pictures, statues of saints and the Madonna that decorate every South Italian home, no matter how poor, had been part of the conversion experience.[5] Thus on the surface at least, the congregation had very clearly assimilated the values of ascetic Protestantism.

The degree of successful assimilation was obvious in many ways going beyond the church architecture. Protestantism is noted among other things for its furthering of a sense of community responsibility. In this sphere, the very fact of the construction of such a substantial church building and its successful day-to-day operation testified as to gains made in the acculturation process. Although mutual aid within the family, where immediate emotional ties are very strong, is common in the South

5. A French sociological journalist, Helena Cassin in *San Nicandro: The Story of a Religious Phenomenon* (London: Cohen & West, 1959) has very vividly described a village conversion in Southern Italy in which, though the conversion was to Judaism rather than Protestantism, the dynamics are the same in that a magico-animistic system of beliefs was given up in favor of rational monotheism. A large portion of the following of the self-styled prophet, Domenico Menduzion, deserted him when it came to throwing out the graven images.

Italian village, great difficulty has been encountered by reformers attempting to secure community co-operation at the village level. However, the parishioners of the Italian Evangelical Church built and maintained their own organization with very little help from outside, not to mention their contributions to church building in Italy. But just because it can become an obsessional pattern in the suburbs, we should not underrate the importance of the capacity for carrying out independent local community activities: it is on this capacity that democratic government is based.

For the parishioners themselves, this capacity was symbolized and perhaps internalized in the process of hymn-singing. This latter activity was attributed very great significance, so that verses were never skipped and very often were repeated. During the collective bursting-out of solid Protestant chorales, the entire congregation stood up straight in a very determined manner—as if it were telling itself that unity could prevail in spite of the factionalizing tendencies that characterize South Italian life. As Alan Lomax has pointed out,[6] choral singing is no more characteristic of Southern Italy than it is of the despotic societies of the east.

A second point which has often been made concerning Protestantism is that its value system and economic ethic are such as to further the growth of the middle-classes and the process of capitalist expansion, the classic work being Max Weber's *The Protestant Ethic and the Spirit of Capitalism*. One aspect of Weber's thesis is that the ascetic and disciplined way of life that Protestantism preaches encourages saving and thus makes possible the expansion of industry. The validity of what he says comes out very clearly when one looks comparatively: while at least in the urban areas of Southern Italy, some persons are able to gain substantial wealth from commercial activity, this wealth tends to dissipate itself over time as a consequence of the natural desires of the flesh. However, the real life consequences of a sucessful internalization of the "Protestant ethic"

6. Alan Lomax, Folk Song Style, *Amer. Anthropolog. 61*, 927–51 (1959).

were quite visible among the parishioners of the Italian Evangelical Church. For the most part poor at the time of immigration, by now the majority own cars and houses, and though still far from the college-educated segment of the population, they had moved into the upper-level working-class or into lower middle-class business and clerical groups.[7] The relation between conversion and social mobility was made very clear in the account of one now prosperous small businessman who told me how he first got "in the spirit" and turned over a great many chairs in the loft after deliberately restraining himself from drawing a knife after a card game offense; this was the first step in his increasingly successful adaptation to middle-class behavioral standards. At the very least, the great majority were steady workers and it is doubtful that any had contributed to the gangsterism and vice that so often accompany the breakdown of traditional social structures.

Thus as expressed in one testimonial, "I thank my savior Jesus Christ that He has given me the will power to put my money in the bank instead of spending it every day on the useless frivolities of the world." The church acted in many concrete ways so as to further the process of mobility from peasant or artisan status towards the middle-class. Beyond any explicit emphasis on saving are the idea of the church as a religious community which is isolated from the world and the taboos on drinking and smoking. The latter served to crystallize and make concrete the idea of giving up immediate pleasures in the interest of future gain, while the former in a more global way served to heighten the self-characterization of the parishioners

7. Unfortunately, I did not carry out any systematic study of socio-economic status. Probably it would show considerable variation within the congregation (held together more by the ethnic link than by socio-economic status as such) with an average level somewhat higher than that of a comparable group of still Roman Catholic immigrants. An additional factor, however, is that average status in Italy, especially for the recent immigrants, was probably somewhat higher than for the mass of landless peasants who have contributed the numerically most important contingent to the mass immigration. For the recent immigrants, backgrounds in the artisanry or the lower levels of the bureaucratic middle-class were common.

as different from the average slum dweller who lives from moment to moment. The immediacy of the threat of "back-sliding" was made quite vivid in a number of sermons in which the preacher made it clear how much of a temptation it can be when friends invite you for a drink at the bar or to play the "numbers" rather than sticking to business.

However, of all the fundamentalist taboos, the one which seemed to arouse the most anxiety in the congregation was that against taking the name of the Lord in vain. This anxiety was revealed in frequent references to "those Italians who call themselves Christians" (i.e., Roman Catholic Italians)[8] and nevertheless do so. But in this anxiety we can see the very heart of the meaning of conversion to these people. In the poorer areas of Italy, swearing is indeed a very characteristic phenomenon, so common that every positive religious image has its negative complement in the form of an oath or obscenity. However, the common use of oaths is not an isolated phenomenon: rather it is tied up with a whole range of others which serve to demonstrate the existence of conflicts within the Catholic framework which in so many respects its participants have outgrown. Related phenomena are a systematic anti-clerical attitude among men— so that they spend a great deal of time in making derogatory jokes about priests and very rarely attend mass as adults—and a sarcastically negative view about higher authority in general.

These attitudes in turn come from open resentment against the authoritarian views which characterize many of the clergy and the widespread poverty about which neither religious nor secular authority does very much—so from the perspective of those who live with it, it looks like an unchangeable aspect of fate. Thus aggression gets turned negatively against the status quo, rather than being utilized in the interest of change: in other

8. In Southern Italy, the word "Christian" is used in a global humanistic way simply to designate man as a creature possessing reason who is different from the beast: this usage dates back to the Middle-Ages when religious pluralism was unknown. However, to this congregation it very clearly signified the members of the church as differentiated from the world, i.e., a group of people sharing common beliefs and behavioral standards.

words, the poorer South Italian Catholics do not like the situation they are in, but aside from emigration, they do not do anything very constructive about it. In sharp contrast, the systematic repression of the expression of negative feelings that characterizes the Protestant group is perhaps the most important token of the fact that in the adoption of a new religious framework, it has indeed found a constructive alternative to the resignation found in the original environment. It is this fact which places the church in the forefront of social change.

However, as a considerable body of social science work goes to prove, it is simply not possible to change all at once in a consistent and unilinear direction. Thus while it is in fact possible to throw away graven images by a conscious act of will, it is not possible to do so without some inner turmoil or without some form in which the past returns even if under another guise. Thus while on the one hand, there were many sharp contrasts between the life-ways of the Italian Evangelical Church and those of Southern Italy, on the other there were many points at which one could glimpse either acute conflicts or important residues of the magico-animistic Roman Catholic tradition. Some of these elements can be focused in a discussion of the prayer period and sermon style and content.

Like all revivalist Protestant churches, this one utilized very openly emotional and collective forms of prayer. In its early history, people "in the spirit" used to turn over chairs in the loft with so much commotion that on one occasion the police were called; in consequence the congregation fired the pastor because of its sensitivity to the surrounding community. By the time of my observation, the manifestations of the spirit were for the most part purely verbal and parishioners very much resented the appellation "Holy Rollers." Nevertheless, the sound qualities and openness of expression in prayer were such as to differentiate it sharply from the more restrained expression of the suburbs. Likewise, the pastor, Sicilian in origin and a person who in the secular world might well have been a successful actor, was by his vivid and rapid verbalization and gesticulation in equally sharp contrast with the sober academic preaching style more common among his suburban colleagues.

It was most clearly in the prayer period that one could see all of the conflicts underlying the solid community spirit and the forward-looking optimism that characterized the singing of hymns. In fact, a kind of bi-polar opposition in values was built into the very structure of the religious service. Immediately after the initial hymn-singing, a sudden and dramatic reversal took place such as to give the observer the feeling of having been suddenly transported from a New England church to a funeral in Lucania.[9] Prayer-period was so individualistic that one's first impression was of a babel of sounds, each voice uttering its own pattern of lament, vehemence, or supplication with no attempt to harmonize with the whole. One of the most conspicuous features was the weeping and supplication of the women, creating a kind of wailing wall impression and contrasting sharply with the determined optimism of the hymns. It seemed to express unutterable grief at the loss of the past—or at the loss of sons marching confidently into the future. Others have to be seen in terms of the phenomenon of speaking in tongues, or the making of verbal utterances which according to members of the congregation could not be given any interpretation on a human level.

Speaking in tongues as a form of religious expression deserves a much more extensive treatment than is possible within the limits of this paper.[10] With respect to the church under consideration, there were two groups of such utterances which did

9. Ernesto de Martino, *Il Lamento Funebrale nel Mondo Antico* (Rome: Enaudi, 1958). In describing the funeral lament which has persisted from Graeco-Roman times until today in Mediterranean rural areas, the Italian anthropologist de Martino, shows how it expresses the very concrete and naturalistic attitude of the peasant towards death, where the focus is on the immediate emotional impact of the loss and its potentially destructive consequences, rather than on the on-going activities which can be carried out by the living.

10. Notably it seems to have an inherent relationship to culture change in that it does not characterize the better established Protestant denominations, but does characterize many change-associated groups. In the New Testament, it can be traced to St. Paul, an advocate of culture change in that it was he who created the most radical break between

not seem so mysterious to the observer. One was the very frequent repetition by women of the phrase *santa, santa, santa* (*santa* = saint), sometimes appearing in the more complex form of a series of indistinguishable words beginning with *santa*, but following a rhythmic pattern and phrase length exactly equivalent to that of *Santa Maria, piena di grazia* . . . or the Hail Mary which is intimately known to every Catholic. It was as if even having thrown away the graven images, these women were simply incapable of refraining from calling on Mary or the saints in moments of grief and trouble. The second concerns some much more aggressively-toned words and phrases, again not quite distinguishable according to content, but which sounded suspiciously like either curse words or like everyday derogatory expressions such as "shut up." Here it was as if the aggression which is so freely expressed in South Italian culture had somehow to return, even within the framework of the religious service.[11]

After fifteen minutes or so of praying out loud, the congregation would again face forwards for more hymn singing. However, within the sermon itself, the bi-polar structure of the service was again revealed. First, the pastor very rarely preached a straightforward and logical sermon following directly from the Bible text. Rather he would start with a text illustrating his major point, and from there proceed to a kind of dramatic role playing or a process of free association which communicated aesthetically rather than logically. Second, elements or views expressed within the sermon sometimes directly contradicted other elements of the same sermon in a way that brought to the fore conflicts related directly to culture change.

Christianity and Judaism by eliminating the requirement that the Christian convert also conform to rabbinical law.

11. To the Latin mentality, this is not as sacrilegious as it can appear from a Protestant point of view. At an annual ritual in the city of Naples which takes place in the cathedral, the blood of the patron saint, San Gennaro, preserved there is supposed to liquefy miraculously as a good omen for the health of the city in the coming year. However, if the miracle is not performed quickly enough for the impatient populace, it has been known to inform the saint of its displeasure with phrases such as "San Gennaro, you stinker," and worse.

An example is a sermon preached on the theme of *il cammino*. *Camminare* in Italian is the common verb meaning to walk; however, in Italy one very rarely hears the noun form which in the religious sense can mean "the way" (of truth). The moral gist of the sermon was that it is necessary to follow the religious way of life or the straight and narrow path that leads to salvation. It began on an affirmative note, indicating that with the proper self-discipline, one can indeed follow a religious way of life. However, about half-way through, the linguistic content of the sermon began to get more and more garbled so that a number of grammatically ambiguous phrases like "the founding of the foundation that was founded" came out. At the same time, the preacher became more and more dramatic in his immediate bodily and gestural expressions, vacillating towards and away from a spot on the floor designated as the "foundation," yelling and waving his arms in a manner reminiscent of the child who has a temper tantrum and simply will not budge from where he is. At this phase, he proclaimed rather plaintively that "we don't want to get left in the middle of the road," with the gestures used by the South Italian who is trying to beg himself off on the grounds of his poverty or misery from some shortcoming vis-à-vis the higher authorities. At this point then, he seemed to be bringing out the other side of a cultural conflict: it is not very easy to follow a new and more disciplined mode of life and the temptation to just sit there and complain about the present, or to remain glued to the past like Lot's wife, is a very real one. Only at the end of this sermon did the preacher again become verbally coherent and adult, in order to proclaim joyfully the promise of paradise in the manner of the returned Sicilian who is able to sit in the sun all day enjoying the fruits of his labor abroad.

Many other sermons also revealed the importance of culture conflict among the congregation: favorite themes during the period of my attendance were the promise of life-everlasting, the unfaithful members of the church, and the foolish iniquities of the young. Each had its referent in a concrete psychological or social problem facing the congregation: many persons did actually leave or threaten to leave the church, mainly in the face of pressures from close kin who had remained Roman Catholic; the ways of the second and third generation young were indeed different from those of the fathers and the spirit of rebellion was among them; the promise of life everlasting did not always seem a very secure one. In the latter sphere, the naturalism of the peasant attitude towards death made for considerable conflict with Protestant doctrine. For the peasant mentality, many pleasures are given in this world in compensation for the sufferings of man, but there is hardly any idea at all of an eternal reward contingent on the morality of one's behavior. The importance of the next world in fundamentalist Protestant doctrine does not appear to be simply a pie-in-the-sky idea that follows automatically from material deprivation, but rather is much more closely related to the degree to which it preaches abstinence from worldly pleasure.

Thus a number of sermons affirmed, but then expressed doubts, about the promise of reward for the just. Moreover, it was in this context that the idea of *spiriti maligni* or evil spirits took on its greatest importance. One sermon preached the Sunday after the death of a parishioner appeared to be a means for dealing with the wave of anxiety which swept the mainly middle-aged and elderly congregation. Drawing a circle on the floor which was again designated as the "foundation," the preacher proceeded to banish the evil spirits from this area of safety by quasi-magical gestures and exhortations. As very often was true on all topics, the sermon seemed to move through a cycle from affirmation to doubt and back to re-affirmation. The same cycle characterized the service as a whole, in that it moved from the upright and determined posture characterizing the initial hymn-singing to the grief and anger discernable in the prayer period (when each person faced backwards, perhaps towards the past) and back to the upright forward-facing position at the end. Thus one can see this particular and distinctive ritual structure as expressing simultaneously new values for the process of change and the undeniable residues of the past.

One way in which the change might be conceptualized is as a present-day re-enactment of the Reformation. In this context, we can next examine the role played by Bible reading in the life of the church. As noted above, the articles of faith put forth the literal interpretation of the Bible as the revealed source of all truth as primary; the importance of the Book was symbolized by the large cut-out Bible above the lectern which was the only ritual adornment. Bible reading and Bible quoting were very obviously crucial foci of congregational life, as were the sale, purchase, and ownership of Bibles of all sorts in both English and Italian, and Bible discussion groups were the activity second in importance to the services themselves. I also commented initially that the meaning of fundamentalism, or Biblical literal-ism, in this context was quite different from when it is a back-wards-moving resistance against the inroads of modern intellec-tual criticism or social and historical interpretation of the Bible. Rather, quite to the contrary, it had one very obviously pro-gressive determinant, namely that these people put so much emphasis on the Book and the process of reading it just because they had only very recently learned to read at all. In the areas from which they came, even today illiteracy rates run up to 25% of the adult population, and at the time of the mass emigration they were much higher. Some persons in the congregation had only learned to read as adults, and a few of the women were still illiterate or only semi-literate.[12] Probably the great majority had had illiterate parents. Thus while we take it for granted that people will read books from age six on, this was simply not the case for them.

But it is around the crucial significance of literacy that we can see in a fresher way the historical meaning of Protestantism in its relation to the present day. As Weber has pointed out,

12. Though such high status value was placed on literacy that they suffered from a continuous embarrassment about it, most of them would not admit to their ignorance, but rather when it came their turn in Bible class, it would somehow turn out that they had forgotten their glasses. Most of them knew the hymn-book by heart and did not need to follow the words anyway.

Protestantism from its beginning has been bound up with the rise of science, industry, and the middle class. However, one key factor on which all of these processes of change depend is the existence of mass, or at least widespread, literacy. To the Roman Catholic Middle Ages, literacy was not nearly the taken-for-granted social accomplishment that it is today: rather the written word, which did not correspond with the spoken vernacular, was a special power which was held in trust for the masses by the priesthood and the secular elite, often to be used for its own ends in order to exploit or to mystify those below. But the Reformation was of course a rebellion against the authoritarianism of the Middle Ages: it was very closely associated with the rise of nationalism and the movement towards translating the sacred Word into the vernacular—so that it would be available to every man who could then interpret its meaning for himself. This of course is a very fundamental step in the direction of human freedom.

Given the very basic social change entailed by the transition from illiteracy to literacy, it is not surprising that it then becomes necessary to take one thing as fixed, namely the content of the Book seen as the revealed source of all truth. Moreover, the actual use made of it in the Italian Evangelical Church was very far from being rigid or doctrinaire. As a social scientist looking from outside, I very often felt that it was by a noting of the selections and individual emphases made among scripture passages that I could come to my best and deepest conclusions about what was going on within the church: the method seemed far better than that of giving questionnaires or asking explicit questions that might call forth artificial or invented answers. Thus, for example, during a period of about two weeks the Italian language Bible class, made up mostly of recent immigrants, discussed the story of Joshua and the battle of Jericho, with great emphasis being put on the number and powers of the helpers that Joshua needed for carrying out the commands given by the Lord. During the same period, a power struggle for leadership roles went on within the group itself between the official discussion leader and several competitors, including one very expressive Sicilian who was more nostalgic for the truly revivalistic days when the spirit first swept his land than he was eager to carry out the sober task of establishment in the United States. Eventually the more teacher-like official leader won out, with many Biblical comments on his chosen role of leading the people towards the Promised Land.

Likewise, the same man, having a higher degree of education, had both of his parents as students. But when we discussed the marriage at Cana, he quite emphatically quoted Jesus: "Woman, what have I to do with thee?" (John 2:4), the statement made by Christ when he miraculously turns water into wine by himself, leaving his mother in the background. The entire group then became quite concerned about the Bible's use of the term "woman," rather than the more reverent "Mother" or "Mary." In the discussion, the leader's actual mother modified the gospel according to St. John to fit her own preference for the greater maternal power that goes with the Latin Madonna cult: "It's a story about Jesus, his mother, and his relatives," she said, turning to me with a whisper and a bit of anxiety. But another change which is closely bound up with Protestantism is the emancipation of the individual, according to his own achievements, from emotional or authoritarian family control. The same tension was revealed in matters pertaining to children. One day the discussion leader brought his son, who was far too young to read, to the class and insisted that he sit up straight by himself holding his book. The entire group, including myself, felt very nervous about this for fear that he would fall; Italian children are continually being pushed or fondled but are very rarely encouraged to do things on their own.

However, the fact of the matter is that all of these very basic advances in the direction of greater freedom and individuality which took place in Western Europe at the time of the Reformation are taking place today all over the world, not only among immigrant residents of American urban slums, but also and even more crucially in the many formerly subservient colonies where only in the twentieth century have people begun to think about nationalism, mass literacy, and industrial development. Just as the middle classes in the sixteenth century became Protestants in freeing themselves from the domination of the aristocracy, so today are a great many persons in the so-called underdeveloped areas—in the Caribbean,[13] Latin America, Africa, and the Far East—becoming Protestants in the course of their attempt to understand and assimilate for themselves the mysterious power based on familiarity with the written word that is now possessed by the powerful industrially advanced nations of the West.

Thus Weber's thesis on the association between Protestantism and the rise of industry is being confirmed from day to day in what is taking place outside of Western Europe and the United States, where this phase in social movement is already in a sense completed. An example concerns the very great "outpouring of the spirit" that took place in 1950 in Trinidad, the richest and most advanced of the islands in the British West Indies. As described to me by a formerly Hindu East Indian pastor, subsequently trained at a Bible school in the Western United States: "Many souls were saved in Trinidad that year— Hindus, Catholics, and souls still lost in primitive superstition and ignorance—it was a truly great outpouring of the spirit and many mighty works were performed by the hand of the Lord." One is reminded of the great American frontier revivals.[14]

But one of the sad facts about such movements of the spirit today is that they are almost completely unknown to the Protestant residents of American suburbs. These latter are indeed introverted, in that their religious energy is either focused only on private life, or it is directed towards the refinement of subtle sectarian differences based on consumption in a world in which material tokens of the Lord's favor have no more meaning because there are too many already. On the other hand, this is not true to the same extent of their fundamentalist brethren: it

13. Michael G. Smith, *Black Puritan,* Department of Extra-Mural Studies, Univ. of the West Indies, Kingston, Jamaica, 1963.

14. These latter, moreover, along with the fact that every pioneer family carried the Book when it went West, can be seen as enormously important determinants of the fact that literacy and middle-class behavioral standards were not lost in the face of the American wilderness.

is these latter that do still have the sense of mission and ministry and are willing to spread the Word to the unsaved. Thus today many Indiana farm boys and former residents of small towns in the South are quietly running small Bible stores or mission churches in various obscure and not very sanitary corners of the world, or helping to educate those who thirst after knowledge in the Bible schools of the United States. Thus they are participating actively in contemporary processes of social change, while the American suburbanites who belong to the richest and most highly educated large-scale sector of the entire world population sit at home, not knowing just how to act morally in the face of the broader problems facing contemporary humanity.

But if the suburban minister wishes to further awareness of the wider human community, to which both he and his parishioners owe a measure of responsibility, one way of going about this is to work towards some sort of linkage with those Protestant movements which are taking place both in American urban slums and in the underdeveloped areas. What the anthropologist can add to the classical and sometimes overly doctrinaire or intolerant kind of mission is the idea of cultural relativity: in order to understand and successfully communicate with other peoples, it is necessary to have some knowledge and understanding of the culture which they possess or have possessed prior to embarking upon a process of change. But the idea of cultural relativity is not necessarily incompatible with the possession of religious faith, as Roman Catholic missionaries have known for many centuries. Nor does it necessarily have to lead to the conservative wish to protect all traditional cultures against the inroads of change, even though many anthropologists in fact have such a wish and thus are inclined to prejudice against missions. Rather it can go along with an affirmation of our own cultural tradition as possessing real and meaningful values which we wish to spread and the belief that with patience and understanding we may be able to spread them at the same time as preserving a fundamental human respect for contrasting life ways.

Moreover, an identification of American suburban Protestants with the fundamentalist movements in the underdeveloped countries seems especially important, if one gives a political significance to religion. For another fact of the matter is that, besides Protestantism, the only system of belief which has proved itself capable of sponsoring industrial development on a large scale is Communism: also encouraging a disciplined life way, the diffusion of literacy, and saving for the future, but on an atheistic and usually less humanistic basis. Communism is the major competitor with our own system for the minds of men in areas which are just beginning to change.[15] But a number of recent unhappy American experiences have gone to show that you cannot help poor and backward nations just by giving them money: what is more important is that they have the education and system of beliefs to be able to do something for themselves. It is in the obvious self-interest of the United States to encourage such nationalistic self-help, which in turn depends upon the growth of solid middle classes in precisely those areas of the world which are most susceptible to Marxist ideology just because society is in fact divided between the few rich and the many, many poor. In such a way we can encourage the strengthening of allies whose values are basically similar to our own—though we would probably not want to interfere with independence wishes or the persistence of more microscopic cultural differences. Such a means of maintaining our present chosen position in the world seems more in accord with both Christian and American values than direct authoritarian control—and most important, a more moral alternative than maintaining this position by means of sheer military force. For in the military sphere, the sect prophecies stating that the end of the

15. Liston Pope, *Millhands and Preachers; A Study of Gastonia* (New Haven: Yale Univ. Press, 1942). For an intensive small-scale study which portrays not only the relationship between Protestantism and industrialization in recent times, but also a microcosm of today's major ideological struggle: when Communists attempted to turn labor discontent in North Carolina in 1929 into revolutionary channels, the churches played a major role in defeating them.

world is at hand can seem uncomfortably close to the reality which has been created by modern science and industry.[16]

Conclusion

In sum, one major way of leading an exodus from the suburban captivity would be the establishment of more meaningful links between the suburban denominational churches and both the central city congregations and the movements of the spirit in the underdeveloped world. From an organizational point of view, the questions concerning how such links could be established are far from being simple ones: a crucial fact is that the selection and training of ministers in the two camps of Protestantism differs in such a way as to make for many divergences of perspective. Today the denominational minister is a specialized professional, while the sect leader is likely to be a self-appointed prophet, a powerful and imaginative man within his own bailiwick, but ill at ease in the alien world outside.[17] However, to the extent that actual channels of contact are created, some meaningful intermingling of spirits should result though we might not be able to predict exactly what kind. In any case, in carrying out the work discussed above, I myself had a profound sense of identification with the other people who were there. Its sources lay both in my own immediate awareness of

16. It is not always certain whether it is the sects or the denominations which have the greatest awareness of contemporary reality. One sermon I heard preached in a Pentecostal church in the West Indies was on the need for moral restraint in the face of the explosive forces now at loose in the world; it began with information on missile launchings at what is now Cape Kennedy.

17. In Weber's terms (see Max Weber, "The Three Pure Types of Legitimate Authority," in *Max Weber: The Theory of Social and Economic Organization,* New York, The Free Press, 1947, pp. 328–29), the denominational minister possesses rational-legal authority, i.e., he achieves his position by passing through standardized training requirements. The sect preacher, in contrast, is usually a charismatic leader, i.e., lacking in formal education, he leads by virtue of whatever immediate personal power and attraction he possesses. However, especially in those groups where other channels of upward mobility are blocked, he is likely to be unusually intelligent. Pope found that the ability of ministers in Gastonia to reach millworkers varied in inverse relation to formal education.

their inner struggles and in their immediate awareness of mine, so that even though I did not phrase my own conflicts in Biblical language, the others did in ways which were very often psychologically accurate. In the Italian-language Bible class, a former resident of an isolated mountainous area said one day: "Jesus said 'love thy neighbor,' but who is my neighbor? . . . it must be the person next to me," and since I happened to be the person sitting next to him, he turned to me with a look of love. (Italian *vicino* which is the word for neighbor also means next to or near.) In the same group, we all followed from week to week the intense suffering of a Sicilian whose mother was dying in Sicily: as is generally true in this area, she was the closest person to him in this world, but at the same time his religious doctrine taught him that, still unconverted, she would burn in hell when she died. At the point of her actual death, he came very close to returning to the Catholic church, but with the real support of the group, he did not do so. And finally, I was led to rethink the meaning of my own liberal Protestant background, in which church affiliation followed automatically from family belonging, rather than being the result of a conscious individual choice made against opposition from outside.

11

The Pentecostal
Immigrants, II

Ritual and Culture Conflict

Bronislaw Malinowski's famous discussion of the circumstances that provoke the elaboration of ritual dealt with fishing techniques of the Trobriand Islanders. From the observation that the Islanders did not employ ritual before making their safe and rather routine lagoon fishing trips, but did, and most solemnly, before the more perilous and uncertain deep-sea ventures, he was led to postulate a general dictum about ritual—that it appears in situations of uncertainty and anxiety.[1] Viewed from this firmly psychological perspective, the function of ritual is not simply circular—that of maintaining a state of equilibrium of which the ritual enactment itself is a part—but progressive,

---

1. Bronislaw Malinowski, "Magic, Science, and Religion," in James Needham (ed.), *Science, Religion, and Reality* (London. 1925), p. 32.

A revision of a paper presented at the Annual Meetings of the American Anthropological Association, November, 1961.

facilitating cultural advance by lessening potential motivational blocks. So far as anxieties from natural sources are concerned, Malinowski's theory contains a verifiable prediction about change: as previously uncontrollable technical factors are mastered, the attached rituals will tend to disappear.

Malinowski did not apply his theory of ritual specifically to the problem of culture change. Such an application is practicable, however, if one attributes to ritual the psychological function of alleviating anxiety, as well as the psychological function of self-maintenance. In this perspective, culture change becomes a kind of deep-sea fishing expedition: the breakup of the prior state of equilibrium gives rise to anxiety and uncertainty, which is thereupon expressed in ritual; and the ritual facilitates in turn the process of "moving ahead" by creating a new meaning-frame of reference through symbolic manipulation. Thus we should expect to find a class of rituals specifically associated with culture change.

There is no doubt that many religious movements are closely associated with culture-change situations. One thinks of the Cargo cults of the Pacific; the modern peyote cults of the American Indian; or the revivalistic Protestantism characteristic of the British working classes in the early phases of industrialization. In the modern world, the spirit which formerly animated British and American Protestant revivals seems instead to be moving among populations more recently drawn into the industrial orbit, as in Africa and the Caribbean area, and among partly integrated immigrant or Negro groups in the United States. Herein is continued the description of a congregation in the last category: the Italian Evangelical Church, which meets in a slum section of an eastern American city, and whose membership consists primarily of South Italian peasants who came to the United States between twenty and forty years ago, converting from Roman Catholicism at about the same time.

Members of the church consider themselves Pentecostals; but for the immigrant group, at least, the major organizational link is with a loose federation of Italian-speaking Protestants in the United States. A summary of articles of faith published in the hymnbook refers to the Bible as the revealed source of all doctrine; to regeneration, or rebirth by faith in Christ, as confirmed by water baptism and by the baptism of the Holy Spirit manifested by speaking in tongues; in the literal existence of the devil, and of evil spirits as his agents; and to the eventual resurrection of the body. In actual fact, the religious style of the congregation differs considerably from that of other local Pentecostal groups. Thus, for instance, in contrast to Negro groups, the congregation forms a solid community in which relatively little effort need be spent by the leaders in deploring backsliding; many men are active participants; and there are few indications of possession or trance, most emotional expression being verbal rather than physical. The English-speaking offspring form a partly distinctive body within the church, having organizational links to the Christ Crusade, from which much of their religious style is taken; the present paper, however, is concerned only with the Sunday morning, and biweekly evening, Italian-language services.

There is considerable emphasis within the immigrant group on the Protestant virtues of thrift, hard work, and this-worldly optimism; in a public testimony, one church member explicitly thanked God that she had religion, and hence had no need to waste money on frivolous entertainment. That this emphasis has led to a fairly successful overt adaptation for most of the members is suggested by the fact that, while the church building remains near the ethnic slum where the parishioners first settled, most members now have to travel long distances by car from outlying and more prosperous working- or lower-middle-class neighborhoods where they own attractive homes. Their status difference from that of the congregation of the nearby Roman Catholic church is seen in, among other things, the fact that the Protestant women wear elaborate hats rather than kerchiefs.

The continued persistence of culture conflict emerges very clearly when one examines the structure and content of the services, in spite of this apparently successful overt adaptation of the members. By a particular alternating sequence of ritual acts, the service actually expresses two sets of values simultaneously;

it does so, as suggested earlier, by maintaining a covert, bipolar, ceremonial structure, the elements of which are drawn not only from the Protestant tradition but also from the Roman Catholic and pre-Christian traditions of the original peasant culture. This bipolarity can be seen in the style and content of the sermons, in the form that speaking in tongues takes, and in the sequence of the service.

On entering the church, which is of extremely ascetic simplicity, members sit quietly facing forward until the precise beginning hour, when all stand for hymn-singing. This activity is taken so seriously that no verse is ever omitted and many are repeated two or three times. The singing is clearly collective and choral, with the melodies drawn from the Protestant repertory. Yet, as we have seen, choral singing is not characteristic of Southern Italy; instead, Southern Italian folk music features solo voices, often harsh and agonized in tone.[2] In spite of the emphasis on choral uniformity and simple hymnal melodies, one will occasionally hear a harsh, dissonant voice during the hymn-singing, quite separate from the melodic and choral stress.

Immediately after the hymns, there occurs the dramatic reversal referred to earlier—for the prayer period, the congregation faces backwards, each member toward his own pew, so that the only stimuli are auditory. Prayer period is so individualistic that any group-patterning by prayer is difficult to discern. The plaintive wailing of the women, clashing noticeably with the rather drab cheerfulness of the hymn-singing, has been mentioned. Within a frame established by a Protestant emphasis on optimism and community solidarity, the prayer period provides an outlet for residues of a highly individualistic-emotive culture, apparently permitting the expression of otherwise tabooed feelings, such as grief for loss of the past, or a sense of finality about death which conflicts with explicit belief.

However, even within the prayer period one can also see the development of new forms of order. One feature is a kind of informal leadership in which one voice will rise above the

2. Alan Lomax, "Folk Song Style," *Amer. Anthropolog., 61* (1959).

others to pray for the common good. For the women, such a role has a Roman Catholic precedent, since in the Italian village one woman might lead a daily rosary; and although specific Catholic prayers are of course taboo, the women's voices often have the intonation of the rosary. For most men, however, active religious participation is a new experience. In Southern Italy men are traditionally anticlerical; they explicitly resent the strongly hierarchical church authority structure, and the near-exclusive religious emphasis on the Madonna figure. That the Pentecostal church, with its emphasis on independent Bible study and discussion, and its lack of formal hierarchy, has a far greater appeal is shown by the fact that so many men are actively involved, rather than simply tolerating religiosity in their wives. For prayer period this means that some men have developed a distinctive style of informal leadership in which they address a kind of supplicating challenge to the Deity by intoning lengthy, aggressive-sounding, vocal recitations. Men more often call on the figure of Signore Iddio, the Lord God, than on the more Madonna-like Christ figure, and one might see this both as a new way of seeking a masculine identification and as a way of challenging the traditional authority structure. In Southern Italy, *Signore* means "Lord" in a secular feudal, as well as in a religious, sense; there, both secular and religious lords are too remote and too elevated to be approached other than through intermediary figures.

A second type of new order, which is revealed fairly regularly on weekday evenings but less in the more male-dominated Sunday services, is a kind of childlike lullaby choral singing. A very simple hymn is initiated by one of the women and taken up in a refrain so that a kind of softer, even gay, community intimacy is created. It is less formal than the initial hymn-singing, and yet creates a more extensive sort of social solidarity than can be found in the South Italian village, where persons other than relatives are linked only in relatively more superficial ways. Sometimes in this mood there is a spontaneous division between segments of the congregation so that counterpoint patterns result.

After prayer period there is another about-face, and the scene again becomes more formal for the more standardized activities of collection and testimonials, interspersed with further hymns. A silent deacon stands at the pulpit to absorb the testimonials, many of which consist in personal reminiscences of conversion experiences of twenty-five or thirty years ago. The style of the testimonials ranges from the more formal and conventional of those who command literary Italian, to the very concrete and personal accounts of those whose mastery does not exceed a local dialect. (Parenthetically, it is worth commenting that participation involves some pressures for change in a purely Italian frame since literacy is highly valued for Bible reading and a common language is to some extent necessary to link persons from different regions.) Some informal leadership roles go to those who do command literary Italian, and although in my experience all the men were literate, some women either admitted begrudgingly to illiteracy or else always seemed to forget their glasses.

In some, although by no means all, conversion accounts the relevance of culture conflict was obvious. I have referred to the very respectable and prosperous small businessman who "got the spirit" after restraining himself very self-consciously from drawing a knife after a card-game offense; the defense of one's honor in a South Italian frame of reference would probably have required aggressive action in such a situation. The perception that, even when expressed within the church, physical aggression is at variance with American social conventions was described to me by one woman who told how the present, highly verbal, pastor was obtained by the congregation after an earlier pastor's excessively demonstrative antics led to an invasion of a meeting by the police. Current parishioners disown the term "Holy Rollers" and insist that they "do not roll."

The final segment of the ritual sequence, except for an additional closing prayer period similar to the first, is the sermon. Within the sermons themselves the bipolar structure can again be identified. Most of them begin in traditional Protestant style, with the reading of a Bible passage selected so as to illustrate some point in moral teaching. Favorite themes during the period of my attendance were the rebellion of the young, the back-sliding of church members, and the promise of life everlasting. In most sermons, the virtue of following the straight and narrow path emerged in one way or another. However, although the Bible reading and initial stages of the sermon could be called preaching (in the sense of a moral lesson), the subsequent stages were often quite different and might better be referred to either as a process of free association, or as a kind of dramatic role-playing that served to act out a number of mutually contradictory attitudes. The effect was intimately bound up with the charismatic personality of the pastor, a man capable of portraying a very wide range of feelings.

Several specific examples may be mentioned. I have mentioned earlier the frequent and garbled references to *il cammino* and *la fondazione del fondamento che fu fondato. Il cammino* is not a term one hears in Southern Italy; it is the noun form of the verb *camminare,* to walk, and, according to context, could be translated as "the way," "the road," "the trip," or "the process of walking." In the course of the sermon in which the pastor maintained that "we do not want to remain in the middle of the road," the accompanying bodily representations were those of a small child who will have a tantrum if compelled to move. On this occasion, the preacher remained in this fixed position for several moments, talking about the Spirit as if it were some kind of cement, holding him immobile, and about how difficult it is to detach oneself from sin, but as if the conventional religious phraseology were secondary to the spatial referent. During this period his voice tone was one of whining complaint, and he mimicked some South Italian gestures which are frequently used in situations where one wishes to beg off for some moral shortcoming. Only at the end did he seem to become verbally coherent and adult once more, gaily portraying heaven as a kind of tourist's Sicily, where the old would enjoy themselves in the sun, leaving the young to their ways of iniquity.

Similarly, in the foundation sermon he began in an exhortative tone, reprimanding the unfaithful who enter the church but do not remain, like women with many lovers. Then, speaking in the high falsetto he often employed after his initial didactic assurance, he began to describe the evil spirits who are ever ready to infiltrate if one does not stay in one place, again making quite concrete the idea of the church as a foundation by designating the same spot on the floor as the foundation laid by God, and showing considerable anger at having to remain there. This particular spot on the floor was repeatedly endowed with various symbolic meanings; on another occasion, the congregation was swept by a wave of anxiety following the death of a member, and the sermon dealt with this anxiety, after a falsetto recitation of the promise of eternal reward for the just, by a kind of casting out of evil spirits in which the same spot served to designate a circle from which they could be banished.

Each sermon thus seemed to consist of one or more cycles running from affirmation, through doubt and regression, and then, finally, to resolution. But in addition, religious style was systematically related to the phase of the cycle: the affirmative phase was most characteristically Protestant in that definite life goals were set up and the faithful were told to expect reward if they followed them consistently, and punishment if they did not. In the resolution phase, the South Italian Catholic elements were predominant; forgiveness for the entire community rather than only the virtuous was preached or implied. In portraying heaven as a sort of tourist's Sicily, the vivacity of the preacher made it quite clear that the Italian capacity for dealing with fate by having a good time in the present had not been lost. In the intermediate cycles, two additional phenomena emerged: the first was a kind of psychological regression, with behavioral manifestations that were inappropriate for adults in either setting; the second was a kind of diffuse anxiety that became linked with out-and-out skepticism or with fear of evil spirits, a fear that seemed more pronounced in this church than it is generally in Southern Italy today. Anxiety and skepticism were revealed by the falsetto voice and by other phenomena such as cognitive incoherence; there were also times when the preacher made statements that, if I heard correctly (they were said very fast, as if to skip over them), amounted to a denial of the most important theological tenets of the group, such as a claim that the devil might win out in the long run, or that the preacher's power vis-à-vis the deity was so great that his moving from the "foundation" would annihilate him.

My initial formulation was that, by its bipolar structure, this ritual is able to combine elements from two distinctive cultural traditions in an aesthetically meaningful way. This formulation, however, cannot wholly account for the intermediate phases of the sermons; for these we might add two further theoretical propositions. The first proposition is that, with the breakup of any cultural equilibrium, a certain quantity of diffuse anxiety becomes unbound and must be dealt with by particular ritual exhortations; this is seen in the fear of evil spirits which had to be cast out by a dramatization that may be considered primitive in the light of either the South Italian Catholic tradition or the present-day Protestant one. Notably, fundamentalist Protestantism accounts for evil with a single personified devil; yet this image, though referred to in formal doctrine, was rarely evoked by the preacher. The second proposition is that the strains associated with culture change are capable of producing psychological regression. Finally, a third proposition might be added: when a cultural equilibrium is undone, diffuse sexual energy, as well as anxiety, becomes part of the conscious field of perception. The evidence for this proposition cannot be dealt with here; but it seems very probable that openly erotic reactions were more prominent in the new setting than they would have been in either traditional framework.

The psychological changes involved in a transition from Southern Italy to the urban United States have been referred to earlier. These have to do with the adjustments required when a resigned and fatalistic peasant group, subject to a fixed hierarchy of social class, and living principally in terms of family ties and immediately available emotional compensations, enters a world in which individualistic achievement and prosperity are possible, but only at the cost of a greater suppression of impulse and a more responsible participation in the wider community. But two specific aspects of this change can be traced in a more detailed comparison of South Italian and American Protestant expectations; both have particular importance for understanding the phenomenon of speaking in tongues, or glossolalia.

Speaking in tongues—making utterances which do not have a consciously understandable meaning to the person who makes them or to his audience—has been characteristic of many phases of Christianity, beginning with St. Paul. But St. Paul was of course an apostle of social change, his missionary activities covering much of the Roman Empire; and his particular contribution to early Christianity lay in his having distinguished it sharply from Judaism by abandoning the law as a ritual structure. The early Christians were taught to revere the gift of tongues, and the same has been true of many sects since, who have claimed to return to the original spirit of the New Testament. Yet glossolalia does not manifest itself among any of the stabler and better established Christian groups. In the Italian Evangelical church being studied, there were no very elaborate discourses in tongues, although these were referred to by members with respect to initial waves of conversion, both in the United States and in Italy. Yet there were several phenomena of the service characterized in these terms: the first were nonsense syllables uttered during prayer period; the second, a particular kind of conclusion to testimonials in which the testifier would sit down while speaking in a seemingly uncontrollable way; and the third, various kinds of audience reactions to sermons, consisting of gasps and brief vocal utterances, accompanied in some instances by minor bodily convulsions.

None of these phenomena was acknowledged to have cognitive meaning understandable on a human level by members of the congregation. But in spite of the stated view of the congregation, it was quite clear that utterances in tongues were not without significance. Because they were conceived of as detached from normal consciousness, it might be possible to conceptualize them as dynamically related to symptoms of hysteria based on a similar pattern of dissociation. According to Freud, the hysterical symptom is a means of expressing a psychic drive which has been excluded from consciousness because of its conflict-generating potentialities. In this framework, we can try to relate specific utterances in tongues to specific intrapsychic conflicts associated with the transition from Italian peasant to American urban society.

The first such conflict concerns aggression. In Southern Italy, there are some situations in which an insult to oneself (or, more often, to the women in the family) requires retaliatory physical aggression in defense of honor. But the major Italian means for expressing aggression is verbal. Techniques for verbal expression of aggression are so highly developed and so frequently used, particularly in cursing and obscenity, that one might say the South Italian value system is a reversible one: for every positive value there is a negative reciprocal. In the religious framework, this reversibility is very clearly expressed, as mentioned before, in the annual ceremonies for St. Gennaro in Naples: if the patron saint does not prove his miraculous powers by liquefying his blood with sufficient rapidity, the assembled populace begins to curse him, even though within the church.

The Protestant ethic, however, requires a far greater inhibition of aggression; here, rather than being directed negatively against the existing system of values, aggressive impulses are ideally channeled toward "constructive" action. In religious imagery, this goes with a representation of God as a figure who is severe but also just—rather than simply appreciating Him when He is helpful and cursing Him when He is not, His children are expected in all events to perform His works with even greater continuity and consistency. For the Italian Evangelical church, one indication of the strains involved in transition appeared in the fact that, while all the fundamentalist Protestant taboos were accepted in principle, it was the taboo on taking the name of the Lord in vain which was by far the most self-

conscious focus of concern. Thus, for instance, strongly con-
demnatory attitudes were frequently expressed about "those
Italians who call themselves Christians" and nevertheless
violated this taboo.

The relevance of the problem of inhibition of aggression to
speaking in tongues appears first in the fact that so many of the
utterances had a sharply aggressive tone. Moreover, one could
discern very close resemblances between the syllables used and
curse words, or everyday verbal abuses. During both prayer
period and sermons, many of the women were prone to uttering
a long drawn out *assai*, brought to a gasping halt with teeth
clenched, as if they were saying "enough, I am fed up with the
whole thing." One testifier, whose thanks to Jesus usually
sounded particularly agonizing, often concluded with an indis-
tinctive babbling which had to be quieted by spontaneous lullaby
singing from the others; again the tone was harsh and aggressive, and the words often reminiscent of curses. The same could
be said for many of the audience reactions to the sermons; sometimes, on a particular difficult point (as when the preacher said
that the true believer must be willing to abandon home and
family to follow in the way of the Lord), one could hear a wave
of response easily interpretable as "damn you, that's impossible."
During testimonials, positive moralistic points of view put forth
on one side of the congregation were sometimes responded to
with what seemed to be "shut-up" sounds from the others. In
sum, these utterances appeared to provide an outlet for a kind
of verbal aggression tabooed in the new culture but not in the
old, the potentially disruptive consequences being handled by the
psychic mechanism of dissociation.

The second focus of conflict concerns the Madonna. While
the ramifications of this are too complex to be adequately
covered here, a major change has involved the renunciation of
the Madonna—who has such crucial importance in Southern
Italy, particularly with respect to the strongly mother-centered
family system. Protestantism may be said to be primarily father-
centered, in that major expectations refer to performing the

Father's works rather than seeking tender maternal forgiveness (though admittedly the figure of Christ does fulfill some of the latter functions). For the Italian Evangelical congregation this modification may have symbolized a loss of female status—having to accept greater independence on the part of children, or to show greater consideration for greater male accomplishments, such as literacy—while male status was increasing. The fact that speaking in tongues occurred more commonly among women may be closely related to this; for men, however, the "rational" side of religious life, especially Bible study and discussion, seemed more important.

The renunciation of the cult of the Madonna signifies the loss of one of those ritual responses so deeply ingrained in Italian Catholic culture—for example, the saying of the rosary, or the calling on a saint or the Madonna in any moment of trouble—as to have seemed immutable. But again, primarily among women during prayer period, one could often hear the word *santa* repeated several times with great intensity, followed by a series of incomprehensible syllables, and ending with a reference to the "blessed Savior." Not only the selected words, but also the timing of the blocking-out, was such as to suggest that the women were making a desperate effort not to say the familiar Hail Mary, substituting nonsense syllables in such a way as to render it unrecognizable. In other words, speaking in tongues may also be a blocking-out phenomenon which appears when a well-known ritual response is incompatible with a current value system. Both with respect to aggression and to the Madonna problem, other slips of the tongue made in sermons or in testimonials or Bible discussions could be seen to have similar determinants.

In sum, I have tried here to apply Malinowski's theory of ritual—that it tends to arise in situations of anxiety and uncertainty—to a limited focus in the study of culture change. The services of the Italian Evangelical church can be interpreted in terms of a particular bipolar structure in which elements from two distinctive cultural traditions are combined so as to create a meaningful whole. Yet it also appeared that, rather than being anchored in a fixed system of belief, this religious group lived with a chronic uncertainty; as the pastor put it on one particularly agitated evening: "I can hear the screams, I can hear the cries, I can hear that life is in doubt." As further confirmation of the view that the ritual is closely bound up with the change situation were a number of indications that it will not continue to exist in this present form after the deaths of the pastor and the senior members of the present congregation; the dropout rate in the second generation is high, and among those who have remained, there is considerable rebellion and the independent use of a new, more conventionally American Protestant religious style. An affiliated church I visited in another city, where the second generation had far more power and major services were in English, was also far more conventionally American and less openly emotional.

But although some classical functionalist propositions may be useful for such studies, it is also true that in order to understand these change-associated religious groups it is necessary to abandon the views that, apart from gross breakdown, cultures necessarily appear as integrated homogeneous wholes, and that the possession of ritual forms necessarily assures psychological and cultural stability. In a recent paper analyzing a case of ritual breakdown in Java, Clifford Geertz[3] has suggested that the problem of change may best be approached by using a kind of dynamic functional model, in which culture, social system, and personality may change in different ways and at different rates of speed, so that they do not necessarily mesh in a coherent fashion. In his Javanese case study, Geertz was principally concerned with failures of congruence between culture and social structure. Here there are similar assumptions, but concerned more with the meshing of personality and culture. The ritual forms are viewed as attempting to resolve—with only partial success—those conflicts which arise as one type of psychic orga-

3. Clifford Geertz, "Ritual and Social Change: a Javanese Example," *Amer. Anthropolog.*, 59 (1957).

nization is replaced by another. It is in this context that the psychological bias of Malinowski's functionalism becomes particularly relevant. At the present time, however, we can increase the effectiveness of his psychological bias by a more thorough employment of psychoanalytic theory, as attempted here in the interpretation of certain ritual phenomena as aggressive, and in the relating of glossolalia to the dynamic mechanisms of hysteria.

chapter 12

Dark Puritan

Dark Puritan is the autobiography of Norman Paul, a Grenadian who lived through a complex series of personal and social conflicts before he achieved his mature identity as leader of an original religious cult. Born on a still paternalistic cocoa estate, he perceives his family, during his childhood, to have been benevolently endowed by nature and the proprietor, but "from after 1914 when everything turn up and change taking place, you had to ask for everything." His mother taught firm conventions of respect backed by reference to a paternal God, but his own father was rarely at home. The closest figures of his early life were his mother, numerous siblings, and

Review of the book *Dark Puritan* by M. G. Smith, Department of Extramural Studies, Univ. of the West Indies, Kingston, Jamaica, 1963, 139 pp. Reprinted by permission from *Social and Economic Studies,* 13 (1964), 329–331.

maternal relatives. Through a maternal aunt, he was introduced to the Biblical culture of the Seventh Day Adventists, but at the same time his grandmother taught him elements of African ritual tradition; thus cultural complexity was early a part of his life. In one sense he became and remained truly literate and Protestant, namely in that he continued the habit of scripture reading throughout his life, putting the written word above demands for conformity with the immediate social community, including the religious one: "I don't look to man to live, I look at the Scripture."

Later life only increased the cultural heterogeneity of his experience. His greatest tragedy was the failure of a marriage with an East Indian woman, in his words more well-read than he. Their bitter quarrels concerned her maltreatment of his prior illegitimate child, his attachment to his mother, and her mixture of subservience and loyalty towards the brother who continued to take an authoritative position over her. This part of the book provides a case study in conflict between two types of kinship system which could not be integrated with each other: her model of monogamy and organized economic co-operation among kin and his matrifocal model with the mother-son tie serving as the main axis of continuity within a much more loosely organized network. At the time of the marriage, both had intents towards change, but notably in time both slipped back to natal attachments and away from the marriage as a unity. It was while sick and alone in Trinidad and soon after the marital failure that Norman Paul was first visited by Oshun or St. Philomena who became the major patroness of his cult.

One of the most notable aspects of this cult was thus that it was centered on a protective goddess figure rather than the Protestant exacting paternal God. In describing his visitations, Norman Paul says, first, that during his illness he knew that, with what he knew concerning the Scriptures, he held God on his right side. However, he then goes on to present a series of myths about women, including St. Philomena, Florence Nightingale, and an illegitimate American Negro girl, in conflict because of her race, whom he closely identifies with himself. Oshun is associated with memories of his mother (with the added complication that she is white) and she directs him in a variety of feminine roles: he is to feed children, separate the clean from the unclean, and in general act in a nurturing and benevolent way towards his fellow man. Moreover, just as Norman had nine siblings, so there are nine African Powers in his visitations. It thus appears that his religious cult is a means of representing an earlier family situation in which his identification was with the mother.

In this respect, one might say that the book has been mistitled since, strictly speaking, Norman Paul is not a Puritan: his symbols come from the matrifocal family in which it appears that the boy's lack of a constant masculine identification figure within the home is compensated by greater toleration for sexual assertiveness outside of it. His lack of a truly Puritan concept of sin appears early in his in-and-out relation to the Adventist church—"while having youth in the body I knew it was the wrong thing. [But at the same time] I thought I could [should] have been forgiven [for an illegitimate child]." In actual reality, his mother forgave him for his philandering, while his more strictly monogamous wife did not: his mother took the illegitimate child away from his wife when she felt it was being maltreated. The idea of maternal forgiveness is much closer to the Roman Catholic than the Protestant view of life, and the cult is in fact replete with Roman Catholic imagery. From Protestantism it takes only the emphasis on scripture, since it says very little about God the Father or his relation to his Son. But this is of course not surprising when we consider his upbringing; rather it seems as if his partial conversion to Protestantism and attempt at monogamous marriage really represented aspirations towards the middle class, but the resultant strains were so great that he slipped back to earlier patterns. In his early life his father was a secondary figure, and so it became in his cult.

The mis-titling need not be considered a serious criticism of the book because Dr. Smith has kept himself so modestly in the background that Norman Paul speaks for himself, and his life can be interpreted in many ways, depending on the perspective of the interpreter. The questions raised concerning relations between personality, family structure, and religious symbolism, and the relations of all three to cultural heterogeneity and change, are exceedingly complex and not easily answered. But the book very clearly shows how useful carefully collected autobiographical material can be for these still untrodden areas, especially when, as is also true for the Puerto Rican Protestant convert worker in the case described by Sidney Mintz,[1] the informant possesses a rich religious imagery. We hope that these two books mark the beginning of a series which will eventually sample adequately the great variety of religious perspectives distributed throughout the Caribbean.

1. *Worker in the Cane,* New Haven: Yale Univ. Press, 1960.

part five

Social Aspects
of Psychoanalysis

In this part Anne Parsons examines the relation between psychoanalytic conceptualization and the problems, dilemmas, and conflicts engendered in the encounter between theory and practice. Chapter 13 presents us with the problems of differential assimilation of concepts in different societies or cultures. It examines how some psychoanalytic concepts are accepted, others more or less ignored, and how the ones that are accepted are subject to subtle differences of interpretation. For example, in France, the concept of "the unconscious" has been assimilated to the Bergsonian concept, and has thus become deprived of its conflictual implications. In the United States also the conflictual aspects of psychic life are given little emphasis, and personality dynamics are understood to mean personality processes more generally.

In Chapter 14 Anne Parsons subjects to serious scrutiny the assumption that psychoanalytically

283

oriented practice has similar therapeutic effects on individuals coming from different social contexts.
Patients coming from a culture significantly different
from that of middle-class American society perceive
the communication received in the therapeutic relationship in quite different ways. What is therapeutic in
one social context may very well be sick-making in
another. This raises a moral dilemma for the practitioner who wants to live up to the normative injunctions of his profession, when these injunctions,
being misunderstood by the patient, may make him
sicker instead of helping him, thus going counter to
the very purpose they are supposed to serve.

In the next chapter Anne Parsons addresses herself
to some fundamental ambiguities inherent in psychoanalytic training. One such ambiguity appears in the
fact that such training is provided for social scientists
on the condition that they will not apply it for the
purpose of treating patients. This brings about the
unusual circumstance that people are being trained in
a discipline with the explicit aim of not practicing
what they are being trained for. Another ambiguity
underlying the philosophy of psychoanalytic training
is that the distinction between the occupational and the
private sphere of life becomes blurred, especially
through the training analysis, and personal attributes
become the measure of professional achievement. This
contrasts sharply with other professions and occupations, where the occupational and the personal spheres
tend to be clearly distinguished from each other.

chapter 13

Diffusion of Psychoanalytic Concepts

Although all problems studied by the behavioral sciences are interrelated, it is nevertheless true that one must make a choice as to the level of analysis most appropriate to a given problem. This is particularly true in regard to social psychology, where it is not always possible even tentatively to isolate social structure from personality and belief systems. To speak of a psychosocial field or of a total personality without further specification precludes a thorough analysis of processes which, it must be admitted, are in fact all-encompassing.

This paper deals with the transmission and distortion of ideas in the framework of social psychology. It is being introduced here on the historical level, without systematically utilizing

This is a translation of the last chapter of Anne Parsons' Ph.D. dissertation, "La Pénétration de la psychoanalyse en France et aux Etats Unis," Thèse pour le doctorat d'Université de la Sorbonne, unpublished manuscript, Paris, 1956.

tools of analysis other than those that link the specific distortions to the elements of a particular historical situation.

I have been much impressed by the part that metaphoric conceptions of the psyche have played, not only in Freudian theory, but also as powerful factors in the distortion of these ideas as they are diffused throughout the culture. For instance, the unconscious, seen as psychic space, plays an important part in the Freudian model, as well as in the French interpretation of Freud's ideas. The unconscious serves as a link between his theoretical concepts and the problems of social ethics which have affected the diffusion of psychoanalysis. One can show how different representations of the same psychic space are related to different theoretical positions. Another crucial representation is that of the Façade and of the Hidden.

There is also a representation of weight which seems to play a part across European thought: the *solid* facts of physiology as against the fantasy of symbolic interpretation. It is even possible to make a scale model, to use Lévi-Strauss's expression, of several currents of European thought in which the spatial conception of psychic life is constant: the conscious is conceived as being above the unconscious and reason is thought to be above affect. A conception of weight is a ploy in the game: there is either a *solid* consciousness, or an illusory consciousness with *solid* foundations underneath.

It might also be possible to situate the reductionist problem in this visual framework. This framework is made of representations common to the European cultures of a given period: they enter into different combinations depending upon the currents of thought in which they find themselves.

The identical visual representations are not present in American culture. There is no widespread representation of the unconscious as psychic space. At the present time one sees a growing use of analogies to machine processes in order to describe the inner world, such as adjustment, ego repair, dynamics (in a particular meaning which shall be specified later). Just as in the terms which refer to biology and behaviorism (growth, purposive behavior), there is the implication of a collective movement within which the discrete units must be coordinated. In contrast to the spatial images of European culture, I believe that images of collective movement are crucial in American culture.

It would seem that for given social groups there are systems of psychic representations based upon different dimensions—space in two or three dimensions, continuous or discontinuous movement with a given orientation within that space, the visual dimensions (as in the representations of knowledge by the image of light) which are shared by the members of these groups and which serve to link symbolically different areas of life to psychological concepts. These representative systems will be more or less integrated. No system would be free of contamination from other systems, but there would be a strain toward inner consistency.

Each of these representations is overdetermined: it has siginificance on several levels simultaneously. To delineate the nonessential fields of reference of each representation, Bally's concept of "the associative field" seems to be useful.[1] The representations of interest here refer on the cognitive level to psychic phenomena and their processes, but the associative fields of the concepts—since they are metaphoric—are extrapsychological. But it is precisely through the process of metaphorical extension that psychological concepts are linked to other conceptual fields: thus the representations of psychic processes in terms of a machine links them to cultural components beyond the field of psychology, and there is a polarization of meaning from several cognitively interdependent disciplines. Or let us take once more the term "unconscious." As metaphoric psychological space it presents itself as a polarization of references to several nonpsychological fields, which involve broad social values closely linked but otherwise independent from the descriptions of a psychic phenomenon. The term unconscious may

1. Charles Bally, "L'arbitraire du signe," in *Le Français Moderne* (Paris, 1940), pp. 193–206: The associative field is "a halo which surrounds the sign, the outward fringes of which dissolve into their surrounding milieu."

mean a residual area about which little is known by psychology; what a given individual fails to understand of his own behavior, but which is susceptible of understanding by a psychoanalyst; what is not systematized, hence of secondary importance; finally, in psychoanalytical theory, repressed impulses. Each one of these meanings has played a part in the diffusion of psychoanalysis in France. It could even be said that this diffusion took place through the significance of the concept of the unconscious which acted as a prism, a nodal point of meaning, and linked the ideas of Freud to general ethical problems.

Similarly, for the semantic coupling Façade–Reality as a representation of psychological phenomena by Freud, it may be understood as evoking a conception of science which searches for the reality behind the visible manifestations, but it may also be understood in terms of social conflict. In the diffusion of psychoanalysis this coupling is utilized most often in the context of a social conflict. In this case it is possible to speak of displacement of the associative field. For Freud the scientific problem is the primary one, but for the others it is the social problem— implied within the same representation.

In analyzing the associative fields of these terms, i.e., the fields to which the statements belong, which in turn influence the conceptions of psychic life, I have attempted to disentangle these strands of meaning. But this disentangling is nothing more than Freud's method of symbolic interpretation, aiming to reduce complex symbols to a series of separate associations. I have transposed his method to the social level, seeking the meanings that are most widespread throughout the society, rather than those that are specific to an individual biography. In the latter context the method of disentangling the symbols is a historical method: the images lead to the understanding of only one case. In contrast, I have searched for a method which could be used for broad theoretical generalizations, and here again I have been inspired by Freud. In his *Science of Dreams*, not only does he use the clinical and historical method, but he also proposes a classification of the symbolic mechanisms which operate in the dream world. Hence, one can bring out similar mechanisms as factors which operated in the distortion of Freudian doctrine. This view is also influenced by Lévi-Strauss's[2] analysis of symbolic processes. The following examples indicate some of the processes. I hope that this outline can point the way to more systematic work of a similar nature.

Displacement

Freud himself, while seeking a mode of conceptualizing psychological processes, imported into psychology terms belonging to other fields, especially from physics and chemistry, but also terms belonging to politics, like the metaphor of censorship. Very often Freudian dynamics are better understood if one remembers the meaning of these terms in the physical sciences. For it is the latter that gives them coherence. But most people who were exposed to the theory in its diffusion did not know the scientific origin of these terms. In his attempt to construct a scientific model of personality, Freud found that each term had for him a double meaning—the meaning which refers to the psychic processes he describes and the meaning which refers to physical science and helps to systematize his thought in dynamic terms.

Let us take the dual concept of repression-resistance. Repression is taken as having two meanings by Freud, one from the starting point of the metaphor of censorship which pertains to politics, and the other originating in the dynamic model which belongs to physics. In the second meaning it is indeed related to repression. The resistance revealed by the patient in analysis, a factor operationally definable, is the index of repression. The two concepts are mutually complementary. But in the process of diffusion the concept of resistance received little stress. The

2. Claude Lévi-Strauss, "L'efficacité symbolique," *Revue de l'histoire des religions,* 135 (Jan.–March 1949), 5–27. I have also used the concepts presented by Lévi-Strauss in his lectures at the Ecole des Hautes Etudes.

concept of repression received the bulk of the emphasis; it made popular sense in that it was related to censorship. This phenomenon seems to be the direct result of a discrepancy in the associative fields. The political field is known to everyone, thus there was no problem of comprehension. This is certainly not the case for terms pertaining to physics. Hence there was distortion by the displacement of the associative field. One field has disappeared and only half of Freud's concept is understood. Part of the arbitrariness orginally attributed to Freud could be explained by this very fact: first it was thought that Freud explained all overt psychic phenomena by means of distortion, without understanding its operational index; second, there was displacement by associations with censorship. Hence, in France, censorship was transformed into *deceit* and gave an interpretative twist to the original theory[3] by linking it to social issues.

In conclusion, we mean by displacement the association of a term to a field other than the one in which it was originally found. This is an oversimplification, since for the metaphoric terms in question here, the problem is not that of the cognitive field to which the term is strictly applied—nobody would have denied that Freud spoke of psychic processes—but that of a complex of metaphoric associations linked by similarity to the cognitive fields in which they properly belong. Thus, certain processes, similar to those described by physics and politics, intervene jointly in the Freudian concept of psychic life: there is a displacement of the associative field when one generalizes from one field while ignoring the other. I have dealt only partly with Freud's concept, for he really describes the displacement of cathexis from one object to the other and I am speaking here only of cognitive processes, but the use of Freud's concept for my purposes seems nevertheless useful.

3. In relation to the term "resistance," Dr. Lacan has remarked in a lecture that the term implies an active struggle. I personally had never conceived of the term in this manner. I had thought rather of the passive resistance of physical matter. It is possible to propose as an explanation the fact that a Frenchman has historical associations in reference to the term resistance which are inexistent for an American.

Condensation

Condensation, as Freud describes it in the most general way, is the mechanism by which the overdetermination of the dream work occurs: Freud remarks that the most striking fact in the analysis of the dream is the discrepancy between the manifest content and the latent content revealed in the course of free association. Condensation would then be the principle of the transformation of the more into the less, or the mechanism whereby the associative field shrinks and follows similarities in imagery. This is in contrast to displacement, which is conceived as a movement within a given associative field. Two types of condensation could be described: (a) fusion by similitude of the cognitive field, and (b) fusion by similarities in the dimension of the representation.

(a) The American interpretation of infantile sexuality is to the point here. All the specificity of Freudian theory has been lost because it has been seen in relation to its object rather than in relation to its content. Thus the theory has been generalized to the total emotional life of the child; there is fusion with a common representation of the child and there is loss of the original content. This sort of fusion characterizes the diffusion of Freudianism in the United States: psychoanalysis is often defined by its object, i.e., emotional life, thus linking its concept to common knowledge. This has left open the road to generalizations which are independent of Freud's thinking.

(b) This can be seen in the literary diffusion of Freudianism in France. Because both Freud and French writers were using a spatial representation of the unconscious, and because the idea of *exploration* was common to both, the writers welcomed Freud's theories. Distortion results from a secondary difference as to the goal of the exploration and as to the content of the unconscious. In Freud the goal is scientific research, analysis of the unconscious, of the elements given by biology or by the analysis of a biography, while for literary writers the term *recherche* has been understood in a broader sense, and the content of the unconscious remained more ambiguous.[4] Hence, certain aspects of Freudian theory were simply excluded from perception or were misinterpreted in terms of other conceptual schemes. In fact there is a loss of content by fusion of Freudian theory with a very broad and indeterminate conception of the unconscious. This fusion takes place through the similarities in the representation.

Reversal Between the Relations of Symbolic Dichotomy

This is most clearly seen in the example of the Surrealist movement. Starting from terms defined dichotomously— "conscious-unconscious," "dream reality"—which oppose each other on the logical and psychological levels, there is a reversal of the ethical valuation, the dream becoming superior to reality and the unconscious superior to consciousness. This is in fact the etymological meaning of the term "revolution": the same terms are kept but the relationship between them is reversed. In this context the concept of "charge" defined by Lévi-Strauss is useful.[5] This term—which belongs to the theory of electric currents—denotes a given quantity that moves between the positive and negative poles. Psychologically, the *charge* would denote a strong affect, since it is polarized at the extremes. It is possible to consider the terms "conscious-unconscious" and "dream-reality" as poles. Among the Surrealists, there is a displacement of a positive charge from the symbol *reality* to the symbol *dream,* and hence an attraction toward Freudian theory. In the latter there is a focusing of attention upon the theory of the dream, since the latter is positively charged. Eventually, there will be second thoughts because Freud, in fact, has not reversed the relations. He wishes to bring back the dreamer to reality.

4. In French, *recherche* has a scientific meaning as in English, but it has also the meaning of *search,* connoting sophistication and romantic coloring.
5. Lecture, Ecole des Hautes Etudes, February 16, 1955.

Similitude of Symbolic Structure

The image of the Façade alluded to earlier, and of the undermining which Freud applied to the description of psychic states, is also found in Marxism. There is a similitude of structure between the Freudian model on the psychological level and the Marxist model on the social level. As a matter of fact, there have been associations between Freudianism and Marxism which could be explained within this same framework.[6] Freud has given an image of psychic life which corresponds to the image that Marx gives of society, and these two images have spread, often for the same reasons. The parallelism was often noticed while Freudianism was in the process of diffusion: one finds sentences such as, "The unconscious in Freud is like the proletariat in a state of revolt," and there are similar comparisons which do violence to the intents of both Marx and Freud. For Freud, who was no revolutionary, there can be absolutely no question of a victory of the unconscious. This can be found in revolutionary movements only by a reversal of the value system of Freudian theory which is encouraged by symbolic assimilation to Marxist theory. The Freudian image of psychic life was perceived in function of its structural resemblance to the social image, and the values of the latter were generalized to the former, thus distorting the Freudian system and leaving aside all its therapeutic aspects. It is possible to say that it is precisely this structural resemblance which on the symbolic level links Freudianism to revolutionary movements.

Similarities of Process

In France the Freudian concept of the unconscious has been assimilated to the Bergsonian concept, thus resulting in a deformation of the dynamic conflict. The Freudian concept of psychic life was simply understood as continuous through time

6. Cf. R. Bastide, *Sociologie et Psychanalyse* (Paris, 1950), Chapter 5, "Marxisme et Psychanalyse."

and not as a constant conflict of opposing forces. In the same way there was in Jacques Rivière and Auguste Marie a concept of psychic phenomena in motion which was foreign to Freud. The whole difference between an in-motion concept of psychic life and one, if not static, at least capable of being categorized, is linked to the specific problem of whether psychic life can be studied scientifically.

In the United States there took place a distortion of the term "dynamic." In Freud this term implies a conflict of forces. The term "dynamic" in American culture is itself a *nexus* of meaning: it is related to the machine, to the concept of progress, and to a highly admired type of personality, to wit the man who accomplishes a great deal through direct action. Hence, for some the term "dynamic psychology" has become equivalent to "progressive psychology" or to "psychology of growth" and the emphasis on conflict has been lost.

In the French and American case there is, at first, an apprehension of certain aspects of the Freudian theory due to the fact that Freud uses a model that systematizes a certain process. Afterwards there is distortion because the processes are not really of the same type; in France they are discontinuous, based upon conflict, while those of Bergson and of American society, even though they differ from one another, are both continuous.

I believe that it should be possible to push this analysis of symbolism much further, by formulating a systematic typology of symbolic mechanisms. It should then be possible, for a given symbolic system, to bring out certain stable patterns, such as the spatial model of psychic life, or variables, such as the concept of movable weight, or the unconscious to be explored as against the harmonious unconscious, as well as an attempt at synthesis based upon this typology.

chapter **14**

Cultural Barriers to Insight and the Structural Reality of Transference *

A number of studies have indicated that patients seeking psychotherapy, or receiving consideration as potentially good psychotherapy patients, are not randomly distributed with respect to social background.[1] From the anthropological perspective, there can be said to be a "culture of psychotherapy" which in the contemporary United States is most frequently found in those urban upper-middle-class

* I am indebted to the Foundations' Fund for Research in Psychiatry and to the National Institute of Mental Health for research support during the period in which the work described here was carried out.

1. L. Schaffer & J. K. Myers, "Psychotherapy and Social Stratification: An Empirical Study of Practices in a Psychiatric Outpatient Clinic," *Psychiatry,* 17 (1954), 83–93. A. B. Hollingshead and F. C. Redlich, *Social Class and Mental Illness* (New York: John Wiley & Sons, Inc., 1958). G. Gurin, J. Veroff, and S. Feld, *Americans View Their Mental Health* (New York: Basic Books, Inc., 1960).

groups that do not possess strongly traditional religious or social values.[2]

Not only is the working-class person less likely to seek psychotherapy on a voluntary basis, but also when for some reason (often because of an encounter with the law) he does fall into a setting where psychotherapy is available, he is less likely to be considered as a patient capable of insight. All other things being equal, the psychotherapist more readily accepts for treatment the office patient who announces himself by saying "I have been feeling anxious and depressed lately; perhaps it has something to do with my submissiveness toward my wife" than the one who says "I gotta nerves, my stomach she hurt alla time," or "I'm not crazy; maybe my wife is because she called the police and had me locked up."

In this paper, I should like to discuss a patient with whom I carried out two years of intensive psychotherapy, whom I shall call Mr. Calabrese. I first encountered him when he was nearly forty, the father of two children, a moderately successful tailor, and just admitted for the third time to a state hospital as a result of complaints made to the police by his wife and her family. His English was adequate only for understanding or for carrying out the minimal requirements of daily life; thus from the first interview we spoke Italian. The language barrier was such that Mr. Calabrese's only close contact within the hospital besides myself was with an Italian-born employee in the tailor shop where my patient quickly began to work. Since the latter was only minimally exposed to the hospital treatment ideology, his case offered a particularly valuable experimental isolation with respect to intensive psychotherapy outside of the culture of psychotherapy. An account of my therapeutic efforts with this patient also serves to illuminate certain aspects of the transference relationship, and of the "structural reality" underlying it. In addition, there are im-

2. P. H. Knapp, S. Levin, R. H. McCarter, H. Wermer, and E. Zetzel, "Suitability for Psychoanalysis: A Review of 100 Supervised Analytic Cases," *Psychoanal. Quart.,* 29 (1960), 459–477. T. S. Szasz and R. A. Nemiroff, "A Questionnaire Study of Psychoanalytic Practices and Opinions," *J. of Nervous & Ment. Disease,* 137 (1963), 209–221.

plications which can be drawn from this case that may well have significance for the treatment not only of working-class patients but of middle-class patients as well.

Mr. Calabrese's social background would, by many of the usual criteria, put him beyond the pale for intensive psychotherapy. An immigrant from an impoverished area of rural Southern Italy, he completed only five years of formal education before being apprenticed to learn his trade. At eighteen he was called up for military service and never after that returned for more than a visit to his native village. On discharge from his four years of service during World War II, he was forced to emigrate in search of work and spent the next twelve years as a wandering bachelor in both Northern Italy and Latin America. He purchased land in Latin America, but failed to carry through with overtures made toward a prospective bride. He then wrote to his mother in Italy that he wanted a wife, and a marriage was arranged with the American-born daughter of a village family. The marriage took place in his native village, and a few months afterward the couple departed for the United States. Not very long after his arrival, Mr. Calabrese was hospitalized for the first time with acute suspicions concerning the fidelity of his wife and doubts as to his paternity of their first child. A quick social recovery was followed by regression, but after the second hospitalization he nevertheless succeeded in effectively supporting his family for three years and producing a second child. The third hospitalization followed an occasion when he became quite angry at home, using obscene language toward his mother-in-law and berating his wife and her family for a variety of deeds which members of her family had supposedly committed, over a period of several generations, in order to cause harm to him and other past and present members of his family. The actual issue, he felt, was that his wife wanted to have nothing more to do with him.

I became interested in Mr. Calabrese because of prior experience in Southern Italy as an anthropologist, and I expected from the beginning that some modifications in psycho-

therapeutic technique would have to be made to fit his distinctive cultural background, which was of course quite alien
to the culture of psychotherapy. I was particularly impressed
by his verbal skill and his richness of political, social, and
religious imagery; intellectually, he was far less submissive than
most middle-class patients in relation to their therapists, and
I considered him to be exceptionally intelligent.

My goals in working with Mr. Calabrese were those which
I would see as governing any psychotherapeutic work, namely,
to help the patient resolve his conflicts within the framework
of meaning relevant to him. Initially I said only that I would
like to go on talking to him in order to get his perspective
on the family difficulties; since he was then vigorously denying
that he was actually as crazy as his wife and the police said
he was, and attributing many of his symptoms to spirits, I
could not very well have expected him to express a wish for
prolonged self-exploration.

On admission Mr. Calabrese was very much afraid of
being transferred to an outlying hospital far from his family,
as had happened in the past through routine bureaucratic
procedure. As a consequence of my request to the administrative physician he was not transferred, a fact which he quite
realistically perceived as the result of my intermediary action
vis-à-vis higher authorities which to him were too distant to
be influenced. Such intermediary action is quite in agreement
with Latin expectations for persons of higher social status and
greater power: both in religion and secular life, the world is
seen as a hierarchy within which those beneath must depend
on the interventions of those above.

The treatment itself can be considered in two phases. The
first I have characterized as the period of crystallization of
positive transference; it lasted for approximately the first ten
months of treatment. The second, which begins with a crisis
phase, can be characterized as the phase of aggression and
progressive alienation. During the first phase, I considered the
therapy successful, with the patient making as much progress
as could reasonably be expected. During the second, I felt

that the therapeutic relationship was deteriorating, and at the point of termination I considered the attempt to have been a failure, in that at the time when I left the hospital for other work, Mr. Calabrese was residing on a chronic ward, on bad terms with his family, and showing no indications of forthcoming discharge or work outside the hospital. My principal concerns in this paper will be with the reasons for this failure.

The Crystallization of Positive Transference

In the initial interview, Mr. Calabrese hallucinated me as a maternal cousin living in France. As soon as his initial blocking disappeared, he showed visible anger directed against his wife and the Chinese, warning me of their untrustworthiness. The anger toward his wife took the form of dramatic mimicry of her gestures and phrases: "You don't want to eat, you don't want to talk, you just sit around the house all day." An initial plan he presented was that they should get divorced. I pointed out that if he was thinking of divorce, he should see a lawyer; contemporaneously he suggested my going to his place of work, where one of his co-workers was a woman who might know a lawyer. This I did not do.

Following a visit home after about three weeks, his anger toward his wife calmed down a great deal. His attitude toward her became one of deferent submission and his plans began to change, e.g., he might go back and live with her, or even if he left the hospital to live and work alone, he would give her most of his salary for support of the children.

During this period Mr. Calabrese's rhetoric was based on three main themes.[3] The first was the jealousy syndrome isolated by Freud as one of the common forms of paranoid psychosis.[4]

3. For further discussion of the defensive use of rhetoric or rapid and persuasive verbalization in South Italian schizophrenic patients, see Parsons, "A Schizophrenic Episode in a Neapolitan Slum," this book Chapter 9.

4. S. Freud, "Psychoanalytic Notes upon an Autobiographical Account of a Case of Paranoia (Dementia Paranoides)," in *Collected Papers,* 3 : 387–470 (London: Hogarth Press, 1956); "Further Recom-

He constantly expressed doubts concerning his wife's premarital virginity and post-marital fidelity, carrying these back to the first moment of their acquaintance when he saw her getting off the plane in Rome and felt that she was not *buona*. *Buona,* or "good," in this context refers to virginity, and in his part of the world the personal integrity of a man depends on his success in preserving the chastity of sister or daughter or on the virginity and post-marital fidelity of his wife.[5] Mr. Calabrese's doubts were not removed by his sister's examining the sheets on the wedding night according to village custom; it appears that he never asked her what she found. Though jealousy is an extremely widespread phenomenon among Latin men,[6] for Mr. Calabrese it was unusually accentuated and repetitive. In the same breath he could accuse his wife of frigidity, and consequently of infidelity, and refer to his own impotence. In one very important quarrel before his hospitalization his wife quite insultingly called him a homosexual. He used the masculine form of *buono* to mean either impotent or homosexual, often with the implication of physical deformity of the male organ.

Much of his rhetoric centered on the phase of his military experience, and in particular one crucial memory of a man who made homosexual advances when he descended from the train in Rome while reporting for duty; this was his first trip away from home. He repeatedly emphasized that since he had passed the army physical exam, he must be a man, and much of the

---

mendations in the Technique of Psychoanalysis: Observations on Transference Love," in *Ibid.,* 2 : 377–391; "Certain Neurotic Mechanisms in Jealousy, Paranoia, and Homosexuality," in *Ibid.,* 2 : 232–243.

5. See this book Chapter 9. Also, L. W. Moss & W. H. Thompson, "The South Italian Family: Literature and Observation," *Human Organiz., 18,* 1 (1958), 35–41. M. Opler, "Dilemmas of Two Puerto Rican Men," in G. Seward (ed.), *Clinical Studies in Culture Conflict* (New York: The Ronald Press, 1958), pp. 223–244.

6. Cf. Leonardo Bianchi, "Paranoia," in *Textbook of Psychiatry* (New York: William Wood & Company, 1906), pp. 570–619. The author, a Neapolitan psychiatrist, delineates a jealousy syndrome which he frequently encountered among middle-aged and elderly men. He says that the man's fears of infidelity usually sound quite convincing to the physician – until he takes a look at the wife. Further exploration usually reveals a loss of potency.

material about his military life, such as his casual contacts with women, was certainly designed to impress me with this image of himself.

A second major theme was the Chinese. This symbol was unique, in contrast to the culturally standardized jealousy syndrome; projection of hostility onto out-groups is unusual in Italy and when it appears in this country it usually takes the form of anti-Negro feelings. To him, the Chinese served as a composite symbol of evil, and his psychic state could very easily be evaluated by the degree to which they dominated the interview. On one level, his representation of the Chinese served to focus primitive oral fears: they were described as cannibalistic, having once eaten 35,000 children. On another, they expressed his role confusion; he commented that since Chinese women wear short hair and the men pigtails, it is difficult to distinguish between the sexes—in contrast to his village where adult women always wear buns.

The third theme was somewhat different in that it was not paranoid in character, but rather testified to the development of at least a modicum of internalized morality. It was revealed in repeated confessions in which his gestures and mannerisms indicated that he was putting me in the place of a priest. The content of what was confessed was always sexual and to a considerable degree incestuous: he would begin by saying that he was an extremely bad man because he had on several occasions touched the vagina of his small daughter, and possibly the penis of his son as well, and from there he would go back to remembering a great number of sexual events from childhood involving heterosexual sex play, relations with animals, and wishes to touch his older sister. Whether consisting in acts or wishes, they were all very clearly seen as wrong; for the last he had expected to be killed by his father.

His confessions were closely bound up with a number of memories from childhood: when he was about eighteen months old, the next sibling died and he did not eat or make a sound for several days; when he was about five (contemporaneously with the death of another sibling) he became seriously ill and could not breathe, being saved only by the happy event of his father throwing him up into the air. When he was about eleven the older sister, with whom he had shared a room, married and left the house, after which he had dreams of a female witch with large breasts coming at him. He had similar dreams during the first phases of his relationship with me. When he was an adolescent, his father told him sarcastically that he was no good (*buono*) and thus should consider becoming a monk.

All of this information and much more concerning his life[7] and beliefs was communicated during the phase which I have referred to as the crystallization of positive transference. Though the explicit content of interviews was quite variable from week to week, there were a number of indications that on a more subtle level Mr. Calabrese was in the process of forming an increasingly meaningful attachment to me. Early indications are found in the fact that he heard voices in English saying "free" and "beautiful," while most of the more insulting voices used either Italian or Spanish. Gradually his initial anger about imprisonment diminished, and he began to see the hospital as a kindly place. After one weekend when he had visited his family, he commented that the world outside was a dangerous place where people are always lurking to kill you, but inside *mi vogliono bene* (they care about me, love me, want the best for me) and "in here I am treated with respect although I am not quite sure if it is respect for me or respect for me as a patient."

During this period I myself was never quite sure what to do about the Chinese, and consequently began to accept a hypothesis proffered by Mr. Calabrese, namely, that after a sufficient lapse of time they would disappear. Their actual, rather vividly portrayed destruction was announced to me in

7. As a biographical sketch: He was the third of seven siblings born after a long interval because of his father's second trip to the United States. The paternal grandfather was a landless peasant, but the two trips abroad enabled the father to purchase a small amount of land and apprentice out his sons as artisans; thus, in its own context, the family was upwardly mobile. Among the five living siblings he was in the middle; it appeared that the oldest brother (a coal miner and father of nine children) occupied the aggressive masculine role, while the youngest, who was the only one who did not emigrate, remained the mother's pet.

the ninth month of treatment after a television program concerning American-Soviet cooperation for disarmament.[8] Prior to this time the content of interviews was increasingly realistic with respect to work and family problems. For a brief period just after the disappearance of the Chinese he showed very acute and open anxiety and expressed fears of self-destructive impulses; he then asked for and was given special protection by the hospital.

During the month of the disappearance of the Chinese, clear signs of positive transference appeared. He retold the oft-repeated story of the fear he experienced at the moment of the Italian-American armistice in 1943, but with a new ending: as before, he referred to a sergeant in his battalion who had been shot from the air just after the armistice, but then added that he himself had been in no danger because he discovered a cave into which he led several companions for safety. The cave ending was told as he disappeared teasingly out of the door at the end of an hour with as genuine humor and gaiety as I had ever seen in him.

Family Structure and Contemporaneous Family Events

At the time of admission, Mr. Calabrese was living in a family unit consisting of his wife, his mother-in-law, and two siblings of his wife, while the only other member of his own family in the United States was an older sister in another city. Thus his admission "delusion," to the effect that he was hospitalized because of collusion between his wife, her family, and the police reflected a structural reality according to which he

8. He frequently used a political framework, and the ideas of American-Soviet cooperation against the Chinese and the 1943 armistice between Italy and the United States symbolized the transference alliance. Always up to date on current events, at the time of the Cuban crisis he felt that the missiles, probably placed by the Chinese, could not harm a strong power like the United States, but might possibly blow up from within, thus destroying Cuba.

was an outsider in a kinship unit which turned solidly against him.

In certain respects the family structure appeared as a matrifocal one, with the strongest links between the wife and her mother and siblings rather than between husband and wife. This provided a particularly conflictual situation for Mr. Calabrese because his values were strongly patriarchal: in describing his own family, he always placed most emphasis upon his father, and the identification with his father extended over a patrilineal line for several generations, so that he knew all the details of his grandfather's and great-grandfather's lives.[9] The nature of this conflict was revealed in one prehospital attempt he made to set up a more independent dwelling for himself and his wife by buying a new house: he was defeated by the matrifocal coalition, and experienced the defeat as a real threat to his identity as *pater familias*. State hospitals indeed contain many men who have been expelled in this way by lower-class families, which are very often matrifocal in orientation.

When Mr. Calabrese was first hospitalized, however, there were only slight indications that he was being expelled; in actual fact during the first ten months of treatment his wife remained in a state of indecision. Mrs. Calabrese was interviewed in her home by my research assistant and visited the hospital several times in order to see the administrative physician or the hospital social worker. Being a Roman Catholic, she did not mention divorce; however, the hospital social worker predicted that

9. Elsewhere (Chapter 1) I have described South Italian kinship as matrifocal in that the boy's strongest positive identification is with the mother rather than the father and the maternal tie very often interferes with marital solidarity. However, both regional and occupational variation may be important in this respect, and most of my informants were from the Neapolitan proletariat or sub-proletariat. For Mr. Calabrese's mountain rural areas, there are indications that the conditions of agricultural labor may make for greater husband-wife solidarity and more emphasis on patrilineal descent: Pitkin ("Land Tenure and Family Organization in an Italian Village," *Human Organiz.*, 18, 1959, 169–173) found this to be true among peasants given land and my data indicates the same for artisans in Naples. Morrill ("The Influence of the Matrifocal Kinship Network in the Italo-American Family," unpublished Ms.) found strong matrifocal kinship links in an Italo-American urban area.

she would abandon her husband since she seemed to be quite capable and desirous of bringing up her family on her own.[10] Her mobility aspirations and high degree of Americanization might lead one to wonder why she married a village man by arrangement; however, the age of the oldest child was such as to leave some question as to whether Mr. Calabrese's paternity doubts were wholly illusory, and an arranged marriage could have been a convenient way of covering an illegitimate pregnancy. She also made it evident that she intended to do "the best" for her husband, provided this did not entail returning to an intimate relationship with him. Her aggressions were veiled with a protective maternal feeling and an apparent reluctance to make the separation final.[11] I had no contact whatsoever with Mrs. Calabrese, since it was decided between the administrating physician, my supervisor, and myself at the beginning of treatment that this would not be desirable.

Soon after the disappearance of the Chinese, Mr. Calabrese brought me two very crucial letters. One was from his older sister, living in another American city, to his wife. In it she berated the wife for calling her brother crazy and putting him away just because she did not want him around; this is the typical response of blood relatives in this society, who almost inevitably stand by their own and against the in-laws at points of conflict. The second was from the sister's husband to Mr. Calabrese himself; it was a very warm and friendly letter in which he said that Mr. Calabrese would be welcome in their

10. Or better, with the aid of her relatives, whose help along with welfare payments made her husband's support unnecessary. Mr. Calabrese doubted that welfare was really a social advance: In Italy, he said, a wife would have to take her husband out of the hospital in order to eat.

11. Cf. T. S. Szasz, *Law, Liberty, and Psychiatry* (New York: The Macmillan Company, 1963). Szasz comments that hospitalization of a spouse in return for deviant acts or failure to fulfill marital obligations is actually a kind of veiled counter-aggression and that defining the deviance or failure as "illness" to be handled by technical specialists has the consequence of legitimizing the acts of one party and illegitimizing those of the other, the distinction being reinforced by law. Mr. Calabrese frequently referred to *la legge* as a social force opposing itself to him. See also, by the same author, "The Concept of Transference," *Intern. J. of Psychoanal.,* 44 (1963), 432–443.

home and he himself would be very glad to help him find work. These letters led Mr. Calabrese to consider the possibility of going to their city. Two difficulties stood in the way of this decision. The first concerned his angry and submissive yet still continuing attachment to his wife: he could not readily abandon his loyalty to his wife and re-evoke that to his natal family, but rather kept wondering whether his wife was right and he was crazy, or whether his sister was right and he was not. The second difficulty concerned myself: he raised the question of what would happen if he did move and then had to be hospitalized again in a strange city where he could not be sure that *mi vogliono bene*. It was within this triadic structure of object relationships, in which the crucial persons in Mr. Calabrese's life were his wife, his sister, and myself, that a very significant crisis in treatment occurred.

Crisis and Regression

During the tenth month of treatment Mr. Calabrese took the important step of finding paid work outside of the hospital. This necessitated a change in the therapy hour, which led to increased anxiety on his part; he also asked about cutting sessions down to once a week in view of a possible termination, which I opposed in line with the general hospital policy of caution on such matters. Before this question could be resolved, and within a week or two of his beginning to work, a sudden crisis descended upon us: Mrs. Calabrese made a formal request to the hospital authorities for the initiation of deportation proceedings, having come to the conclusion that "the best" for her husband would be that he go back home where his mother could feed him and iron his clothes. When Mr. Calabrese began a session by announcing that there were vague rumors around about the law sending people with "chronic disturbance of the mentality" back to Italy, I did not take him seriously. Later, after learning the facts from others, I offered to help him find a lawyer in the event he wished to protest the deportation, but he refused on the grounds that he could not trust the law. An added complication was that all of this happened within a few days of my scheduled departure on vacation. In consequence, he began to regress and lost his job for talking about suicide and the law with a client in the distinguished men's store where he had been promoted to fitter; he was then placed on suicide precautions within the hospital. While I was away, he escaped, but was returned to the hospital after he went to the police voluntarily for protection against two men with whom he considered running away to Florida. When I returned after a month, so did the Chinese.

Although nothing further was heard of the threatened deportation proceedings, Mr. Calabrese showed a completely new and evidently regressive syndrome for about a month following my return. In self-deprecating fashion he took on the gestures and mannerisms of the desperately poor in his country as he begged me for a bit of charity—at the very least to be allowed a place to sleep even if on the floor, and a crumb of bread within the hospital, since he had no other place to go. This syndrome disappeared fairly rapidly when I refused to reciprocate by accepting such an elevated position of authority. There was then a transitory improvement as he again returned to telling me stories of his village, going into long descriptions, with some fairly transparent sexual symbolism, of making olive oil. Subsequently references to the Chinese became an increasingly important barrier to communication, and the real therapeutic relationship began a process of deterioration.

Important signs of this deterioration were his frequent beginning of the interview with the phrase, "I am disturbed in my mentality," and some skipping of interviews or angry failure to end them with his formerly habitual *arrivederci*. Within the interviews, the barrier of respect seemed to have become a thinner one: he would sometimes masturbate during them and he more often hinted that besides cursing the deities, his voices were expressing disrespectful (sexual and aggressive) thoughts about me. Though there were still occasional meaningful exchanges, as when for the first time he showed both tears and

irony on thinking about being abandoned by his wife (momen-
tarily he seemed to realize the hypocrisy of her "I will never
abandon you" with the meaning that she would continue to
visit the hospital every month or two), most of the time we
seemed to be getting nowhere or even losing meanings which
had been present earlier. In the last interview, after twenty
months of treatment, he angrily accused me of failure to help
and expressed the opinion that the things known from books by
people of superior education might not be worth very much.
In the light of his then not very hopeful situation, I was inclined
to agree: it is with the eventual failure of treatment and its
possible explanations that I will be concerned in the next section
of this paper.

Specific Difficulties: Cultural Barriers to Insight and the Structural Reality of Transference

Throughout the course of my work with Mr. Calabrese I
had weekly supervision sessions at the state hospital, and in the
face of the difficulties arising during the second year I also
sought consultation with an experienced psychoanalyst. The
responses I made to Mr. Calabrese reflected my efforts to apply
the recommendations received from these two sources, which
evidently represented the standard approach of psychoanalytically oriented therapeutic practice.

During the first year I refrained from making interpretations
to any appreciable extent, and the situation seemed to carry
itself. During the second year I began increasingly to make
remarks such as "you must be mad at your wife" or "are you
angry at me?" or perhaps even the compound "you feel I am
letting you down just the way your wife has done." I never
felt at ease with these comments, and I suspect that I made
them mainly because of my own uncertainty, which led me to
defer to authorities outside the actual therapeutic relationship.
My remarks never elicited very much in the way of reciprocal
verbal response, and this apparent failure in the "interpretation

of negative transference" gradually began to undermine my confidence.

Mr. Calabrese's behavior in transference showed a repetitive and consistent pattern: whenever he experienced disappointment with me as a feminine object, he either reacted with aggression, which was handled by the mechanism of projection, or he would leave me in spirit in favor of "those men who have desires for other men." This pattern certainly repeated his relation with his wife, just as the homosexuality could be traced back to an unusually submissive and eroticized relation with the father.[12] Presumably the relation to his wife also repeated an earlier pattern toward the mother, of whom his most important memory was that she used to explode with the phrase, "ugly beasts from hell."

However, being able to make these formulations did not in itself resolve the question of communicating them to Mr. Calabrese in a way which would be useful to him. He did not readily make cognitive connections between affects experienced during early life and the emotions and beliefs of adulthood. The notion of ambivalence was similarly foreign to him, and in consequence he had no way of comprehending that "acceptable" hostility could be associated with the fulfillment of required obligations. His attitude of respect (*rispetto*) toward me rendered taboo the direct expression of negative or illicit feelings, and it is doubtful that he ever acquired an idea of "help" as consisting in the willingness of a professional person to talk about one's problems. In general, South Italian men are expected to be reticent about personal and family life.[13] For all of these reasons the cultural barriers to insight proved formidable indeed.

In addition, it was clear that Mr. Calabrese was expecting

12. Every time he referred to his father, or to his unsuccessful attempts to play the patriarch with his son, a passive look of pleasure would come over his face.

13. While two women may discuss marital difficulties with each other, or make ritual complaints about their husbands, even within the close-knit male peer group, references to the family are very infrequent (cf. I. K. Zola, "Observations of Gambling in a Lower Class Setting," *Soc. Prob.,* 10, 1963, 353–361). That Mr. Calabrese revealed as much as he did is in part a symptom of his pathology.

certain gratfications from me which were not legitimate within a therapeutic situation, and in consequence he suffered from continued frustration and anger. It is commonly assumed that such manifestations of a "transference bind" can be handled by interpretation alone, by which it is meant that the therapist points out verbally to the patient that, being inappropriate by the professional norms of the adult situation, his feelings must be unreal or distorted repetitions of feelings which remained unresolved during early family life or in later close relationships such as marriage. The interpretations are seen as inherently curative in that it is taken for granted that once he understands that his feelings are unreal, a realization which is attained by tracing them back to their earlier roots, they will be modified and he will automatically come to lead a fuller and more meaningful adult life.

While in psychoanalytic usage the concept of transference implies that residual infantile drives influence the patient to distort an otherwise neutral or taken-for-granted adult reality, the use of concepts from social anthropology can lead to a different view. In Mr. Calabrese's world, kinship is likely to be the center of existence; among kin one can always be sure of being treated with respect or of receiving help in time of need, while the outside world is an inherently unfriendly and threatening place. Even for an unusually good worker like him, work in itself does not have much meaning; it is simply a means of survival for oneself and one's kin, and surplus wealth will usually go into the fulfillment of kinship obligations (e.g., helping relatives to emigrate).

But Mr. Calabrese was without surrounding kin at the time I encountered him. Presumably, he also was without much motivation for "working" in psychotherapy as an end in itself. Instead he proceeded to re-create his kinship norms by putting me into various feminine slots, beginning from the moment when he hallucinated me as a maternal cousin living in France. Besides being a powerful intermediary with impersonal higher authorities, I therefore became also at various phases a mother or sister figure treated with asexual respect, a wife figure to whom one owes certain obligations which in turn can give rise to anger and conflict, and, by opposition to kinship structure, an outside woman who is by definition a potential sexual object to whom one owes nothing. None of the expectations associated with these roles was by definition infantile, since they characterized adult social interaction in the world which the patient knew. Underlying all of these role representations was his need for an object, and even in wholly psychoanalytic terms, one can see this as a real life need of the adult. Obviously the need for an object does not pass with the Oedipal phase, and in actual fact I was the most available and constant object for Mr. Calabrese. Thus all these considerations together suggest a structural reality for the transference in the patient's adult life: it was a present-day emotion which fulfilled for him a variety of needs arising from a real life gap in kinship structure.

In this perspective, not all of Mr. Calabrese's "inappropriate" behavior need appear as a manifestation of infantile residues, susceptible to being resolved by means of interpretation. Instead his increasing anger and frustration can be seen as the consequence of certain real failures on my part. I did not succeed in realistically defining a role for myself that was legitimate within his cultural frame of reference, nor did I undertake or encourage measures designed to fill the void in his life by helping him establish or reestablish object ties to persons other than myself. Had I done so, relying on a reformulation of certain customary psychotherapeutic approaches by linking anthropological kinship theory with the psychoanalytic theory of object relations, it is possible that a more favorable outcome of my work with Mr. Calabrese might have been achieved.

According to Mr. Calabrese's kinship norms, there were three kinds of women: mothers, sisters, and daughters (these being sexually taboo, and psychologically equivalent to virgin women who are to be protected by men); wives, or women with whom sexual relations are permitted, provided that one accept certain obligations; and bad women, or those with whom sexual relations are permitted without any acceptance of responsibility.

Leaving aside the question of homosexuality, the patient's psychological problem actually consisted in a failure to distinguish clearly between these roles, as when he engaged in nongenital sexual practices with his wife, whom he considered to be bad, touched his daughter on the vagina, or had incestuous thoughts about his sister, or sexual ones about me. In fact one way in which one can look at schizophrenia is to say that it simply represents a failure to internalize the incest taboo and thus securely establish cultural sublimations or distinctions between categories of social objects.[14] From this perspective, my task with Mr. Calabrese could well have been that of enabling him to reinternalize the distinctions made by his environment with respect to various categories of women (and men). The confusion which added to his sense of guilt and frustration might then have been lessened, with the result that he might have been more readily able to form legitimate adult object relations based on mutually understood reciprocal expectations. In this framework the particular kind of object relationship would not be crucial—by his norms he could have lived with his sister, provided that he could have repressed his sexual feelings; his wife, provided that a balance of reciprocal obligation could have been worked out; a woman encountered in the street who would have simply satisfied his physiological needs, or with one or more men, provided that he could have achieved the degree of sublimation characterizing peer-group friendship. The crucial consideration was that of channeling instinctual drives within a culturally meaningful and reciprocating frame, rather than simply letting them appear in unstructured confusion as they did in the therapeutic relationship.

14. In neurosis, by contrast, sublimations are present although there may be inhibitions of legitimate adult genital expression. In many primitive societies schizophrenia is seen as the consequence of violating the incest taboo. The Navaho, being matrilineal, see it as a consequence of brother-sister incest and refer to it as moth disease: as the moth is attracted blindly to the flame, thus destroying himself, so may brother and sister be blindly attracted to each other, thus destroying the kinship distinctions which make them people rather than animals.

Reevaluation: An Alternative Approach

The following is a hypothetical formulation of what I might have done to bring a greater degree of structure into the treatment if I had responded differently to a number of the communications actually made by Mr. Calabrese himself.

On an early occasion I failed to follow his suggestion that I should help him find a lawyer in order to obtain a divorce. During the subsequent session it seemed that our relationship had been put in doubt, probably as a consequence of this failure to act according to expectations which I had initially established. The same difficulty appeared at a number of later points, as when he was routinely transferred to a chronic ward after about six months in the hospital and I failed to do anything to stop it. On both occasions I failed to fulfill one expectation which was not only legitimate (because related to my higher social status) but also quite asexual: namely, that I would carry out concrete and practical actions on his behalf. Since he in fact could not control the impersonal legal and administrative forces governing his fate, these expectations were completely reasonable.

I dealt with both of these issues by attempts to elicit material about his "feelings" after the questions of action had simply been bypassed. But it is doubtful that my comments were motivated solely by humanitarian interest in *his* pathology; rather they served very conveniently to cover the ambiguities built into *my* role as an outsider in the hospital, not always certain of the extent to which I could ask for favors or violate rules of procedure.[15] One may thus query whether the taboo on giving concrete help to patients in institutional settings is designed to serve patients' interests, or whether it may rather be

15. Earlier I had carried out a considerable amount of research concerning South Italian schizophrenics (this book, Chapters 3 and 9) as an anthropologist, and in this role had not hesitated to secure as many social perspectives on the patient's life as possible by means of extra-hospital visits. However, initiating individual therapy, I felt it important to give at least some acknowledgment to the professional conventions of psychiatry which usually restrict field investigation.

a device for simplifying the role of the therapist within the institution.

When I did nothing about the matter of lawyers, Mr. Calabrese got over his explicit anger in a day or two and the issue simply dropped out of sight as he again became respectful and submissive toward me in transference, just as in reality he again became respectful and submissive toward his wife. However, we can see here the first seeds of pathology within the treatment itself. He was sacrificing his point of view for mine with too great ease and dealing with the consequent aggression by means of projection.

A second and more complex episode concerned the relation between his sister, his wife, and myself. At the beginning of the second year, he said one day that his tailor friend had visited his sister in her city, and then he remembered an earlier occasion when I had picked up a letter thrust under my office door as we entered, and he had thought that this was a card to give me permission to go to his sister's city. I replied that this had probably been when he was thinking about going to visit his sister, but that I remembered he had decided not to go. His reply to me was "definitely I decided not to go," and he then wandered off into past history about his sister which had already been repeated several times. This concluded the genuine exchange since I returned to a properly sanctioned interest in infantile sexuality.

When we had discussed the possibility of a visit to his sister, he had *not* actually decided *not* to go; my response thus represented something of a distortion. Rather, the subject had simply been dropped because of the deportation crisis and my vacation. Reinterpreted in the perspective of the structural reality of transference, his state of indecision at the time pointed to a fluctuation of libido between three feminine objects: his sister, his wife, and myself. But in the same perspective, the vacation regression itself takes on a different meaning: since he was subsequently in fact precipitously abandoned by both his wife and myself, the sister was at that time the most realistically available choice. A better retrospective interpretation of his remarks would thus be to say that he was suggesting indirectly that I get in touch with her so as to help him to compensate for the double loss; I again disappointed him by failing to understand, thus implicitly telling him that he had decided to build his life around me instead, and encouraging his choice to stay in the hospital. For this is in fact the decision he made, partly as a result of his image of the hospital as a place where *mi vogliono bene,* in contrast to the in fact very lonely outside world. Of course I did not tell him directly that this was the best course for him; but by the simple fact of failing to deal constructively with the available alternatives, this is what I encouraged him to do. In effect I persuaded him to build his emotional life around me, even though I knew quite well that there were inherent limitations to the satisfactions which such a choice could bring him, and that after a given period of time the relationship would have to come to an end.

Thus, if I could redo the treatment, I would from the beginning have recognized the realistic bases of the transference attachment and would have carried out a number of measures designed to cope with the problem of how Mr. Calabrese would fill the void once it ended. Such a plan would have required an abandonment of the dyadic isolation of the therapeutic relationship, at least after an initial period in which this isolation did appear to have had a positive value. The first and most obvious device would have been to hold interviews, either alone or in conjunction with the patient, with both his wife and his sister. Among other things, this would have clarified the definition of my own role far better than any words: a woman who is interested in knowing a man's wife and his sister is much more easily assimilated to the image of "the good one" than a woman who appears to be avoiding them.[16]

This procedure could have been based on my knowledge both of his social environment and the life possibilities it offered

16. I believe that one aspect of the transference bind was that in actual fact I felt guilty about what I was doing; I had resided in Southern Italy long enough to understand the norms according to which, while a man and a woman may joke in public even about sexual matters, there is something inherently suspicious about isolated private contacts.

and on my knowedge of his personality structure as derived from psychoanalytic concepts. Four possibilities emerge, each of which contains certain potential advantages and disadvantages. First, it was possible that his marriage could have been reestablished, with some of the more obvious difficulties resolved, and that he could then have simply returned to his prehospital situation; second, he could have taken up residence with his sister, with at least some hope that in her environment he might have found a new woman as a permitted sexual object; third, he could have returned to his village to stay with his mother and lead the life of the returned *Americano;* and fourth, he could have again taken up his premarital wandering bachelor existence. With respect to each possible life course, I could have made certain predictions in advance, drawing upon both anthropological and psychoanalytic formulations: that his sister, being blood kin, was more likely to treat him as a person than his wife; that he was more likely with the money and prestige of the *Americano* to find a new woman in his native village than near the hospital with his broken English and the law against him; or that any relationship with a woman was likely to contain some difficulties because of his homosexual impulses. No prediction could have been made as to the future with complete accuracy, both because the realization of any life course would depend on others as well as Mr. Calabrese and because any human biography contains an irreducible element of uncertainty and chance. However, I could have utilized these schematized possibilities as a framework for organizing the treatment, testing each possibility in turn against its workings in reality.

If it should have proved impossible to reestablish the marriage, we would at least have had this as a concrete fact brought into the range of therapeutic confrontation and could then have gone on to further alternatives. Among other things a direct confrontation of the question of divorce or separation would have made it possible to see that Mr. Calabrese had more of a chance to take the upper hand in the matter, rather than remaining passive. With my support and encouragement he might actually have contacted a lawyer for working out matters such as financial arrangements and continued visits with his children.[17] Simply the possibility of taking a more active role in separation should have augmented his masculine self-esteem. With a separation underway, we could then have turned to the most readily available substitute for his wife, namely, the sister. The fact that she did not visit spontaneously or write him directly indicates some degree of alienation, for which his incestuous thoughts point to the deeper cause. However, Italian immigrant relatives sometimes stay away from hospitals simply for fear of impersonal bureaucracies or because of language difficulties. Such fears could very easily have been resolved by a note from me saying that it was important for her to visit in order to discuss her brother's future. If such a visit had taken place, it would have raised the hope that we could arrange a trial visit for the period of my vacation. As a matter of fact his thinking of this idea himself (after I had, according to established procedure, given him warning of the coming abandonment) was about the most constructive thing he could have done, especially since vacations for their own sake are almost completely unknown in his world, where people travel only to visit relatives.

But one important fact in his failure to carry through any plans was that, being bound by the law, he was not a free agent; a visit would have required clearance from hospital authorities which in turn would have required some action on my part. His sister's concrete presence would have been the best possible persuasive device. In this sphere as well there was no guaranteed success: but even with respect to the deeper incest problem, actual contacts with the sister would have given us something mutually understandable to work with. It did not do very much good for me to point out the existence of infantile

17. The Roman Catholic religion might have been an unsurmountable deterrent to formal divorce for both parties; however, alternative possibilities such as an informal or legalized separation were available which would not have necessarily been incompatible with his finding a new mate. See the discussion following.

sexuality, but a few well-timed challenges, such as "What are you going to do about it if you have bad feelings about your sister, so that she doesn't call you crazy and get the police?" might have had more effect.

A failure with respect to his sister would still not have exhausted the possibilities, for we still could have gone on to consider others. His wife's idea of a return to the village in fact was not at all inappropriate, though it would have been preferable for him to return in his own good time with a bit of money in pocket, rather than being ignominiously deported by the authorities as suffering from "chronic disturbance of the mentality." Among other things, due to his father's death, the family situation had radically changed since his departure, so that he might have been able to secure some of the maternal attentions he missed in earlier life. And for all I know, his uncle was still holding a plot of land in Latin America waiting for him to return to farm it. Again, I could not with any certainty have predicted what was likely to happen to him in any of these lives, nor could I have been certain that he would not again have been picked up by the police for incautious verbalizations about the Chinese. The essential point is that almost any of these possibilities, even if not totally successful, would have been better than the life of a chronic patient on a back ward.

The fact that I failed to help Mr. Calabrese more realistically with the problems of his life can be seen as something much more than a minor flaw in my treatment technique; rather, its consequence was that he chose to remain in the hospital simply because, being actually dominated by the law, there was not very much else he could have done without more active intervention on my part. Moreover, at first this must have seemed to him by far the best alternative, since outside there was only a non-kin alien world in which he feared that men were lurking to kill him. There were moments in treatment, especially about the time of the disappearance of the Chinese, when I thought that the logic of transference would lead to the point where he would grow a new and stabler personality, as if recapitulating with a better outcome the earliest phase of object internalization when the mother's image becomes a part of the self.[18]

Rather than propelling a deep-lying personality change, however, the transference relation seemed more and more to disintegrate in consequence of its real-life adult frustrations and ambiguities. It thus seems a badly oversimplified view to interpret the symptoms which appear in transference binds as consequences of infantile repetitions alone. One could glibly talk about "infantile masturbation" with respect to some of Mr. Calabrese's unaesthetic actions of the second year; one could talk as well of the innate aggressiveness of the "paranoid personality." However, both his earlier history and many aspects of the therapeutic interaction itself contraindicate the view that he had simply never gained control over primitive drives: his aggressiveness at first took the quite socialized form of an impressive rhetorical display, and intitialy he found it quite possible to maintain an attitude of respect and trust in me. Thus both the manifestations of sexual drive, which the Italians refer to as *il fatto materiale,* and the progressive diffusion of aggression throughout his personality can just as easily be seen as consequences of anomie, or the breakdown of cultural forms, as of a mechanical "repetition compulsion" which acts independently of any external referents. But the cross-cultural ambiguities of the therapy itself were such as to increase the degree of anomie rather than to aid in the consolidation of structure. As Mr. Calabrese quite acutely observed, though I spoke his language, it was not with the profundity of a person born in his country.

Wider Conclusions

My aim in this paper has not been just to present the therapeutic history of a single case, but rather to use this history as material to illuminate some much broader questions concerning the culture of psychotherapy and therapeutic technique. In

18. Around this time, pleasurable memories of going on pilgrimages with his mother and other women appeared, along with a use of expressions like *Madonna mia* which was very rare for him.

these conclusions I shall be concerned with the methods of treatment best adapted to the working-class patient, with the potential contributions of social science to psychotherapeutic practice, and with the culture of psychotherapy and the treatment techniques conventionally used within the middle class.

One need not despair of the feasibility of adapting psychological treatment modes to the working class. I would certainly not be in favor of substituting organic treatment on the grounds that only upper-status people have internal feelings, as is sometimes implied when they are viewed as having more highly developed "introspective" capacities. Rather the most appropriate form of working-class treatment appears to be the brief interventionary type of psychotherapy, the goal of which is to get the patient back into a viable social situation where he will not start the downward course that leads to imprisonment, Skid Row, or chronic back-ward hospitalization. Such treatment is also called for from the pragmatic point of view, since the limitations in professional resources characterizing most working class treatment centers are unlikely to be quickly overcome, and it seems more equitable to give brief and well-planned interventionary treatment to all than to start a few on an uncertain course of analysis interminable while leaving the rest to the mercies of bureaucracy![19]

Up to the present time, psychiatric use of social science has largely been restricted to studies of the treatment setting itself. But while such studies may be helpful for understanding patients during the course of treatment, they say little about how patients come to a treatment setting or what they will do when they leave. With respect to the latter questions, by far the most useful available material has to do with the patterns of kinship and family dynamics, which have been studied systematically for a great variety of cultures. Matrifocal kin patterns, in which the relation of the male to the family unit is more

19. The treatment philosophy of the state hospital where I saw Mr. Calabrese was in fact very much influenced by psychoanalytic models; however, the actual consequence was that a favored few received intensive treatment, while the rest received lower prestige drugs, milieu therapy, or nothing very much at all.

peripheral than in the middle class, are of course a particularly crucial focus of study for working-class psychopathology; in the Caribbean area matrifocal patterns have been well studied by anthropologists,[20] and these patterns may very broadly characterize marginal urban industrial as well as ex-slave and landless peasant groups.[21]

Since social anthropology is a discipline which deals with social structure and conscious mental representations, it may well be relevant not only to the treatment of lower-class patients, but of middle-class patients as well. A further potential use of social anthropology in the latter context lies in its capabilities for cutting through some of the overly idealistic representations of the culture of psychotherapy—that is, the sum total of shared social meanings and communication patterns which characterize those who believe that the path to salvation lies in a self-conscious understanding of personal feelings.

For those who believe that simply getting the patient to talk and attend therapy sessions is in itself worthwhile, it is important to emphasize the very great difficulties which can arise. When working-class patients receive intensive long-term psychotherapy there is a high probability that the motives of the therapist will be misunderstood. Such difficulties are not peculiar to my case. During the same period I observed several analogous situations of "transference bind" involving psychiatric residents and second-generation Italian women. In more than one such case I felt that the patient was induced to stay in the hospital because of the transference attachment. In another instance, while the staff was discussing the "transference fantasies" of a young Sicilian girl who claimed to have been raped, her irate brothers were after local politicians to protest the insult to the honor of the family that the complaint entailed. Although in South Italian hospitals, when families fear such a dishonor-

20. Cf. W. Davenport, "The Family System of Jamaica," *Soc. & Eco. Studies,* 10 (1961), 420–454. M. G. Smith, *Kinship and Community in Cariacou* (New Haven: Yale Univ. Press, 1962). R. T. Smith, *The Negro Family in British Guiana* (London: Routledge & Keegan Paul, Ltd., 1956).
21. Cf. Morrill, *op. cit.*

able loss of virginity, the medical staff deals with the problem by means of a vaginal examination, in this case no one except the gardener ever understood the social meaning of the situation.

Beneficial results going beyond what can reasonably be expected from brief interventions might be achieved by introducing certain changes in the therapist's mode of treatment. Such changes would entail bringing the patient's intimates actively into the therapeutic situation and structuring the therapeutic work in such a way as to organize a sequence of possible alternatives for his post-hospital life, each one being taken up in such a way as to lead to a reality decision within a framework of normative expectations familiar to the patient. A treatment plan of this sort could be considered as a form of *intensive* psychotherapy, in that to carry it out successfully would require at least two years' work. A more accurate term for this sort of approach is *active* psychotherapy, since the primary focus would be on the patient's reality situation rather than simply on interpretation of affect and its mechanisms. But in the minds of many persons, perhaps in particular the most sensitive and well-trained psychotherapists engaged in intensive work, the idea of active psychotherapy is likely to strike a negative chord. The discussion which follows will center on the reasons for this particular devaluation and their anchorage within the culture of psychotherapy. By this route we can approach the question of the implications of this particular case for middle-class as well as working-class patients.

ACTIVE TREATMENT

By active treatment, I mean that the therapist is actively concerned with the patient's possibilities for social reciprocity within the context of his own life, not that an attempt is made to provide a life for the patient within the context of treatment. The therapist should help the patient to seek his gratifications within the range of relationships socially available to him. The patient is then bound by the social norms of his environment, whatever these happen to be. This is not by any means a form of psychotherapy that manipulates complex personality dynamics in favor of a limited or specific goal. Nor is it similar to the dramatic role-playing with the patient undertaken by John Rosen[22] or Mme. Sechehaye.[23] I do not believe that one can actually provide love or reciprocate the patient's projected roles; for one thing this may confuse the needs of the adult and the residual ones of the child, and for another it may act so as to increase the potentialities for transference binds or treatments interminable, since real life gratifications received in therapy can always act so as to increase the patient's involvement in it and his detachment from the realities of his life.

Active therapy requires far more rapid and complex assimilation of knowledge on the part of the therapist than the purely interpretive communication of well-known psychodynamic formulations. Likewise the inclusion of third persons in the treatment increases its complexity and thus its unpredictability. These considerations may help to explain why it tends to be viewed with caution. It requires, furthermore, the expenditure of far more energy on the part of the psychotherapist, and perhaps in many ways can require greater technical skill. However, for precisely these reasons one could say that it should have the higher valuation. An active effort, even if it entails an element of risk, can in the long run be more satisfying than sitting behind a desk day after day listening to human misery without the conviction that one is doing very much about it.

Active psychotherapy means, furthermore, that it is the responsibility of the therapist to know about his patient's social norms and to consider them as crucially relevant to the treatment process. What would contrast such active treatment with many of today's conventionalized techniques would then be the view that the psychotherapeutic relationship is only one part of a total social context. Active psychotherapy would in turn require the systematic use of social science, not just as a means for understanding "therapeutic communities," or for "testing

22. J. Rosen, *Direct Analysis: Selected Papers* (New York: Grune & Stratton, Inc., 1953).
23. M. A. Sechehaye, *Symbolic Realization: A New Method of Psychotherapy Applied to a Case of Schizophrenia* (New York: International Universities Press, 1951).

hypotheses," but rather as a means for describing the great variety of social patterns which exist in our melting-pot society. Moreover, since this society is constantly changing, the problems of patients in psychotherapy, and of those who see them as well, more commonly concern a lack of normative structuring or cultural anchorage than a simple conflict between a fixed social order and illicit instincts that push against it. An active psychotherapy would accordingly also have to be concerned with the formulation or reformulation of social norms.

For such an active therapy, the therapeutic problems would always be precisely the same as the one I defined for work with Mr. Calabrese, namely, to help the patient to come to terms with his own conflicts, and his own necessity for choice, within the framework of social meaning which is relevant to him: its basic rule would be that the therapist should always talk to the patient in his own social vocabulary, and never attempt to initiate him into the language of psychological research by means of alienating interpretations about his personality mechanisms. Among early psychoanalysts, Ferenczi[24] stands out for his open advocacy of active technique; more recently Erikson has been particularly concerned with questions of adult identity choice, and in the increasingly systematic family studies[25] we can see the use of concepts about real social structures, rather than the use of vague "culturalist" or "interpersonal" ideologies. However, the fact remains that the most widely diffused conceptual and ideological bases of psychotherapeutic work to-

24. S. Ferenczi, "On the Technique of Psychoanalysis," in *Further Contributions to the Theory and Techniques of Psychoanalysis* (London: Hogarth Press, 1950), pp. 177–189. Ferenczi seems to have initiated his modifications of classical technique mainly because of an acute perception of the kinds of superficiality and boredom which can occur within the psychoanalytic situation itself when the analyst does nothing but encourage the patient's verbal flow: in this, he was far less bound by theory than Freud. See also, by the same author, "The Further Development of an Active Therapy in Psychoanalysis," in *Ibid.*, 16 (1920), 198–216. Also S. Freud, "Katharina," J. Breuer & S. Freud (eds.), *Studies on Hysteria* (New York: Basic Books, Inc., 1957), pp. 125–134.

25. Theodor Lidz, Stephen Fleck, and Alice R. Cornelison, *Schizophrenia and the Family* (New York: International Universities Press, 1965).

day can very easily lead to a distorted view of man in which his early psychological development and his internal affect are abstracted from normative structuring and cultural form, or from the situational demands of life, and are seen simply as "objects" of psychological research.

THE TREATMENT HIERARCHY

One of the principal determinants of the tendency to under-value active psychotherapy can be found in the present-day treatment hierarchy. The psychoanalyst at the top of the hierarchy carries out a form of treatment which is generally centered on feelings alone or on a search for "deeper" levels of the personality. In the most orthodox Freudian practice the search for feelings tends to be rather exclusively focused on sexual impulses or on the early years of life, but essentially the same view characterizes much less orthodox or neo-Freudian practice as well. By contrast, those treatment forms which center to a greater extent on immediate reality problems in the patient's life tend to be perceived as the province of, or to be relegated to, personnel who rank lower on the status hierarchy. Thus the bright college student with minor neurotic problems, whose life is taking care of itself, will be seen on the couch by the psychoanalyst, while the chronic schizophrenic who lives alone in a rented room will be handed to a social worker for "support" or "help with reality problems."

However, as with all status hierarchies, the values underlying this one can be reversed in valence when an outside observer takes a critical role, and one can begin by asking whether or not there might be something strange about a system of values that puts reality in such a secondary position.[26] In actual

26. In case discussions, one often hears it said, "Well, maybe some of what the patient says is reality," with the implication that while his affect is by definition distorted, perhaps some real event or injustice did elicit it. The view whch I have tried to present with respect to the breakdown of cultural norms is rather that no affect ever arises except in consequence of a real social stimulus; individual differences and reactions which can be called pathological then relate only to intensity and mode of expression.

fact, the social worker often gets the most difficult cases—persons with grossly disorganized lives and bizarre libidinal impulses showing in visible form—while anything but a few hysterical symptoms in a bright young college girl can be considered too difficult for the beginning psychoanalytic candidate. However, to the extent that she accepts the current status hierarchy as a valid one, the social worker will consider the province of her own work to be the more superficial or lower-valued "reality" one and in consequence keep her hands off her client's "deeper" conflicts, lest her psychoanalytic superego give her a spanking.

There is a corresponding hierarchy of patients or clients: those who turn to the welfare department have worries about the rent, while those who turn to psychoanalysts usually are much freer for engagement in refinements of feeling. However, the greater victim of exploitation may in actual fact be the middle-class or wealthy patient[27] who goes to the psychoanalyst, in particular if the latter uses an extreme of passive technique; some psychoanalysts fulfill their role requirements by the simple process of saying virtually nothing at all. It takes far more energy for the witch doctor to manipulate his ritual implements. A reversal of values would be such as to put on top the active treatment in which the therapist does something for the patient and expends energy in the process.

THE CONCEPT OF NEUTRALITY

A second and perhaps deeper reason for contemporary avoidance of realistic object relations and social norms in the patient's adult life has to do with ethical considerations

27. Though this is often considered a matter too indelicate for discussion, it is worth noting that the economic problem of psychoanalysis is by no means limited to the poor: at current rates, full psychoanalysis takes from twenty-five to fifty per cent of an upper-level business or professional income, and many analysts do not hesitate to extend the treatment five or six years or to prescribe a second analysis if the results of the first are disappointing. None but other-worldly sects among religious institutions practicing tithing as a way of insuring financial security for those whose job is salvation has ever appropriated anything like this proportion of individual wealth.

underlying the concept of neutrality. Insofar as the aim of the concept of neutrality is to leave matters of choice to the patient, and to prevent the therapist from approaching the role of God who made man after his own image, its ethical basis is of course quite sound. It is important to note that in my active plan for Mr. Calabrese I did not mean that *I* should have decided whether he was to live with wife, sister, mother, or alone. My task would only have been to clarify each possibility, its advantages and limitations, leaving all questions of actual decision to Mr. Calabrese himself, and to those who were close to him.

Though to the scientific observer interested in theory, incestuous impulses may be seen neutrally, in every known human society they in fact are characterized as bad. In attaching a value judgment to them, as I did when I spontaneously referred to them as "bad feelings," I was simply speaking in terms of the frame of reference Mr. Calabrese knew, which was also that of all humanity excepting only psychoanalytic theorizers. The same was true for the seductive attempts toward the children: he himself felt these to be sinful and they probably were in fact a major reason for his being expelled from the family scene.[28] In failing to comment more actively and judgmentally on sins which to him in a very real way appeared as sins, I helped to increase his psychological uncertainty and flux, rather than providing badly needed ego controls. In retrospect, I believe I was siding with unrestrained instinct rather than with his moral mind.

Similarly, my emphasis on Mr. Calabrese's hostile feelings toward his wife created a conflict between my permissive attitude concerning negative feelings and his norms, which said that even if a marriage is difficult you keep quiet about it in order to

28. In Naples, while murder may under certain circumstances be considered quite justifiable, the man who has sexually assaulted a child becomes an irrevocable social outcast. [This is based on a "morality of reciprocity." While some kinds of murder can be considered, from the point of view of the actor, as setting right a wrong, the overpowering of children, sexually or otherwise, is an act of unilateral abuse of power.—*Ed.*]

preserve the institution of marriage as such. In more general terms, simply discussing feelings without reference to the particular normative structures which govern them in the mind of the patient can lead to an undermining of the norms or an acute conflict between them and participation in the treatment itself. Consequently, the "neutral" therapist does not remain outside value conflict, but increases it, or helps to create a kind of social anomie in which feelings appear without regulating devices. It thus seems more truly neutral to accept at face value the patient's conscious norms, whatever these happen to be, and not allow them to drop out of sight.

Moreover, social science can also contribute a great deal to the development of psychotherapeutic technique along these lines. Many trained psychotherapists today can talk about homosexuality, perversion, bestiality, and fantasies of murder and rape without a blush, but when it comes to questions of personal value or religious belief, reactions of blushing, embarrassment, and avoidance begin to appear. This evidently points to a kind of sociological primitivism: it is as if the therapist believed that confrontation of the patient's norms is in fact equivalent to agreeing with all of them or trying to convert him to one's own. This, of course, is far from being the truth. Social scientists have known for a long time that norms and values can be investigated and considered just as objectively as affects and drives. All I would have had to say to Mr. Calabrese in this respect was that I knew his religious belief was for him a real deterrent to divorce; but I also knew that sometimes couples do separate informally in Italy and that also some couples do divorce after they have been in America for a long time, because here people are quite different and it is sometimes harder to get along. Again the choice would have been his, but I could have pointed out the various legitimate or semilegitimate channels available in his environment for resolving marital difficulty. In this I would have emphasized the same official norms as the priest, so as to avoid putting him in conflict between two authorities. But I could have done so with much greater flexibility, since my task was dealing with a particularly conflictual individual situation, while that of the priest is to reinforce the norms themselves, since he serves as a representative of a larger social institution.

The most important way, however, in which my posture of neutrality was not a true one was that it gave Mr. Calabrese implicit encouragement to stay in the hospital because of the isolating attachment to me that followed from my failure to consider more consistently and objectively the range of external possibilities that were open to him. But this is also probably the commonest and most dangerous kind of violation of neutrality in contemporary psychotherapy: rare is the analyst who, when confronted by the patient with three or four alternative possibilities for his future, only one of which is compatible with the continuation of treatment, judges the question in a purely neutral fashion with respect to relative merits for the patient's life. An extreme result of the usual form of therapeutic "neutrality" is the patient, not uncommon today, who moves from analysis to analysis, building both an emotional life and a system of values around the treatment process itself, always in search of a still undefined Absolute in the personal understanding of feeling. This latter patient is of course one of the most fully initiated members of the culture of psychotherapy and so brings us to the question of active treatment for the middle class.

NORMATIVE STANDARDS AND THE PROBLEM OF INSIGHT

A study carried out by several members of the Boston Psychoanalytic Institute revealed that 50 per cent of the patients accepted as control cases are psychologists, social workers, or social scientists, i.e., close professional affiliates of the budding psychoanalyst himself.[29] The fact that such a selection was not

29. P. H. Knapp, S. Levin, R. H. McCarter, H. Wermer, & E. Zetzel, "Suitability for Psychoanalysis: A Review of 100 Supervised Analytic Cases," *Psychoanal. Quar., 29* (1960), 459–477. The same study also discovered that not being married or having difficulties in getting along with the opposite sex were the major presenting complaints; it thus shows very clearly the extent to which psychoanalysis has come to replace religion as today's solution to the problem of object deprivation.

the conscious intent of the Institute makes the study particularly valuable as an index of the latent importance of "speaking a common language" in evaluating a patient's capacity for insight. However, this fact introduces a new and complicating variable, namely, that when people speak the same professional language, there is always the danger that they will agree on the validity of certain perceptions of interpretations mainly through a process of consensual validation which has no real referent outside itself. Thus "insight" need no longer be a personalized matter; it may become simply a new kind of status acquisition according to which a social worker, for example, begins to speak the erudite language of the psychoanalyst after the manner of the *Bourgeois Gentilhomme*. This kind of consensual validation may provide a new sort of cultural barrier to insight, different in kind from Mr. Calabrese's cognitive failure to understand the psychotherapeutic situation, but not necessarily different in its confusing effects.

Another source of confusion results from the values governing psychotherapy, and the failure to distinguish between acceptance of these values and "insight" on the part of the patient. Thus the patient's wish to remain in treatment in the hospital becomes a token of insight, while his AWOL attempt, whatever its individual motive, comes to be defined as an expression of unchanneled instinct. But while this problem is most accentuated within the psychiatric hospital, because of the degree to which the lives of patients are controlled in reality, it also much more broadly characterizes the culture of psychotherapy, e.g., in that it selectively reinforces certain kinds of verbal communication as opposed to other conceivable values.

It is obvious that psychiatric patients sometimes do need to be hospitalized, and there is reason to believe that the treatment they receive is likely to be most effective if it occurs in the setting of a "therapeutic community" where attention is also given to teaching and research. But the patients in such a setting are most likely to want freedom and concrete solutions to the problems of their lives, while staff members may be concerned with carrying out their various teaching and research enterprises.

Among other things, the therapeutic community provides a captive audience for the teaching of psychotherapy to residents, and since long-term psychotherapy is most emphasized today, this in itself may lead to an emphasis on long-term hospitalization without any prior proof that this is the type of treatment that is most helpful to patients. Likewise, research motives may lead to an emphasis on "uncovering" without much consideration for whether the patients feel better or worse after they have been "uncovered." On the psychological plane, the therapeutic community today may be doing the same thing as the old-fashioned hospital, which felt entitled to undress its patients in order to search for lice. This again is a problem which characterizes the culture of psychotherapy as a whole. It supports and maintains certain generalized social values, but perhaps to a far greater extent than is ever admitted these values are determined by research, teaching, and other career-maximizing motives of the psychiatric profession which conflict, rather than harmonize, with the immediate needs of patients, who want help that makes sense within the framework of their own lives.

Since the normative pressures exerted by the professional structure and research interests of contemporary psychiatry serve to isolate certain naked features of personality from the ordinary social clothing of norms, social reciprocity, and the material requirements of life, the norms of psychotherapy are likely to end up either with the kind of idealistic bias exemplified by the patient who continually searches for an Absolute in the pure understanding of feelings, or with the kind of amoralism which turns the uncovering of lice into a positive goal. Conceiving of feelings experientially, both views appear as a new kind of alienation from the humanism which would say that the only valid goal of treatment is to help people to live better lives than they would without it. According to the latter conception, therapeutic progress can be measured only by reference to values that are external to the treatment process itself.

It thus seems worthwhile to start afresh in trying to define insight in such a way as to make it unnecessary to initiate patients into the culture of psychotherapy and to teach them the language of psychiatric research. A psychotherapist obviously cannot assume that all of his patients are operating according to the same normative standards. The essence of our own society is its very great diversity of social values and norms. But what he can do, to a much greater extent than is commonly done today (except by those who systematically consider family process), is to take it for granted that patients do have structures of object relations and specific behavioral norms that are independent of the therapeutic situation itself.

Applying an anthropological viewpoint, it appears from my work with Mr. Calabrese that the cross-cultural ambiguities of the therapeutic situation were such as to accelerate a movement toward anomie, or a process of breakdown in the cultural forms which in all well-integrated societies serve to channel expression of instinct through patterns that are reciprocally understood by those who participate in them. In Mr. Calabrese's case, in spite of his individual pathology, we can very clearly see the outlines of the traditional forms which did not accord either with his internal impulses or with the changes in his reality situation following from emigration. However, the more typical psychotherapy patient today, and the more typical psychotherapist, is not Mr. Calabrese himself, but rather his son or his grandson. That is to say he is a person who is no longer bound by particular traditional patterns, but rather may be very ready to admit to "hostile impulses against father figures," precisely because nowadays it is legitimate for sons to depart from the values of their fathers.

Thus one of the major functions of the culture of psychotherapy is to fill a cultural gap: lacking inherited norms and values for structuring life, many persons have turned to a study of psychological processes, utilizing psychological models which have been abstracted from social norms. While such an effort may produce valuable scientific results, it is doubtful if the scientific study of psychology in itself can answer questions about how to live. The patterns of the European peasant village, the Jewish ghetto community, or the solidly Protestant New England or frontier small town no longer suffice for today's complex urban and suburban world. In the long run individuals cannot avoid questions of choice and personal commitment, nor the question of how to fill the voids of anomie which have been created by rapid social change. The largely unmet need of individuals for new cultural forms, adapted to the contemporary world but still meaningfully linked to their cultural predecessors, may in fact be a crucial determinant of the overly idealistic preoccupation with words about the psychological development, feelings, and past histories of individuals. But the void of anomie cannot be filled without the invention of genuine cultural forms. And these cultural forms cannot be created nor derived from scientific concepts alone—nor from any set of concepts which assume only an atomized individual.

Perhaps the most important lesson to be learned from my two years' work with a poor immigrant tailor who did not understand the culture of psychotherapy, but instead was bound by a system of traditional values and expectations which were in many ways incompatible with it, concerns not the specific problem of treatment for the working class, but rather the more general one of limitations existing in the culture of psychotherapy itself.

chapter **15**

*On Psychoanalytic Training for Research Purposes**

It is widely taken for granted today that persons engaged in any academic or hospital research employing psychoanalytic concepts or touching on clinical questions should have psychoanalytic training. But, because of the high cost of the full psychoanalysis involved, many research workers are unable to undertake such training, however useful it might be to them professionally. In recognition of this fact, a number of

* I am indebted to Drs. Rose Coser, Theodore Lidz, Sidney Mintz, David M. Schneider, and Thomas S. Szasz for critical comments on earlier versions of this paper, and to the Foundations' Fund for Research in Psychiatry for the fellowship on which my observations are based. The responsibility for all views expressed is my own.

foundations currently follow the practice of giving fellowships that either pay directly for a didactic analysis or include the expectation that the recipient will be in analysis as part of a larger program. Here I should like to set forth the view that, although the needs on which it is based are unquestionably real, this practice is in actuality much less desirable than it appears at first glance.

I shall begin by observing that, as currently organized by the American Psychoanalytic Association, psychoanalytic training gives priority to the candidate's personal analysis rather than to educational work in seminars or apprenticeship in dealing with patients; though standards exist in these latter areas, they are both more variable locally and more loosely formulated than the essential criteria of progress in analysis, achievement of insight, and working through of personal problems that are now used as standards for professional advance. This is especially true for the nonmedical candidate who does not take a control case. I shall try to establish the fact that, as a consequence of this approach, contemporary analytic training blurs the distinction between public and private spheres that generally characterizes modern societies; it is on this point that my discussion will center.

By its very nature, psychoanalysis is concerned with matters pertaining to private life. From one standpoint, it is a new way of dealing with some very old problems. Starting from some ideas about early personality formation and the influence of early family relationships on the child, it deals, in the treatment of adults, with the more intimate feelings and social relationships in private life or with the more intimate facets of public ties with colleagues and authority figures. Every neurosis, according to Freud, is the outgrowth of difficulties in one single sphere of life. In other times and places, the same difficulties have been dealt with by other means: In the primitive society, the magical practitioner may prescribe a love potion for the person unable to attract the one he would like to attract; and in the Roman Catholic world, the confessional serves as an outlet for conflicts concerning the family and sexuality. The French anthropologist, Claude Lévi-Strauss,[1] has said that the magical practitioner and the psychoanalyst have in common the fact that they attempt to cure intrapsychic disorder by the manipulation of words or symbols. (In this respect they both differ from the physician, who manipulates physical organs of the body.)

However, he points out, the two part company sharply on another dimension. The primitive practitioner provides for the patient a myth or a ritual having a standardized social content. The psychoanalyst, in contrast, acts merely as a catalyst while the patient creates his own individual myth by the recovery and integration of personal memories. Thus psychoanalysis is an appropriate mode of treatment for an individualistic age. Unlike both the magical practitioner and the priest, who represent particular kinds of social or moral order, the psychoanalyst does not make decisions of value for his patients and, ideally, does not act as an agent of social control. In this sense, the rapid growth in his prestige and importance, especially among those contemporary groups which no longer adhere to any dogmatic religious or moral tradition, is only one aspect of the general trend toward a greater separation of public and private spheres of the personality. Formal social controls in the modern world tend to be restricted to public spheres, such as behavior on the street or on the job; and, especially in the complex social organization of the modern city, such matters as behavior within the family, sexual morality, and private attitudes about public authority are increasingly viewed as matters of individual concern.

General Problems in Psychoanalytic Training

It is in this context of progressive social differentiation and individualization that psychoanalysis has evolved as the major modern competitor for the healing role. However, the paradoxical fact of the matter is that psychoanalytic training, just

1. Claude Lévi-Strauss, *Structural Anthropology* (New York): Basic Books Inc., 1963).

because it is not based on a built-in separation between public and private spheres, runs counter to the same social trend that has most furthered the diffusion of psychoanalysis. The training analysis, as Thomas Szasz has pointed out,[2] differs from the purely private treatment situation in one very important respect. In private treatment, the patient can reveal his innermost thoughts and feelings without any risk of undesirable consequences in the real world, for nothing he says in analysis goes beyond the analyst. In the training analysis this is not the case, for the analyst can communicate with the authority body that determines the candidate's status in training. Thus the candidate does not possess the guarantee of medical confidence that applies to every private patient. This means that the authority of the training analyst is very unusual by the standards of modern societies because it covers the entire personality rather than certain specified public segments of it. The result is that matters pertaining to private life may have consequences in the public sphere and vice versa; in this respect, analytic structure resembles that of totalitarian societies in which children may be expected to inform the authority figures of their parents' deviations from ideological conformity.

The research foundation exemplifies the more common authority pattern in democracies. It possesses authority because it can both make grants and reject applications; thus the careers of persons in research work depend upon its actions. However, while it can reject an applicant either because he is incompetent or, as sometimes happens, because it does not understand or agree with his views about research, in either instance it is presumably concerned only with one segment of his total personality, namely his capacities and motivation for research. Moreover, this segment is a public one in that any person who honestly does research publishes his work so that it can be evaluated by qualified and interested others. In most instances, the research foundation simply does not know how the applicant

2. Thomas S. Szasz, "Three Problems in Contemporary Psychoanalytic Training," *AMA Arch. General Psychiatry* (1960) 3 : 82–94. See especially pp. 87–88.

feels about his parents or his marriage, or even what images of research foundations he happens to have on bad days.

In contrast, the training analyst does have access to these spheres. This means that matters other than work capacities or qualifications can play a part in the selection and training of psychoanalysts. Many institutes, for example, are suspicious of unmarried candidates, and homosexuality is usually a reason for outright rejection. In actual fact, then, training standards are such as to reinforce the psychoanalyst's role as representative of a specific moral order—even though Freud's scientific humanism preached objectivity concerning all forms of human behavior, and even though the psychoanalyst is ideally not an agent of social control. Both of the criteria mentioned above are congruent with suburban American upper middle-class family standards, which, while not exactly Puritan in the old-fashioned sense, do put a great deal of emphasis on early marriage and child-bearing and in many respects agree with the Latin peasantry that there is something highly sacred about the relationship between a mother and her child. But of course, as social anthropology has shown, a great variety of cultural solutions has been offered for the universal facts of sexuality and reproduction, and many can be found within the wider metropolis.

The reason given by psychoanalysts for using private criteria in training is, of course, that since the analyst deals professionally with private life, his own private life is relevant to his role. However, it is possible to disagree with this view while emphasizing the necessity of objectivity to the analyst's professional work. If a homosexual has so little objectivity about his own problem that he is unable to understand or to deal with the conflicts of his patients, which, statistically speaking, are most likely to be heterosexual, then he would presumably make a bad analyst and should not be admitted to training. However, such difficulties should show up in work with patients which can be publicly evaluated—that is, in supervision; and, just as many practicing homosexuals are good writers, teachers, or businessmen, there seems on the face of it no reason why a homosexual who can clearly distinguish between his own feelings and those of others cannot be a good analyst. By modern standards, his private life should still remain his own business provided that it does not interfere with his public role.

The ambiguities inherent in the professional use of personal psychoanalysis have played a role in psychoanalytic politics from the beginning. In the early days, the epithet "unresolved transference neurosis" was very commonly hurled in situations of intellectual disagreement between analyst and analysand. This tendency is perhaps less pronounced today because American community-centred modes of reconciling differences have to a considerable degree replaced the authoritarian patriarchalism of Freud. Moreover, the difficulties of the training situation have not gone completely unnoticed by psychoanalysts,[3] who have established a number of informal rules for dealing with the complications that arise from the social overlap between the training analyst and the candidate. Thus, in the more orthodox circles at least, there is an implicit taboo on inviting the two to the same party, on the grounds that their interaction should be restricted to the analytic sphere, thus establishing some privacy around this. Many training analysts also voluntarily refrain from communicating specific details of the analysand's life that might, if divulged to colleagues, have social repercussions.[4] Most important, nearly all of the institutes have by now restricted the very great power of the training analyst by the committee

3. See, for example: Clara Thompson, "A Study of the Emotional Climate of Psychoanalytic Institutes," *Psychiatry* (1958), 21 : 45–51; Martin Grotjahn, "About the Relation Between Psycho-analytic Training and Psycho-analytic Therapy," *Internat. J. Psychoanal.* (1954), 35 : 254–262; Sacha Nacht, "The Difficulties of Didactic Psychoanalysis in Relation to Therapeutic Analysis," *Internat. J. Psychoanal.* (1954), 35 : 250–253. The difficulty of these writings is that, except for Thompson, the main concepts used are those of transference and countertransference, which are technical terms referring to infantile affects and not designed to deal with problems in adult social structure. However, all seem to agree that the didactic analysis is less likely to be successful than the ordinary personal one; it is thus surprising that the organization of training has remained so long unchanged.

4. Thomas S. Szasz, "The Problem of Privacy in Training Analysis," *Psychiatry* (1962), 25 : 195–207.

system, which means that crucial decisions on admission and on promotion or dismissal are made by collective bodies.

In spite of these rules and modifications, the fact remains that analytic training involves a collective control over private life. Moreover, while the committee system lessens to some degree the power of the training analyst, it may in other respects make for greater ambiguity in the professional use of personal psychoanalysis. A common practice today is for career decisions to be made by a committee on the basis of global impressions communicated by the training analyst. For example, the training analyst may report that the candidate is either making satisfactory progress toward insight or failing to do so, that he is either resolving his problems or showing unconscious resistance, and so on; and the committee is guided by this information in deciding whether or not a candidate should be admitted to seminars, given a control case, and the like. But because, with the institutionalization of psychoanalysis, a number of its technical terms have taken on value connotations, this method of arriving at career decisions may, in effect, increase the arbitrariness of judgment by creating stereotypes of the "good" and the "bad" candidate. Thus if the training analyst reports "unconscious resistance," he may simply be saying that he does not like the candidate or that the candidate does not agree with him. The ultimate source of the judgment still lies in the private sphere because it is based on what the candidate says on the couch. When global judgments are batted around by the members of a committee, each of whom may have his own personal or theoretical reasons for trusting or distrusting the judgment of the training analyst, the degree of arbitrariness can increase still further. It is not impossible for the private personality of the candidate to be turned into the battlefield for social conflict within the institute; and, as Grete Bibring has pointed out,[5] the committee system can be used as a shield for the abdication of personal responsibility.

While most of these difficulties have their impact primarily

5. Grete L. Bibring, "The Training Analysis and Its Place in Psycho-Analytic Training," *Internat. J. Psychoanal.* (1954), 35 : 169–173; 171.

on the candidate, there are others that are more significant for the training analyst. In all fields of human endeavor, the thinking undergoes a natural course of change over the years; as a consequence, many of the ideas of the older generation, which were radical in its day, are regarded by the younger generation as outmoded or just too obvious to be interesting any more. In most fields, however, the psychological impact of such differences on the older generation is modulated by conventions of respect which govern what one says in public to authority figures. The graduate student who feels that his professor is sometimes a bit of an old fogey keeps his view to himself or divulges it only to his peers. But if the psychoanalytic candidate has such thoughts on the couch, he is supposed to express them because in analysis one says everything that comes into one's mind. If he does not, he is violating the basic rule; but if he does, he is being disrespectful to the analyst. Erikson has said that no organizational rules can entirely contain the destructive and creative spirits freed by the combination of the personal, the professional, and the organizational that goes into psychoanalytic training.[6] Certainly one potentially destructive opening lies in the very unusual absence of conventions of respect based on distance. No matter how conscientiously the training analyst tries to analyze his own reactions, he is likely to be affected by continual exposure to hostile comments from rising competitors. This, in turn, can lead to a certain hardening of position, and one might expect a predictably greater conservatism of ideas and technique among training analysts than among others in the profession. Since training analysts have the greatest prestige and in a sense act as official guardians of traditions, this makes for a slower rate of change in psychoanalysis than in other scientific fields.

Many of these difficulties are of such a nature that they can operate against the values of increasing competence and knowledge. It is unlikely that they will be corrected by purely remedial measures, such as the establishment of new types of

6. Erik Erikson, *Young Man Luther: A Study in Psychoanalysis and History* (New York: W. W. Norton & Company, 1958) pp. 152–153.

committees or increased bureaucratization of procedure, unless the most significant axis of structure—namely, the public use of private criteria—is modified. The one currently available proposal for accomplishing this has been advanced by Szasz, who would separate public and private spheres by institutionalizing strict rules of confidentiality for the didactic analysis, thus restricting evaluations determining the candidate's status as candidate to the public spheres of seminars and actual work with patients.[7] Such an arrangement would lessen the role-strain of the training analyst, who would then be free to devote his attention solely to the private life of the candidate without having to guard tradition at the same time. It would also greatly decrease the role played by "good" and "bad" candidate stereotypes by strengthening the status of more subtle and refined types of performance judgment—for example, the candidate has understood or failed to understand the seminars on instinct theory or dream interpretation; he is detailed and sensitive or sloppy and boorish in his case presentations; he works well or does not work well with homosexual, depressed, schizophrenic patients, and so on. All of these standards are directly relevant to the candidate's capacities for becoming a good psychoanalyst. This cannot be said with equal truth of such matters as personal happiness in love, inhibition or emotionality as character traits, or conformity or opposition in relation to authority figures that lie behind the analyst's judgment as to whether or not the candidate has successfully worked through his problems.

Special Problems of the Research Worker

These considerations bear upon general questions of psychoanalytic training that are of interest to everyone. However, at the beginning of this paper, I raised the more specific question of the advisability of giving fellowships to research workers for psychoanalytic training. This, of course, touches

7. See footnote 2; pp. 89–91.

on the controversial subject of the current nonmedical programs, and it is these that I should now like to discuss. The nonmedical programs represent a compromise solution of the conflict existing within the American Psychoanalytic Association between those who wish to restrict psychoanalysis to a status entirely within medicine and those who feel that other disciplines, such as psychology and the social sciences, have potentially valuable contributions to make. In the larger perspective, this conflict can be seen as part of the emergence of a society in which various aspects of the healing role, including both practice and the ideas which govern it, will be divided around among a series of disciplines, all of which are concerned with the study of man as he is rather than with any pre-established doctrine about him—medicine, biology, psychology, sociology, social anthropology, and even empirical philosophy. For the moment, however, there is a great deal of very real social conflict concerning who is allowed to do what and to whom, with the greatest power and prestige going to medical psychoanalysis. But of course the rush of psychologists and social scientists into psychoanalytic training (and into hospital research) represents a wish to share in the business of soul-saving. Much of what is called research today consists in various attempts on the part of these formerly academic disciplines to emerge into the world of action.

However, the great difficulty of the current compromise is that it has produced an institutional structure within which the political motives of those who wish to preserve a restrictive hierarchy against potentially expansive change can very easily outweigh either scientific or humanitarian considerations. Presumably any research worker who enters psychoanalytic training has three goals: To acquire concepts and methods that will further his own work; to make original contributions to the development of psychoanalysis; and to secure for himself whatever benefits he can from psychoanalysis as a therapeutic technique. The first two of these goals lie within the public sphere; the third is a private one. The realization of the public goals depends on the existence of a professional climate promoting a free and reciprocal exchange of ideas, while the realization of the private one depends on the immediate human consideration which the research worker receives from his psychoanalyst. The actual social structure of psychoanalytic training is such that it very often operates against the realization of all three goals.

The free and reciprocal exchange of ideas is likely to thrive best in an open society comprised of competing status equals. However, in the psychoanalytic training situation, the status of the nonmedical candidate is formally defined by the American Psychoanalytic Association as a subordinate one; and, while local institutes vary considerably in this respect, restrictive policies are likely to create restrictive climates. The term itself, which says that anyone else is something less than a physician, establishes a negative role definition, and the research worker who enters psychoanalytic training must begin by signing a pledge that he will never present himself as a practicing psychoanalyst. The pledge thus informs him of what he cannot do rather than what he can, and its existence points to a climate of mistrust.

In the course of training, the nonmedical candidate may encounter further barriers to the full understanding of psychoanalytic concepts and practices in the fact that his fellow candidates are taking control cases and discussing clinical material to which he may not have direct access. The importance of these barriers, however, differs widely depending on the local institute; and both the increasing participation of nonphysicians in hospital work and the newly initiated research candidacies are steps which promise change. But, at the present time, the procedures governing the research candidacies are still restrictive in that they are still based on a hierarchical model that starts with the medical psychoanalyst. The effects of this hierarchy can go beyond consideration specifically related to practice in that the status gradient can play an important part even in theoretical discussions concerning the groundwork for future modifications in technique. To take an example, some Freudian psychoanalysts regard the concept of culture as a "superficial" one, relevant perhaps to some external layers of the personality but not to the deeper levels which operate in the origins of neuroses. On a scientific plane, this view may have a certain validity: One can say, for example, that cultural representations are embodied in the individual ego, and the ego is the portion of the personality which is influenced by reciprocal social exchange or by cumulative historical tradition, while the id is not. However, the view that the concept of culture is superficial can also be used in defense of the higher status position of orthodox psychoanalysis; thus in such theoretical discussions the psychoanalyst may simply be asserting that the anthropologist's work or ideational perspective is less important than his own.

To the extent that the anthropologist accepts such a lower status, the second aim may be frustrated as well as the first. By way of illustration, I shall postulate a hypothetical healing profession in which the top honors go to anthropology. To the psychoanalyst, the fact that the patient is a second- or third-generation immigrant, that he is the first person in his family to live in a sophisticated urban area, or that he is devoutly religious or an atheist is likely to appear of secondary importance; the primary or most common focus in psychoanalysis is rather on the effect of past developmental phases on the adult personality, conceptualized in a way that is independent of sociocultural membership. In contrast, the anthropologist (or an anthropologically trained psychoanalyst) would most immediately select for analysis the aspects of the patient's personality that do relate to sociocultural membership. Thus he might say that many persons turn to psychoanalysis today because they are suffering from anomie, or a lack of cultural forms, a condition that is causally related to social change. His therapy would then take the direction of a search for cultural forms that are viable for the present, rather than any intensive examination of the past. The difference in emphasis could be a very concrete matter of therapeutic technique. For example, in the case of a second-generation East European woman of Jewish origin complaining of depression when faced with her child, the psychoanalyst might ask how she felt about her mother, while the anthropologist might ask how she plans to replace, in the new suburban environment in which she lives, the ritual structure or the close community network with which she was brought up. It is hard to deny that feelings such as love and hate have great significance in all human environments; however, the problems of social change in our own present environment can hardly be called superficial ones, and the social scientist might confront them more directly than the psychoanalyst.

The anthropologist could also make novel contributions to the organization of psychoanalytic education. In today's world of increased travel and international communication among professionals, it would not be wholly impracticable to include a year's field work, based on anthropological models, as a customary stage in psychoanalytic training. This would make the concept of culture a concrete and vivid one to the budding psychoanalyst, and it would require of him a degree of fluidity in adaptation to new social situations that does not necessarily follow from prolonged and near-exclusive involvement in a well-known professional structure. Quite possibly such an innovation could even do a great deal toward resolving some of the problems facing psychoanalysts today. For example, expectations concerning analysis interminable might dissolve in the face of the Latin attitude that "everybody's got troubles, but you might as well enjoy life anyway"; or a confrontation with traditional forms of respect and reciprocity might help the psychoanalyst in learning to deal with some of the normative breakdowns that occur within the often ambiguous and unstructured analytic situation. But the institutionalization of this kind of suggestion can follow only from the institutionalization of a positive role for persons who might make it.

The third aim of the research worker, which he shares with both the private patient and the psychoanalyst in training, is to secure the therapeutic benefits of treatment. However, the present structure of psychoanalytic training is such that this aim may be frustrated as well, and it is in this respect that the blurring of the distinction between public and private spheres becomes most crucial. Anyone who enters psychoanalysis has the expectation, whether or not it is clearly formulated in this way, that he will be treated as an individual person and understood as such by his psychoanalyst. Precisely because the most important aspects of the analysis pertain to one's private life, the analytic situation requires an isolation from the conflicts and rivalries that characterize the public social stage. The present-day system in which the didactic analysis is the fulcrum of training, and in which its content can be transmitted to the authority body that both determines the candidate's status in training and rules on matters of general policy concerning who shall be trained, does not favor this kind of isolation of private conflict.

The institutional focus on private personality first makes it possible for both candidate and institute to avoid defining his professional role. On the one side, the institute may not be interested in the candidate's work at all, but only in the degree to which he is able to "work through" his conflicts. The emphasis placed on this point is likely to be seen by the candidate, whether rightly or wrongly, as the expectation that he will give up any critical or divergent views he might have; and if this is the institute's only interest, one can reasonably ask why it does not simply refer him as a patient for private treatment. On his side, too, the candidate may engage in a kind of cheating on the public sphere by initiating training not because of a clearly thought-out professional commitment, but simply in hopes of resolving private difficulties with financial aid from a research foundation and the excuse that he does not really have these difficulties but is only furthering his work. But if he is interested primarily in resolving his own difficulties in life, and only secondarily in professional acquisitions or contributions, then he himself should seek private treatment; otherwise he also is helping to blur the distinction between public and private spheres.

The consequences that can arise within the didactic analysis itself from these ambiguities are more serious still, and they may have as their effect the undermining of the analysand's professional and personal identity. Far from understanding the candidate as a person, the analyst may utilize his analysis to propagandize his own title to truth, and the analysis then becomes influenced by the status gradient that is built into the situation. The analyst may, for example, stereotype aspects of the candidate's identity in his interpretations, either because he does not understand them or because they represent a threat to his own. Thus the research worker's questions become a sign of "intellectualization," or the anthropologists's assertion that the values of other cultures are sometimes preferable to our own becomes an "inability to accept" the life he was given. Such "interpretations" transform positive identities into negative ones. Though the analysand may also use stereotypes and unfair techniques, as when he puts his anger into the form of a counter-analysis of the role of the analyst, the situation is a highly asymmetrical one in that the analysand is expected to reveal all of his private insecurities to the analyst, who need not reciprocate in kind. As a consequence of this status gradient, the effects of social conflict within analysis are qualitatively different from those that attend the same type of conflict in public competition with others. The difference is again that psychoanalysis involves the total personality, while public competition involves only particular segments of it.

The present-day situation of the nonmedical candidate can thus be summarized as one in which it may be very difficult for him either to learn or to teach and in which the possibilities of social conflict entering into the analytic process are such that, rather than becoming more productive or creative as the result of analysis, he may become less so. Such a situation obviously calls for change. In the remainder of this paper, I shall be concerned with the directions that such a change might take.

The first and most obvious solution would be simply to turn psychoanalysis into an open and independent profession, giving full qualifications as psychoanalyst to anyone who has satisfactorily met its own standards of training. One would then expect persons to choose their careers, whether in teaching, research, or practice, according to personal talent and inclination, each contributing original perspectives according to any other specialized knowledge he might have. Such a solution would have many advantages. Most important, it could free psychoanalysis to follow its own special competence without ties to the often divergent and conservative (by comparison with what can be learned from continuous contact with living social and psychological material) perspectives of either organized organic medicine or the academic behavioral sciences. It could, in a more pragmatic vein, greatly shorten the length of training by admitting qualified persons with the B.A. degree and making the training period contemporaneous with either medical school or graduate school work combined with hospital or other clinical apprenticeships. This solution would be in accord with much of current European practice. It would also be in accord with the teaching of Freud, who himself hoped for an independent psychoanalytic institute that would combine various disciplines using direct observational methods and who believed that anyone who had completed psychoanalytic training merited the title of psychoanalyst.[8]

However, in spite of a consistently strong opposing minority, the American Psychoanalytic Association has repeatedly and with considerable feeling voted against the adoption of lay analysis in the United States. There may be some valid arguments in support of this position, but they do not re-

8. See Sigmund Freud, "The Question of Lay-Analysis: Conversations with an Impartial Person," *Standard Edition of the Complete Psychological Works 20* : 177–258 (London: Hogarth Press, 1959). "Preparation for analytic activity is by no means easy and simple. The work is hard, the responsibility great. But anyone who has passed through such a [two-year] course of instruction, who has been analyzed himself, who has mastered what can be taught today of the psychology of the unconscious, who is at home in the science of sexual life, who has learnt the delicate technique of psycho-analysis, the art of interpretation, of fighting resistances and of handling the transference—anyone who has accomplished all this is *no longer a layman in the field of psychoanalysis*" (p. 228; italics in the original). It is also important to remember in plans for the development of future generations of psychoanalysts that the contributions of lay analysts such as Anna Freud and Erik Erikson have been very great ones.

late to the knowledge of medicine[9] since psychoanalysis is a healing technique which manipulates words and symbols rather than physiochemical organs of the body.

The argument most commonly advanced by the opponents of lay-analysis is based on the fact that psychoanalysis in America, in sharp contrast to European psychoanalysis, is closely linked with psychiatry and hospital practice. This link has been a major factor in the rapidity with which psychoanalysis has gained widespread social recognition in this country. It has given psychoanalysis a set of pre-established social forms for legitimatizing itself—for example, the legal concept of privileged communication covering physicians—and has also limited its potentialities for gyration into an esoteric cult.

A second argument often advanced against lay-analysis concerns the undeniable differences that exist between persons who are trained in research or academic thinking and persons who are clinically trained. For the most part, nonmedical candidates have come from the university world, which has a different subculture from that of medicine. Since subcultural belongingness, by definition, goes with a complex organization of personality response and social expectation that cannot be altered overnight by a course of formal training, it is true that the most competent of professors may have difficulty in dealing with patients and may not be particularly inclined to try. However, the medical subculture as well has its limitations when it comes to psychoanalysis. Thus the highly precise kind of observation and technique that is learned in medical school can be dysfunctional in the psychological realm, and the physician who turns to psychiatry may have to face the charge that what he is doing is "not scientific" because psychological standards of verification differ from organic ones. The low prestige of psychiatry

9. An important fact is that when a question of physical illness arises in the mind of a psychoanalyst, he almost always refers the patient to another medical specialist. It is also a fact that no one who is not a physician, but who is interested in carrying out psychological treatment, would object to a requirement of periodical physical examinations for the patient in order to insure against the possibility of falsely perceiving an organic malfunction as a psychological one.

within the general field of medicine may account for a great
deal of the defensive emphasis within psychoanalysis on its
status as a medical discipline. Yet, having the more complicated
and uncertain task, psychoanalysis should be able to stand on
its own two feet.

Moreover, two factors make the present situation radically
different from that which existed when the American Psychoanalytic Association first formulated its policy on lay-analysis.
The first is the greater demand for psychoanalysts, coinciding
with a decline in medical school applications and an increase
both in medical specialization and in the demand for general
medical care; though this is a consideration which the postwar
rush of applications may have concealed, psychoanalysis may
be facing serious recruitment difficulties. The second is the increasing trend toward apprenticeship programs and field interviewing in the universities, as a result of which graduate students in psychology and the social sciences today are far less
cloister-bound than were their counterparts of a generation ago.
Both factors point to the desirability of broadening the base
of candidate selection.

There is also ample reason for the psychoanalyst who feels
very strongly that practice should be restricted to physicians to
favor improvements in status for the nonmedical candidate. The
main reason why all of the specialty research roles are negatively defined is precisely that the question of lay-analysis has
usually dominated the thinking of the American Psychoanalytic
Association about all admissions to training. But the status of
research workers is not linked to the question of lay-analysis by
any necessity. Rather, it would be quite possible to give separate
but equal roles to persons whose careers run parallel to that of
the psychoanalyst. But, as officially defined at least, the present-
day nonmedical programs exist in order to train persons in
other specialties who will bring psychoanalytic concepts into
their fields. In actual fact, this is an imperialistic rather than
egalitarian conception since it assumes only that psychoanalysis
should influence other fields and ignores the necessary parallel
assumption that psychoanalysis itself should also be influenced

from outside. No specialty which takes its claim from science can in the long run avoid facing competitive challenge. Thus in the interest of enriching its own culture, psychoanalysis should admit a variety of persons from other fields who will play positive roles within it. In this respect, the most important consideration is not the nature of the roles these persons play, but the minimal condition that they be truly equal.

The idea that outsiders will absorb concepts to be used in their own work rests on the assumption that they are entering unfamiliar territory which they will explore with naive curiosity. But the success of psychoanalytic colonizing efforts has been such that this assumption is an unsound one. In reality, it is difficult today to find a Ph.D. or a Ph.D. candidate who, if he has any interest at all in personality, does not know the meaning of repression, denial, projection, regression, and the Oedipus complex quite independently of formal psychoanalytic training. A second assumption, also imperialistic in nature, is that in almost any field in which the candidate's work may lie, psychoanalytic training will be helpful to it. But, while specific acquisitions from psychoanalysis have led to genuine innovations in other fields,[10] this view neglects or greatly underestimates the importance of specificity in technique. In order to do research, one must learn research techniques; in order to carry out anthropological field work, one must learn anthropological methods and go to the field. The learning of psychoanalysis, therefore, does not automatically qualify the student for work in every domain.

It thus seems that reciprocal culture contact with other disciplines is far more important for psychoanalysis today than any further colonizing efforts on its part. Among other things, while it is difficult to find a graduate student in any of the human sciences who cannot define denial, repression, and pro-

10. See, for example, Géza Róheim, "Dream Analysis and Field Work in Anthropology," in *Psychoanalysis and the Social Sciences* (New York: International Universities Press, 1947, pp. 87–130. Róheim shows how the anthropologist may greatly increase his understanding of primitive dreams by the collection of free associations from informants. Here the technique adapted from psychoanalysis is a specific and usable one.

jection, it is very easy to find an accredited psychoanalyst who has no idea at all of what social scientists mean when they talk about norms, the differences between primary and secondary groups, kinship structures, and anomie. Yet psychoanalysts deal with these phenomena every day in their work. Thus the paramount need today may be for social science teaching within the psychoanalytic institutes. The role of the teaching specialist, therefore, would be the first and most obvious role in which the outsider could make genuine and positive contribution to psychoanalysis. A concrete step toward its institutionalization might be for the American Psychoanalytic Association to abandon its present policy of restricting active membership to physicians, so that any graduate of an accredited institute would automatically acquire full membership with voting and transfer rights regardless of his professional origins. Along with this should go the expectation that the person who is qualified and seriously interested will eventually come to teach institute seminars in his own specialty as it touches on psychoanalytic work and to participate in the institute's educational planning and in its selection of future candidates in his area of competence. A change of this sort would mark the beginning of a cumulative tradition of reciprocal exchange and the end of the imperialist era.[11]

Secondly, while the claim that psychoanalytic training automatically equips the candidate for any kind of work is a dubious one, it should at least equip him for playing a role in psychoanalytic research. It is in this respect that the newly initiated research candidacies mark a crucial step, especially insofar as they may help define psychoanalytic research as differentiated from the research of the academic behavioral sciences and point up areas of knowledge in which psychoanalysis today requires more than the random contributions of a few unusually gifted individuals. Thus the second meaningful way in which the out-

11. Outsiders have on occasion played active roles in psychoanalytic education. However, without a cumulative tradition, arrangements which work at one point in time are likely to fail once particular individuals move on or lose interest.

sider can acquire a positive role is by participation in psychoanalytic research. In this effort, as well, one can hope that the anthropologist, whose focus has always been on the description of complex patterns, will be able to make a special contribution, more immediately understandable to the practicing clinician than that of the methodologist who insists that only the highly formalized or quantitative project merits the title of research.

Were the role of the teaching or research specialist to become fully institutionalized within psychoanalysis, it should be possible to create a truly collaborative effort at cultural enrichment on a nationwide basis that would not require a policy change with respect to lay-analysis or any substantial modification of the link between psychoanalysis and psychiatry.[12] However, if the necessary minimal changes cannot be effected, my view is that psychologists and social scientists should either take special care to work out genuinely reciprocal arrangements with the local institute on a contract basis, thus insuring themselves of a work role that is independent of personal psychoanalysis, or refrain altogether from entering training programs sponsored by the American Psychoanalytic Association. For the fact of the matter is that the present nonmedical programs are actually company unions; they admit psychologists and social scientists to training, but only on condition that they subordinate their own interests to those of the established management. The labor movement learned early in its history that it could not get very far with company unions. Moreover, for a candidate to enter didactic analysis as the subordinate rival of the psycho-

12. In "A Questionnaire Study of Psychoanalytic Practices and Opinions" (*J. Nervous & Ment. Disease* [1963], *137* : 209–221), Szasz and Nemiroff found that of the members of the American Psychoanalytic Association who returned their questionnaire, 65 per cent were willing to consider psychoanalysis as a social science (p. 213, question 22). If this sample is a representative one, it should be possible to raise the status of social scientists by reform from within the American Psychoanalytic Association. Moreover, 39 per cent favored giving full psychoanalytic training to persons with Ph.D.'s in anthropology; 52 per cent for psychology; and 34 per cent for sociology (p. 213, question 23). The return rate was 56 per cent, which is high, but one might expect persons with the more favorable attitudes toward research and social science to return a questionnaire.

analyst is comparable to a labor union organizer turning to the boss for help in his quarrels with his wife, or a Negro leader of the NAACP in a Southern town deciding that his own soul could best be saved by the pastor of the segregated white Baptist church. Neither the union organizer nor the Negro leader is likely to do any such thing. But the nonmedical candidate is expected to expose his entire private life with no guarantees at all that the exposures will not be used against him. It is therefore necessary that he himself insist on some guarantees.

In conclusion, I should like to refer back briefly to the views on the social role of psychoanalysis presented earlier in this paper, for they serve to point up the very great need for reforms in psychoanalytic training that will further research and creative thinking in a variety of disciplines. I commented in this connection on the importance of interprofessional competition today as part of the growth pangs of an emerging society in which various aspects of the healing role will be divided among subspecialties in the study of man as he is. That such a role should have its roots in medicine is in certain respects desirable, in that medicine has a long tradition of healing based on special access to private life and a number of rules which act against the misuse of the power that goes with it. Equivalent rules are only at present beginning to be formulated in psychology and the social sciences as these fields emerge from the ivory tower; recent preoccupations in both with questions concerning the ethics of handling research data are indications of their change in status. Many persons think that the most important problem in this emergence process concerns rules governing practice. However, it is also possible to take the view that questions concerning practice are secondary to those concerning the ideology or system of beliefs and values that governs those doing the practicing. There are many different arrangements that can operate to assure a reasonable level of competence and ethical behavior among practitioners, and the choices among them are primarily pragmatic. However, no human activity is ever governed by external rules alone. Rather the nature of practice, along with the effectiveness of the rules, depends on what is in the minds of the practitioners. But this in turn, of course, depends on education and research.

Moreover, now that psychoanalysis is being asked to create a new kind of religious role, based on empirical knowledge rather than dogma, it is also being asked the questions about meaning and value that used to be asked of magical practitioners and priests, not to mention the new questions that have arisen in our epoch: Is there any meaning to our existence going beyond the individual life? What should I do with the individual life that I have? Should I follow the traditional ways of my parents or grandparents, or should I adopt quite a different manner of living? What kind of sexual standards should I have? What is the meaning of love? Is our world likely to disappear in an atomic holocaust? Psychoanalysis has on the whole refrained from giving doctrinal answers to such questions—for example, if you work hard, are faithful to your spouse, and vote the straight Republican ticket, then the world will remain safe for democracy while you go to heaven. The fact that it has done so is what puts it well within the more sophisticated currents of the modern world. Though it often takes on the characteristics of a religious sect, this is not in actuality what it is. At the same time, the dangers of retreat into a defensive and narrow ideological position are very great for the medical psychoanalyst who suddenly finds himself faced with a role requiring far more education in the deepest sense of the term than the narrow technical competence required of the physician who removes an inflamed appendix or administers penicillin to a feverish patient. Current psychoanalytic practices provide many indications of such a retreat. The most important of these is perhaps the fact that the criteria of cure in psychoanalysis are for the most part purely private ones; considerations of social value play a definitely secondary role. But personal insight is a totally valueless commodity if it cannot be utilized in some socially meaningful way.

It may be exactly this kind of defensiveness that Freud forecast when he referred to the anxiety characterizing his medical colleagues at the thought of any change in traditional role patterns and expectations.[13] However, since psychoanalysis does have the religious role, whether or not it has asked for it (and psychoanalysis itself has done a great deal to encourage global rather than specific disease concepts of neurosis), it must find some means of dealing with the questions addressed to it in this role; otherwise the new society that is emerging will be an extremely neutral or valueless one. If it is to do this and at the same time avoid either dogmatic answers or totalitarian publicizations of private life, it must have the help of intellectuals whose cooperation, in turn, depends on the freedom given them to think and to criticize within the system of procedures governing practice.

But the sad fact of the matter is that, while most American intellectuals are in some way interested in psychoanalysis, official psychoanalysis at least is far less interested in intellectuals. A case in point is that there is no American-born, American-trained intellectual of the stature of an Erikson or a Rapaport who is closely affiliated with psychoanalysis today. This is the broadest issue behind all of the current conflicts over psychoanalytic training for persons engaged in research; and it is doubtful that these conflicts can be resolved by any system which insists on total subordination of research interests to the requirements of present-day practice.

13. See footnote 9.

INDEX

Index

Adaptability
  cultural, 134–35, 146–47; *see
    also* Culture conflict
  to Protestant ethic, 265
  psychological, 146
Admiration of sexual development,
  30–32, 44
Africa, 207, 243, 258, 264, 279;
  see also Zande society
Aggression, 24, 220, 277, 305
  of analysand, 309, 314, 319
  childhood, 30, 32, 45, 46–47
  cultural expression of, 249,
    252, 268
  defenses against, 146
  inhibition of, 273–74
  masculine, 94
  of paranoid schizophrenics,
    179, 185, 207–8, 224, 233
  parental, 30, 42

in schizophrenic's family, 100,
  111–12
of ward patients, 154–55, 172
American family dynamics, 69
  of matrifocal Negro family,
    52n, 87–88
  Oedipus complex in, 53–54,
    57–59
  of schizophrenics, 99–102
American mental patients, 49
  intensive therapy for, 296–319
  paranoid delusions of, 101,
    103n, 107, 143–44, 146,
    204–7, 209–11
  psychiatrically hospitalized,
    100–2, 123–34, 139, 142,
    151–73, 179, 204–7
  schizophrenic episodes of,
    225–30, 232–36

American mental patients (*cont'd*)
   schizophrenics, 99–102, 116–
      17, 142, 149
   specific life patterns of, 137–
      50
American Psychoanalytic Associa-
   tion, 335, 343–44, 349, 351,
   354
   membership policy of, 353
Anal culture theory, 44, 59
Anella (Davino), 20–21
Anger (rage), 166, 209, 224, 254
   of patient, 299, 302, 310–11,
      314, 348
   male, 29, 46
   taboo on perceiving, 42–43,
      79–80
Anomie, xiii, 36*n*, 145, 345, 353
Anglo-Saxon, 160–62, 165–67,
      173
   therapeutic, 319, 328, 332–33
Antagonism, *see* Hostility
Anthropology, function of, 242–43
Anticlericalism, 18–20, 249
Anxiety, 59, 101, 116, 172, 178,
      221, 356
   behind witchcraft, 186, 188–
      91, 196–97
   due to male identification, 95
   neurotic vs. psychotic, 228*n*
   oedipal, 5, 57
   parental, 148
   over religious taboos, 249
   after symptoms disappear, 303
   underlying ritual, 263–64,
      270–71
Asexuality (desexualization), 34,
      45, 140
   in culture complex, 18, 23–24
   of father-daughter relation-
      ship, 49
Associative fields, 287–88, 290–91
Athens, Greece, 145
Authority figures, 13, 28, 149*n*,
      261*n*
   father as, 36–40, 44, 51, 61,
      115–16, 136–37, 147–48
   mother as, 34–36, 43–44, 53
   in training analysis, 337, 341,
      347

Authority relations, 117, 144, 298
Authority structure, Neopolitan,
      67–97
   acceptance of authority, 82–
      83, 84–85
   case histories of, 89–92
   continuity within, 68–69, 76–
      77, 93
   empirical evidence of, 70–86
   peasant, 68–70
Autistic schizophrenia, 102
Avellino, Italy, 180–81
Avoidance, *see* Taboos

Balinese Character (Mead and
      Bateson), 59
Bally, Charles, 287
Bateson, Gregory, 59, 236*n*
Behaviorism, 59–60, 286
Benedict, Ruth, 213
Bergsonian theories, 293–94
Bianchi, Leonardo, 300*n*
Bible, 245–46, 252, 258*n*, 275, 279
   reading of, 255–57, 268–69
Bibring, Grete, 59*n*, 340
Bonaparte, Marie, 145
Boston, 100, 125–26, 180–81, 191
Boston Psychoanalytic Institute,
      329–30
Boston Psychopathic Hospital, 183
Boston State Hospital, 125
Brown, G. W., 167
Bureaucracy, impersonal, 164

Cameron, Norman, 207
Camorra, 24, 94, 95*n*
Capriciousness, prepsychotic, 105,
      107–8, 112–13, 230
Caribbean area, 258, 264, 281
   matrifocal patterns in, 321
Cassin, Helene, 246*n*
Catholicism, *see* Roman Catholi-
      cism
Caudill, William, 231*n*
Censorship, 289–90
Central city, *see* Slums
Chaperonage, 23, 32, 50, 91

enforcement of, 70
problems of, 218, 231
Character disorders, *see* Psychopathic personality
Charge, psychic, 292
Church, ethnic, *see* Pentecostal immigrants
Class, *see* Social class
Committee system, 339–40
Communion, First, xii, 31–32, 54
Communists, 199, 204–6, 260
Comparative method, 99
Competition, 55, 355
    in schizophrenic's family situation, 107–8, 111–12
    See also Jealousy; Rivalry
Condensation, 291–92
Conflict, 142, 192, 224, 262, 357
    over authority, 67, 69, 75–76, 82–86, 90, 92–93
    between sex instinct and family continuity, 58
    Catholic solution for, 336
    culture, *see* Culture conflicts
    of disturbed adolescents, 136–39, 141, 147
    financial, 27–28
    Freudian theory of, 293–94
    ideological, 206–7
    intrafamily, 24–26, 143
    intrapsychic, 62
    oedipal, 38–41, 56
    physically violent, 88–89
    prepsychotic, 217–18, 223, 232–34
    in religious practice, 245n, 249–52, 273–75
    of schizophrenics, 100, 107, 206–9
    social, 288, 340, 343, 347–48
    therapy for, 328–29
Confusion, 185–86, 301, 311–12
Conscious, concept of, 286, 292
Coppola, Carlo Felice, 228n
Courtship complex, xi, 18, 46
    authority structure underlying, 70–71, 80, 83–86
    described, 20–24

father-daughter relationship in, 39, 41, 48–52
    importance of, 35
Courtship problems, 218, 230–32
Cultural complex, xii; *see also* Courtship complex; Madonna complex; Nuclear family complexes
Cultural relativity, 259
Cultural values, 165–66, 169, 348
    mobility as, 124
    security as, 58–59, 166
    spread of, 259
Culture concept, 344–46
Culture conflicts, 146–47
    over inhibited aggression, 273–74
    over Madonna, 274–75
    of religious immigrants, 252–54, 263–77
Cursing, *see* Swearing

Dark Puritan (Paul), 278–81
Death, 218, 227–28, 254, 262
    as focus of witchcraft, 188–89, 196
    of parents, 48–49, 55, 74, 208
    in pentecostal belief, 266
    psychosis precipitated by, 103, 105, 110, 139–40, 208
    rate of, 161
    remarriage after mate's, 26
    of siblings, 301
    sorrow over, 37, 74, 216, 235
    See also Suicide
Defenses, 5–6, 233–34; *see also* Denial; Displacement; Projection
Delusions, x, xii, 100
    psychoanalytic definition of, 178
    religious, 47
    See also Hallucinations; Paranoid delusions
De Martino, Ernesto, 235, 251n
Denial, 156, 178, 352
    ethic based on, 233
    of mental illness, 170, 172

Denial (*cont'd*)
  of oedipal feelings, 5–6
  paranoid, 184, 187*n*, 200
Dependency, 62, 129
  as cultural value, 231–33
  as life pattern, 135–36, 146
  schizophrenic (symbiotic),
    102–3, 109–14, 117
Depersonalization, 209, 236
Depression, 62, 154, 216, 218,
    342, 345
  community, 241
  with mental illness, 142, 156–
    57, 182, 225
Desexualization, *see* Asexuality
Destructive impulses, 235–36; *see*
    also Self-destructive im-
    pulses
Discipline, 91, 112, 138
  in mental institutions, 155,
    165
Displacement, 289–90
  oedipal, 6, 9, 46–48
  in witchcraft, 190, 198
Dissociative syndrome, 225–26
Docility, 141–44, 147
Dreams, 117, 182, 302
  appearance of dead people in,
    227–28
  of incest, 5, 11–12
  interpretation of, 288–89, 291
  symbolic, 292
Drifters, 130–32
Drive theory, 211, 273
Dyadic relationships, 104–7, 110–
    11, 117

Education level, 127, 217
  influencing delusions, 205,
    207, 209
  of ward patients, 158, 171–72
Ego, 102, 178, 235–36, 286, 327
  control of, 150
  cultural representations in, 345
  development of, 103
  psychotic, 186, 197, 201
Ego functions, 201–2
Ego ideal, 54, 58

English mental patients, 151–73,
    225
  atmosphere of hospitals for,
    154–55
  number of discharged, 167–68
English revivalism, 264
Erikson, Erik, 324, 341, 349*n*, 357
Evans-Pritchard, E. E., 187–88,
    190
Evil eye, 186–87, 191–93, 200
  paranoid belief in, 179, 181–
    82, 184, 186, 192–93
Evil spirits, 254, 264, 270–71
Evolutionary anthropology, 6
Exclusive dyads, 104–6, 110–11,
    117
Expressive symbolism, x, 175–236
  cognitive element of, 188–89,
    194–95, 197
  dual character of, 189
  imagery as, 184, 204–11
  in schizophrenic episode, 212–
    36
  in witchcraft and delusion,
    177–203

Façade, concept of, 286, 288
Family complexes, *see* Nuclear
    family complexes
Family disintegration (break-
    down), 105–6, 115–16
Family disorganization, 87–88
Family dynamics, 1–120
  American, *see* American fam-
    ily dynamics
  "folding in" in, 102
  intimate, 59
  of Italian families, 15–32, 43–
    56, 67–120
  source of conflict outside, 85
  of Trobrianders, 3–15, 19*n*,
    60
  underlying creative achieve-
    ment, 55–56
Family roles, 44–45
  authority, 77–78, 89–94, 97
  fully institutionalized, 49–50

importance of maternal, 28, 89–90, 91
of schizophrenics, 105, 109
separation of, 25, 29, 77–78
specific life patterns and, 141, 143, 148
Fantasies, 11, 32, 147n
Madonna, 45, 51
oedipal, 13, 46–48, 52–54
schizophrenic, 100, 218, 227–28
transference, 321–22
Father-child relationship, discontinuous, 48–52
Father-daughter TAT responses, 72, 83–86, 116n
on Oedipus complex, 38–41
Father-son TAT responses, 36–38, 54–55
on authority structure, 72–77, 82, 86
Feeding, 77
forced, 30, 136, 159, 164
Ferenczi, Sandor, 324
Fleiss, Wilhelm, 55
France, 286, 288, 290–92, 293–94
Freud, Sigmund, 356–57
Freudian theories, 6–11, 236, 273, 324n, 338–39
of anthropology, x
of delusion, 187, 193
diffusion of, 286, 288–94
of lay-analysis, 349
neo-Freudian, 325
of neurosis, 335
of Oedipus complex, 4, 6–9, 11, 43–45, 49, 54–59
of psychosis, 156, 197, 299
See also Infantile sexuality; Instinct theory; Trauma theory
Functionalism, 276–77

Gangs, function of, 94
Geertz, Clifford, 276
Glossolalia (speaking in tongues), 251–52, 266, 272–75, 277
Gratification, 112–14, 156, 322–23

Greek national character, 145
Grief, *see* Sorrow
Guilt, 101, 167, 312
oedipal, 41–42, 44
over rebellious wishes, 75
schizophrenic, 114, 222

Haiti, 207
Hallucination, 226
auditory, 179, 184–86, 219–20
of ward patients, 158–60, 172–73, 299
Hebraic tradition, 56–57
Hollingshead, A. B., 123–25, 132–33, 164
Homans, G. C., 115
Homosexuality, 138, 342
of analysts, 338–39
childhood experience of, 48
of hospitalized patients, 156–57, 300, 309, 316
in paranoid delusions, 200, 211
of schizophrenics, 100, 117, 150, 235
taboo against, 57
Honor ethic, 215, 233, 236
defense of honor, 268, 273
family honor, 23–24, 50–51, 321–22
Hospitalization, psychiatric, *see* Psychiatric hospitalization
Hostility (antagonism), 309, 327, 332, 341
toward authority, 76n, 78–79, 81–82
latent, 95
oedipal, 6, 9, 39, 44, 54–56
paranoid, 221, 223, 229
witchcraft and, 178, 197–98
Hysteria, 62, 277, 326
Freud's studies of, 11–12, 57, 273

Id, 197, 236, 345
Identification, 58, 83, 224, 230, 261
conflicted, 217–18

Identification (*cont'd*)
  in cultist religion, 279–80
  cultural, 193, 199, 202
  with feminine values, 46, 51
  with higher status group, 27
  masculine, 8–9, 12–13, 48, 93,
    95, 97, 267, 304
  negative, 92
  same-sex, 52, 54, 56, 75
  of schizophrenics, 103*n*, 106,
    107, 113, 118, 200
Idenitity, 324, 347–48
  formation of, 150, 205
  renewing of sense of, xi
  of schizophrenic, 100–1
  search for, xiii, 76
Illegitimacy, 35, 87–88, 105, 210,
  305
  cultist religion and, 279–80
  legal recognition of illegiti-
    mate child, 27
Imagery, 29, 56, 286–87
  in paranoid delusions, 184,
    204–11
Imbedded dyads, 106–7
Immigrants, 100, 345; *see*
  also Italian-American im-
    migrants; Pentecostal immi-
    grants
Inappropriate affects, 228–29
Incest (incestuous impulses), 83*n*,
  198, 301
  as obscenity, 19
  in schizophrenic's history,
    105, 116, 117, 150
  therapeutic approach to, 327
  unsublimated, 40, 49–52, 61,
    312
  See also Oedipus complex
Incest taboo, 9–14, 312
  Freudian study of, 11
  Italian, 48–49, 115, 118
  of Trobrianders, 4–5, 7, 9–
    12, 14, 19*n*
Industrial society, 36*n*, 173, 264
  attitude toward mental illness
    in, 170
  discontinuous nuclear family
    in, 96

family function in, 15–16, 69
  job-orientation of, 166
  role differentiation in, 162–64
Infantile sexuality, 6–7, 10
Inhibition, 50, 105*n*, 232, 342
  of aggression, 273–74
  drive, 45
  muscular, 30
  neurotic, 39–40
  schizophrenic, 108–9, 230, 234
Insight, 335, 340, 356
  cultural barriers to, 308–12
  normative standards and,
    329–33
Instability, family, 107–8, 111–12
Instinct theory, 8–10, 59, 211, 213
Instincts, 235; *see also* Ego; Id;
  Superego
Internalization, 247–48, 301, 312
  of authority, 36*n*, 38, 40–41,
    44, 53, 61, 76, 82
  superego formed by, 45–46
Irish-American immigrants, 100
Irrational beliefs, 178
Ischia, Italy, 209
Isolation, 231
  pathogenic, 102, 108–9, 146,
    150
  for therapy sessions, 315, 347
  of ward patients, 155, 157,
    160–73
Italian-American immigrants
  intensive therapy for, 296–
    319
  pentecostal, *see* Italian Evan-
    gelical Church
  schizophrenic, 100–2, 142,
    145–50, 180–86
  specific life patterns of, 135–
    50
  witchcraft beliefs of, 180–86,
    191–96, 200–1
Italian cultural complexes, 43–56,
  61–62
  elaboration of two major, 15–
    24
  family structure underlying,
    24–32, 43
  orthodox complex vs., 55–59

Italian Evangelical Church, 244–
62, 264–76
architecture of, 246
power struggle within, 256–
57
prayer period of, 250–52,
254, 266–67, 272, 274–75
sermons preached in, 252–54,
266, 268–72, 274–75
testimonials in, 268, 272,
274–75
theology of, 244–45, 255,
264–65, 271
Italian mental patients, xii
intensive therapy for, 296–
319
paranoid delusions of, 101,
103n, 107, 180–86, 191–96,
200–1, 204–5, 207–11
psychiatric hospitalization of,
100–2, 104–9, 117, 123–
34, 139, 142, 151–73, 179,
204–5, 207–9, 220–24, 232–
33
schizophrenic episodes of,
103, 106, 212–36
schizophrenic's family dynamics, 26, 47–48, 98–120
specific life patterns of, 137–
50

Java, 276
Jealousy, 21, 299–300
disfigurement due to, 215–17,
228–29
oedipal, 9–11, 13, 47, 49, 55–
57
prepsychotic, 105, 107–8,
112–13, 217–18, 229–30
Job orientation, 166, 310
Joking pattern, *see* Anticlericalism; Courtship complex
Jones, Ernest, 3–9, 11–12, 14
Judaism, 56–57, 252n, 272, 345–
46

King, Stanley H., 154

Kinship, 243, 279, 310–12, 353
Italian, 19, 24
Malinowski's study of, 4, 7–
8, 14–15, 59–60
patrilineal, 57
Kluckhohn, Clyde K., 187–88,
190, 198

Lambo, T. Adeoye, 207
Latin America, 297, 318
underdeveloped countries of,
243, 258
Lay-analysis, 348–51
Lévi-Strauss, Claude, 63, 178, 286,
289
on magic and analysis, 336
Lidz, Theodore, 117, 142, 144,
148
Literacy, 255–57, 258n, 260, 268
Lomax, Alan, 247
Love, 57, 209, 323, 342, 346
former object of, 201
maternal, 36, 42, 77, 79
romantic, 52

Madonna complex, xii, 45–47, 68,
95–96
courtship complex comple-
menting, 20, 22–24, 51–52
described, 16–19
mother-son relationship like,
41
Madonna cult, 246, 257, 274–75
Magic, 171, 207, 210, 298
fortune-telling, 153
in lower-class belief system,
215, 227–28
in pentecostal religion, 254
practitioner of, 335–36
in traditional Catholicism, 17,
166, 246, 250
See also Religion; Witchcraft
Mahler, Margaret, 102
Male peer group, 46, 94–95, 148n
family structure and, 25, 27–
29
patterns of, 18–20, 23
of schizophrenics, 136

Malinowski, Bronislaw, 3–12, 59–60
  theoretical influence on, 10
  theory of ritual of, 263–64, 277
Manic-depressive psychosis, 157
Marie, Auguste, 294
Marital skew, 117, 142
Marriage, 297, 327–28, 338
  authority structure and, 71, 80, 91
  cousin, 102, 106, 114–15
  culture complexes meet in, 23–25
  after elopement, 218–19, 232
  ideal of monogamous, 87, 279
  life pattern of, 136, 139–40, 142–44
  paranoid fears concerning, 210
  in pathogenic subculture, 131–32
  responsibility in, 129–30
  of schizophrenics, 102, 104–9, 114–15, 117
  status based on, 93
  See also Courtship complex
Mars, Louis, 207
Marxism, 293; *see also* Communists
Matrifocal family, 52–53*n*, 304
  authority structure of, 94–95, 96–97
  pathological, 320–21
  religious cult based on, 279–80
  specific life patterns of, 141, 148, 149*n*, 150
Matrilineal societies, 90, 92–93, 312*n*
  Oedipus complex in, 4–6, 14
Mead, Margaret, 59, 213
"Meaning, spread of," 195
Menduzion, Domenico, 246*n*
Mental illness (psychopathology), 121–73
  case histories of, 137–44, 180–86
  incest as indication of, 49, 312

  social attitude toward, 170–71
  of victims of witchcraft, 202
  See also American mental patients; English mental patients; Hysteria; Italian mental patients; Neurosis; Paranoid schizoprenia; Psychiatric hospitalization; Psychoanalysis; Psychopathic personality; Psychotherapy; Schizophrenics
Messenger, John C., Jr., 243
Milieu therapy, 173
Mintz, Sidney, 281
Moscovici, S., 199
Moses and Monotheism (Freud), 57
Moss, Leonard W., 68
Mother-child relationship, 58, 89
  as axis of family structure, 48
  pathogenic, 148
  See also Oedipus complex
Mother-daughter TAT responses, 72, 80–82
  on Oedipus complex, 33–36, 53–54
Mother-son TAT responses, 41–43, 72, 77–80
Motivation, x, 32, 97, 264, 337
  behavioristic approach to, 59
  psychiatric, 321, 331
  subjective, 177–78
  "unconscious," 189–91
  for work, 135, 163, 310
Murray TAT, *see* Projective test material
Myers, J. K., 124, 149
Mythology, 5, 10–11, 14; *see also* Penitence myth; Religion; Witchcraft

Nadel, S. F., 190
Naples, Italy, 61, 145, 207–9, 252*n*, 327*n*
  cultural complexes in, 15–17, 19, 24
  history of, 214–15

mental institution in, 152–54, 160–61, 165, 167–69, 173
religious ceremony in, 252*n*, 273
See also Neopolitan family; Neopolitan slums
Navaho Indians, 187, 198–200, 312*n*
Negroes, 264–65, 301, 355
family dynamics of, 52*n*, 87–88
as urban migrants, 242
Neopolitan family, xi–xii, 15
family dynamics of schizophrenics, 104, 107, 115–16, 118
parental authority in, *see* Authority structure, Neopolitan
projective test material on, 33–43
structure of, 26–28
Neopolitan slums, xi, 32
culture complexes in, 16, 24
schizophrenic episode in, 212–36
Neurosis, 335, 339, 345, 357; *see also* Hysteria
Neurotic symptoms, 141, 186
physical violence as, 62
street phobia as, 22
New Haven, Conn., 124–25, 133
New York City, 243
Normative context, 213–14
Nuclear family complexes, 53–54
family structure beneath, 24–32, 43
Oedipus complex as, 4, 7–8, 10

Object relations, 311–12, 329*n*
oedipal, 8–10, 12–13, 33
Obscenity, *see* Swearing
Occupational level, 128–33
Occupational status, 92–93, 135–36
Oedipus complex, xiii, 3–66, 352
genetic hypothesis of, 12–14
Italian vs. orthodox, 55–59

Jones-Malinowski debate over, 3–12
projective test material on, 33–43, 53–55
psychosexual development and, 31–32
unsublimated, 47–52, 61
See also Incest
Opler, M., 100
Oral culture theory, 44–45, 51, 59, 62

Paradox of progress, 161–62
Paranoid delusions, 177–211, 303–304
abstract and concrete images in, 184, 204–11
case histories of, 101, 103*n*, 107, 143–44, 146, 179–86, 191–96, 200–1, 204–209, 219–24, 226–29
institutional (ideological), 204–6, 210
persecuting agent in, 201
of ward patients, 156, 158–59, 172–73, 204–9
Paranoid language, 189, 202
Paranoid personality, 319
Paranoid schizophrenia, 142, 170, 299; *see also* Paranoid delusions
Paranoid symptoms, 139, 209; *see also* Paranoid delusions
Parent-child relationships
as structural axis, 26–27, 48
See also Father-child relationship; Mother-child relationship; Oedipus complex
"Parenti," 16
Parsons, Talcott, 3*n*, 166
Passivity, 32, 50, 179, 316–17
Patriarchal societies
authority structure in, 68–69, 96–97
eating patterns in, 28
Oedipus complex in, 4, 6, 43, 48, 57–58
Paul, Benjamin, 187*n*

Paul, Lois, 187*n*
Paul, Norman, *Dark Puritan*, 278–81
Paul, St., 251*n*, 272
Peer groups, *see* Male peer group
Penitence myth, 17, 80, 95–96
Penitence response, 41–42, 45, 78
Pentecostal immigrants, xii-xiii, 239–77
    church of, *see* Italian Evangelical Church
    culture conflicts of, 252–54, 263–77
    foreign missions of, 259
    geographic origins of, 242–43
    speak in tongues, 251–52, 266, 272–75
Perella, Angelina (pseudonym), 180–86, 191–96, 200–1
Personality, 59, 200, 214, 335, 345
    as cultural phenomenon, xii, 61, 236
    disorganization of, 147, 185–86
    prediction of, 10
    psychopathic, 61–62, 149, 156
    public and private, 336–40, 342, 347
    schizoid, *see* Schizoid personality
    scientific model of, 289
    total, 285, 348
    weakness of, 173
Phallic admiration, 30
Phallic phase, 44–45
Phallic wishes, 46
Physical contact, 156–57
Pitkin, Donald, 67*n*, 68
Pleading, repetitive, 155–56, 164, 170–71
Polygamy, semi-institutionalized, 27, 92
Pope, Liston, 260*n*, 261*n*
Posturing, 157
Present-oriented society, 159–60, 172
Primary family ties, 24–28, 92–93
Primitive societies, 22, 335–36

symbolism in, 178, 187–89, 194*n*, 195, 198–200, 336
Projection, 301, 309, 314, 323, 352–53
    in delusion, 178, 193, 204, 229
    in witchcraft belief, 199
Projective (TAT) test material, 116*n*
    on authority structure, 70–86, 89, 92, 93–96
    on Oedipus complex, 33–43, 49, 53–54
Propaganda, 199, 201–2
Protestant ethic, 165, 247–48, 265–66
    inhibition of aggression in, 273–74
Protestant Ethic and the Spirit of Capitalism, The (Weber), 247
Protestantism
    history of, 255–56, 258
    See also Pentecostal immigrants; Puritanism
Provincial Hospital of Naples, 152, 160–61, 173
Psychiatric hospitalization (ward patients)
    intensive therapy during, 296–319, 329–31
    of schizophrenics, 100–2, 104–9, 117, 179, 183–85, 204–9, 220–24, 232–33
    See also Ward society
Psychoanalysis, 146, 178, 190, 213–14, 277
    beginning of, 11, 55
    crisis in contemporary, 60
    cultural values evolved from, 58
    diffusion of, 285–94, 337
    rejection of, 199
    training (didactic), 335, 337–42, 347, 354–55
    See also Freudian theories; Infantile sexuality; Instinct theory; Social psychoanalysis; Trauma theory

Psychopathic personality, 61–62, 149, 156
Psychopathology, *see* Mental illness
Psychotherapy (treatment), 98–99, 206, 240
  active, 322–25
  culture of, 295–96, 298, 319–22, 329–33
  within mental institutions, 159–61, 164, 170–73, 296–319
  neutrality in, 326–29
  for working class, 295–333
  See also Insight; Psychiatric hospitalization; Psychoanalysis; Transference
Psychotic episodes, *see* Schizophrenic episodes
Puerto Ricans, 242–43, 281
Punishment, *see* Discipline
Puritanism, 58*n*, 235, 278–81, 338

"Quiet and good" pattern, 112–14

Rage, *see* Anger
Rapaport, David, 14, 357
Reality, 322–23, 325–26
  diffusion of concept of, 288, 292
  of transference, 308–12, 314–15
Rebellion, 218
  against authoritarianism, 256–57, 276
  of family scapegoat, 138, 141
  against parental authority, 34, 38, 40, 44, 46, 51, 54–55, 73, 75–77, 84–86, 91
Redlich, F. C., 123–25, 132–33, 164
Reformation, Protestant, 243, 255–57
Regression, 270–71, 352
  during treatment, 297, 306–8, 314
  of ward patients, 157, 160

Religion, xi–xiv, 102, 237–81, 328, 329*n*, 345
  as culture complex, 15–20
  fundamentalist, 245, 255, 258–60, 271
  as hierarchy, 298
  pentecostal, 239–77
  personal conflict over, 206
  Puritan, 58*n*, 235, 278–81, 338
  religious cults, 264, 279–80
  religious delusions, 47
  revivalist, 244–45, 250, 257, 258, 264
  of suburban church, 239–41, 258–61
  therapy as new, 240, 356–57
  value systems from, 165–66, 199, 240–41, 246
  See also Anticlericalism; Judaism; Madonna complex; Mythology; Protestantism; Roman Catholicism
Remarriage, 26–27
Repression, 172, 289–90, 352
  oedipal, 9, 14, 45–46, 47, 49, 55, 61
Resistance, 289–90, 340
"Rissa di Donne" (drawing), 89
Ritual (rites), xi–xii, 59, 159, 336, 346
  anxiety underlying, 263–64, 270–71
  bipolar, 268–71, 275–76
  culture conflict and, 263–77
  Lenten, 18
  of male peer group, 20
  oedipal wishes symbolized in, 31–32
  ritualized pleading, 155–56, 164, 170–71
  witchcraft and, 188, 192
Rivalry, 28, 112, 347; *see also* Competition; Jealousy
Rivière, Jacques, 294
Roberts, B. H., 124, 149
Róheim, Géza, 352*n*
Roles, 185–86, 236, 354
  confusion over, 301, 311–12

Roles (*cont'd*)
  family, *see* Family roles
  of psychoanalysis, 355–57
  of religious ministers, 242–43
  of therapist, 313–14, 348
  of training analyst, 342, 344,
    351–52
  of ward patients, 162–64,
    168–69
Roman Catholicism, 249–50, 252,
    258, 265, 317n
  confession in, 335–36
  in cultist religion, 280
  history of, 256, 259
  of immigrants, 242–43, 248n,
    254, 262
  magico-animistic, 17, 166,
    246, 250
Rosen, John, 323

San Gennaro ceremony, 252n, 273
Sapir, Edward, 210, 213, 214n
Scapegoating, 137–41
Schizoid personality, 62, 111–14,
    146
  opposite of, 230
  paranoid, 319
Schizophrenic (psychotic) episodes,
    103, 110n, 212–36
  case history of, 214–30
  cultural context of, 230–36
  death causing, 208
  recovery from, 106
Schizophrenics, xii, 179, 312, 325,
    342
  hereditary, 114–15
  peer-group ties of, 136
  specific life patterns of, 142,
    145–50
  ward behavior of, 152–53,
    160, 167–73, 204–5
  See also Paranoid schizo-
    phrenia
Schizophrenic's family dynamics,
    98–120
  case histories of, 100–3, 105–
    9, 117
  family size, 112–14, 149

marriage in, 26, 102, 104–9,
    114–15, 117
  mother-son dynamics, 47–48
Schneider, D. M., 115
Schreber case, 187
Sechehaye, M. A., 323
Security, 29, 58–59, 166
Self-destructive impulses, 179, 303,
    307; *see also* Suicide
Seventh Day Adventists, 279–80
Sibling rivalry, 112
Sicily, 70, 100, 103, 269–70
  family honor in, 23–24
Singer, J. K., 100
Slums (central city), 146
  ethnic church in, 239–44; *see
    also* Italian Evangelical
    Church
Social change, 76, 237–81, 346
  church as agent of, 250, 259,
    268
  culture change, 264, 271, 275,
    281; *see also* Immigrants
  in rural areas, 70
  in transition to literacy, 256
  in underdeveloped countries,
    257–61
  See also Social mobility
Social class, x, 271
  as aspect of mental illness,
    100, 123–34, 149
  church organization along
    lines of, 240
  lower-class ethic, 215
  within mental institutions,
    164–65
Social control, 336, 338
  extrafamily agents of, 90, 94n
  mechanism of, 77, 80, 83–84
Social inertia, *see* Anomie
Social mobility, 107, 248, 258
  impediment to, 48, 136
  of mental patients, 124–26,
    133
Social psychoanalysis, x, xiii-xiv,
    60–63, 295–357
  cultural barriers to, 295–333
  failure of, 299, 308–12
  importance of, 60–61

language barrier to, 296, 316–
17
new ethics of, 326–27
psychoanalytic training for social research, 334–57
in therapeutic community,
330–31
Social (community) responsibility,
240–41, 246–47, 259
Social roles, *see* Roles
Social status, *see* Status
Social workers, 325–26
Socialization, 29–32, 112, 149
Sorrow (grief), 42, 79, 92, 235–
36, 266
over death, 37, 74, 216, 235
Stainbrook, Edward, 231*n*
Standards, *see* Value systems
Status, 93, 298, 330
adult, 91
aspirations for, 216–17, 230
church-sect, 245
extrafamilial, 27–29
hierarchy of, in treatment,
325–26
immigrant, *see* Immigrants
loss of female, 275
occupational, *see* Occupational status
of pentecostal immigrants,
248, 255*n*, 265
of training analyst, 342, 343–
45, 347–48
of ward patients, 157, 158,
165
Sublimation, 312
of oedipal feelings, 47–48, 51,
55–57
*Suburban Captivity of the Church-
es, The* (Winter), 239–41,
244
Suicide, 35–36, 185
Superego
cultural definition of, 61–62
as internalized maternal authority, 34, 36*n*, 45–46
Superstition, *see* Magic; Witchcraft
Surrealism, 292

Swearing, 18–20, 46, 297, 307
prohibition of, 249, 252, 273–
74
Symbiotic schizophrenia, 102–3,
109–14, 117
Symbolism, 6, 27–28, 59, 301
expressive, *see* Expressive
symbolism
oedipal, 31–32, 54
in pentecostal religion, 270
psychoanalytic, 13–14, 286,
289, 292–94, 336
Szasz, Thomas, 337, 342, 354*n*

Taboos, 32, 44–47, 57, 157, 309,
311
courtship 21–22, 46, 50, 85–
86
incest, *see* Incest taboo
modesty, 31
of perceiving anger, 42–43,
79–80
in psychoanalytic training,
339
religious, 245, 248–49, 267
on therapeutic help, 313–14
Tausk, Victor, 188, 193
Tentori, Tullio, 68
Thematic Apperception Test
(TAT), *see* Projective test
material
"Themes, interpretation of," 207
Thompson, Walter H., 68
Transference, 57, 295–333, 339
discovery of, 60
negative, 309, 314
positive, 299–303
transference binds, 310, 319,
321, 323
Trauma, sexual, 48
Trauma theory, 10–12, 59, 146
Trinidad, 258, 279
Trobriand Islanders, 3–12, 14–15,
19*n*, 60, 116
kinship system of, 4, 7–8, 14
rituals of, 263
Tubercular-genic character, 145–46

Uncertainty, 275–76
Unconscious, 234, 236
  diffusion of concept of, 286–88, 291–94
  role of, in witchcraft, 189–91
United States, xi, 198, 303, 349–50
  culture of psychotherapy in, 295–96
  diffusion of psychoanalysis in, 286–87, 291, 294
  See also American mental patients; Immigrants; Navaho Indians; Negroes
Untouchables, 156

Value systems (standards), 147, 240–41, 304, 328–33
  cultural, *see* Cultural values
  hospital, 159, 172
  maintenance of morals in, 95–96
  normative, 329–33
  Protestant, 246–48, 254, 265–66
  rejection based on, 199
  for therapy, 325–26, 338, 355
  See also specific values
Virgin Islands, 210
Virginity, 94*n*, 137, 139, 210, 311, 322
  as a given value, 54, 56

perception of, 300
respect for, 21–24, 46, 49, 61
Von Mering, Otto, 154

Waelder, R., 188, 193
Ward society, psychiatric, 139, 142, 296
  intrahospital anomie, 160–62, 165–67, 173
  pathogenic subculture of, 123–34
  ward social structure, 151–73, 206
Warmth, 29, 58–59, 141
Weber, Max, 165, 247–48, 255–56, 258, 261*n*
Weinstein, Edwin A., 210
West Indian immigrants, 242
Winter, Gibson, *The Suburban Captivity of the Churches,* 293–41, 244
Witchcraft, 177–203, 207, 302
  agent of, 188–91, 195, 197–202
  nonpathological belief in, 180, 187–88, 195
Worker in the Cane (Mintz), 281

Zande society, 187–89, 194*n*, 195
Zuni Indians, 199